KICK *Diabetes* ESSENTIALS

THE DIET AND LIFESTYLE GUIDE

Brenda Davis, RD

Book Publishing Company
Summertown, Tennessee

Library of Congress Cataloging-in-Publication Data

Names: Davis, Brenda, 1959- author.
Title: Kick diabetes essentials : the diet and lifestyle guide / Brenda
  Davis, RD.
Description: Summertown, Tennessee : Book Publishing Company, [2019] |
  Includes bibliographical references and index.
Identifiers: LCCN 2019021050 | ISBN 9781570673764 (pbk.)
Subjects: LCSH: Diabetes—Popular works. | Diabetes—Diet therapy—Recipes. |
  Self-care, Health—Popular works.
Classification: LCC RC660.4 .D384 2019 | DDC 641.5/6314—dc23
LC record available athttps://lccn.loc.gov/2019021050

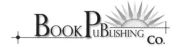 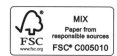

We chose to print this title on paper certified by The Forest Stewardship Council® (FSC®), a global, not-for-profit organization dedicated to the promotion of responsible forest management worldwide.

Cover and interior design: John Wincek

Printed in the United States of America

Book Publishing Company
PO Box 99
Summertown, TN 38483
888-260-8458
bookpubco.com

ISBN: 978-1-57067-376-4

24 23 22 21 20 19   1 2 3 4 5 6 7 8 9

> Please note that the word "diabetes" in this book refers to type 2 diabetes unless otherwise indicated.

Contents

To my father, the late John Charbonneau; my mother, Doreen Charbonneau; and my brother, Andy Charbonneau. Growing up in a home filled with love and laughter is a gift that I will always treasure.

My dad was my superhero—always there when I needed him, with wise and carefully thought-out advice and unfailing support.

My mom is my angel on earth—a beautiful, positive spirit, deeply devoted to family, and constantly inspiring creativity, character, and compassion.

My brother is my most cherished lifelong friend—loyal, caring, and generous—the kind of brother who stands with you through all the joys and tears of life.

With love and a grateful heart,

Brenda

Foreword

The case for using plant-based diets to reduce the burden of diabetes and improve overall health has never been stronger. Type 2 diabetes can be prevented, arrested, and even reversed with plant-based diets; we've known this since the 1930s.

The effectiveness of plant-based diets was long assumed to be the result of weight loss. However, in the 1970s, a research team proved that even with no weight loss, plant-based diets were effective. In one study, plant-based diets reduced insulin requirements by about 60 percent, and half of the participants with diabetes were able to eliminate insulin completely—and they were forced to eat so much that they did not lose weight! How long did this take? Only sixteen days! Since the 1970s, research has continued to accumulate, proving that healthy plant-based diets are the most powerful medicine we have to treat type 2 diabetes.

There is a stepwise drop in insulin resistance and insulin-producing beta cell dysfunction as more and more plant-based foods are added to the diet. In the Adventist Health Study-2, people eating a semi-vegetarian diet had a 31 percent lower diabetes risk, those eating a lacto-ovo vegetarian diet had a 57 percent lower risk, and those eating a 100 percent plant-based (vegan) diet had a 62 percent lower risk when compared to similar health-conscious omnivores. People eating a standard American diet obtain only about 12.6 percent of calories from whole plant foods, which could help explain why North Americans are experiencing an epidemic of diabetes.

Plant-based diets are not just effective for the prevention and management of diabetes but also for the prevention of its complications. One of the most devastating complications of diabetes is kidney failure. Kidney function tends to decline at a steady, inexorable rate in people with diabetes. However, when people switch to a plant-based diet, kidney decline is stopped in its tracks. Plant-based diets also simultaneously treat cardiovascular disease, the leading cause of premature mortality in people with diabetes and the number one cause of death for men and women in the United States. The advantages of eating plant-based diets also extend to a reduced risk of cancer, the second leading cause of death in the United States.

Kick Diabetes Essentials is a gold mine for people with diabetes. It is packed with solid scientific evidence, practical guidelines, and carefully constructed recipes. Brenda Davis is my favorite go-to dietitian. You can rest assured that you are in very capable hands.

Michael Greger, MD

Acknowledgments

Many thanks to the outstanding team at Book Publishing Company: my exceptionally skilled and insightful editors and advisors, Cynthia Holzapfel and Jo Stepaniak, and the entire Book Publishing Company team, particularly Bob Holzapfel, Anna Pope, and Michael Thomas. It is a privilege and a joy to work with such talented and dedicated professionals.

Heartfelt appreciation to my cherished writing partner of twenty-seven years, Vesanto Melina, and her partner, Cam Doré, who are a constant source of support and wisdom. Thank you, Vesanto, for your delicious recipe contributions: Green Giant Juice, Spiced Creamy Barley Bowl, Apple Pie Oats, Smokin' Lentil Soup, and Healing Greens, Beans, and Vegetable Soup.

Deepest gratitude to my recipe testers and dear friends Margie Colclough, Lynn Isted, and Daneen Agecoutay. You were committed to getting every recipe to the highest rating, and the results are simply outstanding. Thank you so much for your attention to detail, your willingness to test and retest, and your incredible generosity. Your contribution is invaluable, and readers will reap the rewards of your efforts for many years to come. Special thanks to Margie for coordinating the effort and for your continued love, support, and brilliance; to Lynn for your unfailing dedication to this task and your determination to get every recipe just right; and to Daneen for your culinary expertise and for contributing the delicious Creamy Dill Dip, Creamy Dill Dressing, and Nut Parmesan recipes.

Many thanks to special friends who provided support with recipe and taste testing: Sheanne and Dan Moskaluk, Sonya Looney and Matt Ewonus, Art Isted, and Stacey Agecoutay.

With sincere appreciation to my cherished colleagues John and Sally Kelly, Michael and Alese Klaper, and Wes Youngberg, who have provided advice, support, and inspiration over many years.

With love and respect to my treasured friends Andres, Lily, and Carlos Vallejo for sharing their inspiring stories and for their astute advice, generosity, and delightful companionship.

Last but not least, many thanks to my family, who provides endless love, encouragement, and support: my beloved husband, Paul Davis; my cherished children, Leena Markatchev and Cory Davis; their spouses, Nayden Markatchev and Josie Mengmeng Jiang Davis; my precious grandchildren; my dear mother-in-law, Linda Davis; and my sister-in-laws, Peggy Davis and Jaclyn Labchuk.

Unmasking a Metabolic Monster

Diane always dreamed of being a svelte woman—long, lean, and graceful. But as beautiful as she looked on her wedding day, at five foot three (160 cm) and 127 pounds (57.6 kg), svelte she was not. Each of her three pregnancies blessed her with a little seven- to eight-pound bundle of joy and cursed her with an intractable seven- to eight-pound sack of potatoes that stuck to her hips like glue. By age fifty-six, Diane was teetering on the edge of obesity at 168 pounds (76 kg). She considered herself reasonably health conscious—she ate low-fat yogurt, granola, and tuna sandwiches on brown bread. She limited herself to one glass of red wine with dinner and only occasionally indulged in sweet treats. She walked her dog daily and did Pilates twice a week. So when Diane's doctor told her that she had type 2 diabetes, she was blindsided. She knew something was up, as she was chronically thirsty, constantly hungry, and more tired than usual. She lost five pounds (2.3 kg) in a month without even trying. This tickled her silly, since her most diligent diets were never that successful. What eventually led her to the doctor, and to this dreaded diagnosis, was a stubborn bladder infection. Diane wondered what this meant for her future. Would she be on medications or, worse yet, insulin injections for the rest of her life? Would she end up on dialysis? She thought of her mother and her aunts, uncles, and cousins who also had diabetes. Maybe her diabetes was the inevitable consequence of bad genes.

Perhaps you can relate to Diane's story. If so, you're in good company. Diabetes now affects one out of every eight adults in the United States (12–14 percent of the population), an increase of twelve times since the late 1950s. By the time you're sixty-five, your chances of having diabetes are one in four. In addition, an estimated 37–38 percent of American adults have prediabetes (a condition that can lead to diabetes). This means that 49–52 percent of American adults have either diabetes or prediabetes, and the rates are even higher for Hispanic Americans and Native Americans.[1,2]

WHAT IS DIABETES?

Diabetes is a group of diseases characterized by high blood glucose (sugar) levels. If you have diabetes, your body fails to produce enough insulin and may also fail to properly use the insulin it produces. Insulin is the hormone you need so your cells can convert glucose (a sugar that's the body's main source of fuel) into energy. Insulin does this by attaching to receptor sites on your cells (like a key in a lock) and sending signals to open the gates so glucose can enter the cells. When insulin isn't present or doesn't do its job, sugar accumulates in the blood, resulting in high blood sugar (hyperglycemia). Some sugar also spills out into your urine. When diabetes was first discovered, it was diagnosed by tasting a patient's urine. If it tasted sweet, this was a sign that death was imminent. Fortunately, the prognosis changed dramatically with the discovery of insulin in 1921.

There are three main types of diabetes: type 1, type 2, and gestational diabetes.

Type 1 Diabetes

Type 1 diabetes is an autoimmune disease. The body mistakes the cells in the pancreas that manufacture insulin (beta cells) for foreign invaders and generates chemicals to destroy them. The insulin-making machine is disabled, so little or no insulin is produced. In some cases, a person's genetics could be responsible for this condition. In others, viral infections or environmental contaminants may trigger this abnormal immune response. A third possibility is that certain food proteins that find their way into the bloodstream are the culprits. These proteins are so similar to pancreatic beta cell proteins that the body attacks both. Specific types of dairy protein fit this bill, and introduction to whole cow's milk at a very early age appears particularly problematic, especially in infants and children who are genetically susceptible.[3]

Type 1 diabetes was formerly referred to as *juvenile-onset diabetes* or *insulin-dependent diabetes mellitus* because it occurs mostly in children or young adults. However, adults over the age of thirty occasionally develop type 1 diabetes. This type of diabetes is called *latent autoimmune diabetes in adults* (LADA) and is sometimes also referred to as type 1.5 diabetes. Adults diagnosed with LADA are often not overweight and have little or no resistance to insulin (the body is able to use insulin when it is present). They also often have a slower rate of beta cell failure and thus may not need insulin as quickly as younger individuals with more aggressive disease. LADA is more common than previously recognized, accounting for an estimated 2–12 percent of diabetes in the adult population. Individuals with LADA can be distinguished from those with type 2 diabetes by the presence of autoantibodies (antibodies that are directed against one or more of the body's own proteins) associated with type 1 diabetes.[4]

People with type 1 diabetes rely on daily insulin injections for survival. It's possible for people with type 1 diabetes to develop type 2 diabetes if their body becomes insulin resistant. Only 5–10 percent of people with diabetes suffer from type 1.

Type 2 Diabetes

Type 2 diabetes is a disease of insulin resistance and reduced production of insulin by the pancreas. While either of these metabolic abnormalities can result in full-blown type 2 diabetes, in the majority of affected individuals, both are present. Insulin resistance is a condition in which the body's cells are insensitive or resistant to the insulin it produces. In other words, insulin is made, but it can't do its job moving glucose into cells or it does the job inefficiently. The natural consequence of insulin resistance is elevated blood glucose. The pancreas responds by putting out more insulin, which shifts the beta cells into overdrive. Insulin resistance is generally present for many years prior to the diagnosis and is a key feature of prediabetes.

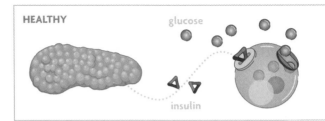

The pancreas produces insulin, which opens the gates to cells to make full use of glucose in the blood.

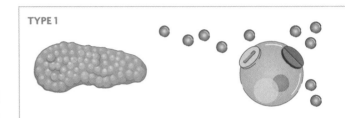

The pancreas fails to produce insulin, which must be injected daily in order for cells to make full use of glucose.

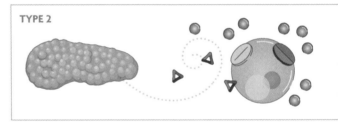

The body develops a resistance to insulin, leaving the cells unable to make full use of glucose, resulting in high blood sugar.

What commonly triggers the progression to type 2 diabetes is that, in addition to insulin resistance, the insulin-producing beta cells begin to fail and the amount of insulin produced declines. This failure may well be the result of beta cell exhaustion. By the time a person is diagnosed, insulin production has commonly diminished to about 50 percent of normal, although in some individuals insulin production remains high. Although insulin resistance tends to remain relatively constant over time, a steady decline in insulin production generally continues if changes in diet and lifestyle are not made.[5,6]

Type 2 diabetes was once known as *adult-onset diabetes* or *non-insulin-dependent diabetes mellitus,* as it was a disease that occurred almost exclusively in adults. Although exceedingly rare prior to the twentieth century, today type 2 diabetes is a global epidemic and accounts for 90–95 percent of all diabetes. While type 2 diabetes was once unheard of in young people, it now accounts for 20–50 percent of diabetes in youth.[7] Although type 2 diabetes is the focus of this book, people with type 1 diabetes will find many of the dietary strategies useful for them as well.

Gestational diabetes

Gestational diabetes is a temporary condition during pregnancy that is often resolved with the birth of the infant. Its incidence has risen from 3–5 percent of pregnancies prior to the twenty-first century to 5–10 percent today.[8] An estimated 50 percent of women with gestational diabetes go on to develop type 2 diabetes.[9]

HOW IS TYPE 2 DIABETES DIAGNOSED?

 ype 2 diabetes may be suspected if you experience the following common symptoms of the disease:

- Blurred vision
- Fatigue
- Itchy skin
- Pain, numbness, or pain in extremities
- Polydipsia (constant thirst)
- Polyphagia (increased hunger)
- Polyuria (frequent urination)
- Recurrent infections
- Slow wound healing
- Sudden, unexpected weight loss

Some people with type 2 diabetes don't experience obvious symptoms. In such cases, the disease could be discovered by chance at an annual checkup or because of an unrelated condition. Long before you're diagnosed with type 2 diabetes, prediabetes has been present for some time—often for several years. Prediabetes—also called impaired glucose tolerance (IGT)—is a condition in which blood sugar is elevated, but not elevated enough to be classified as diabetes. This is not a benign condition, as chronically elevated blood sugar damages the body and increases the risk of many chronic con-

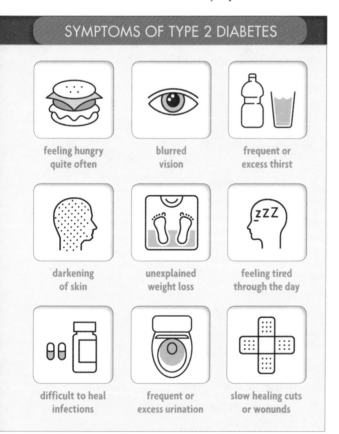

SYMPTOMS OF TYPE 2 DIABETES

feeling hungry quite often

blurred vision

frequent or excess thirst

darkening of skin

unexplained weight loss

feeling tired through the day

difficult to heal infections

frequent or excess urination

slow healing cuts or wounds

ditions. If your doctor or health-care provider suspects diabetes or prediabetes, special tests will be ordered. The following are the four tests most commonly used to confirm a diabetes or prediabetes diagnosis:[10]

1. **Fasting plasma glucose.** After a fast of at least eight hours (nothing by mouth except water), your blood sugar is tested. Your fasting blood glucose results will determine whether or not you have diabetes or prediabetes. See the table below:

DIAGNOSIS	FASTING PLASMA GLUCOSE
Diabetes	126 mg/dL (7.0 mmol/L) or higher
Prediabetes	100–125 mg/dL (5.6 to 6.9 mmol/L)
Normal	60–99 mg/dL (3.3 to 5.5 mmol/L)

2. **A1c (or HbA1c).** This is a blood test that provides information about your average blood sugar levels over the past two to three months. It measures the percentage of blood sugar attached to hemoglobin (the oxygen-carrying protein in red blood cells). The result is reported as a percentage, as shown in the table below:

DIAGNOSIS	A1c
Diabetes	6.5% or more
Prediabetes	5.7–6.4%
Normal	Less than 5.7%

3. **Oral glucose tolerance test.** This test measures how well your body uses sugar. You fast overnight and then drink a sugary liquid (glucose dissolved in water). Your blood sugar is then measured periodically over the next two hours. Interpretation of the results are shown in the table below:

DIAGNOSIS	ORAL GLUCOSE TOLERANCE TEST AT TWO HOURS
Diabetes	200 mg/dL (11.1 mmol/L) or higher
Prediabetes	140–199 mg/dL (7.8-11.0 mmol/L)
Normal	140 mg/dL (7.8 mmol/L) or less

4. **Random plasma glucose.** This is a random measure of your blood sugar level at any time during the day, irrespective of the time of your last meal. A random plasma glucose level of 200 mg/dL (11.1 mmol/L) or higher suggests diabetes.

DEVASTATION BY DIABETES

Insulin resistance, rising blood sugar, and diabetes come with a dreadful physiological price tag. Living in a milieu of excess glucose, your tissues become awash in a syrupy fluid. The sugars stick to proteins, bridging spaces between connective tissue layers. Arteries stiffen, the lenses of the eyes become less flexible, internal wiring malfunctions, and aging accelerates. Every body system is affected, and the consequence is a metabolic meltdown. As a result, people with diabetes have a two- to threefold increase in risk of mortality compared with those who do not have diabetes.[11] The devastation wrought by diabetes is responsible for a myriad of complications.

Cardiovascular Disease

According to the American Heart Association, about 84 percent of people age sixty-five or older with diabetes die from heart disease or stroke. Adults with diabetes are two to four times more likely to die from heart disease or heart failure than adults without diabetes. This is thought to be because people with diabetes have more hypertension; higher levels of cholesterol, triglycerides, and blood glucose; increased rates of obesity; and tend to be less physically active.[12,13] Deaths from cardiovascular disease also occur at earlier ages than they do in people who do not have diabetes.

Peripheral Artery Disease (PAD)

An estimated 10–20 percent of people with diabetes suffer from peripheral artery disease (PAD), with its incidence increasing with age. This condition is marked by narrowing of the arteries to the legs, stomach, arms, and head caused by atherosclerosis. Diabetic foot ulcers resulting from PAD are also a common complication, with 12–25 percent of people with diabetes being affected in their lifetime.[14]

Peripheral Neuropathy

Diabetes can damage nerves and cause pain in the limbs, especially in the legs, feet, and hands. This impairs feeling and makes it easy to miss small injuries that can become infected. If left unchecked, peripheral neuropathy can lead to serious infections. Diabetes is responsible for about 60 percent of nontraumatic, lower-limb amputations among adults age twenty or older.[15]

Kidney Disease

In 2011 and 2012, the prevalence of chronic kidney disease in American adults with diabetes was 36.5 percent, and diabetes was the main cause of kidney failure in 44 percent of new cases.[15]

Cancer

Diabetes is positively associated with overall cancer risk, particularly cancers of the pancreas (1.94 times the risk), colon (1.38 times the risk), rectum (1.2 times the risk), liver (2.2 times the risk), and endometrium (2.1 times the risk).[16] In a 2018 American study, people with diabetes had a 47 percent greater chance of having colorectal cancer (CRC) than individuals without the disease. Although the increase in CRC risk was not significant in people age sixty-five or older, the odds of developing the disease in those younger than sixty-five were nearly five times greater than those without diabetes.[17]

Cognitive Dysfunction

Vascular dementia and Alzheimer's disease are frequently seen in diabetes sufferers. One recent meta-analysis (combined findings) of seventeen studies involving close to two million individuals reported that participants with diabetes had a 1.54 times increased risk of Alzheimer's disease.[18]

Other Conditions

Diabetic retinopathy, a complication of diabetes that involves damage to the retinal blood vessels, is the leading cause of blindness in American adults. It's estimated to impact over 25 percent of Americans with type 2 diabetes.[15,19] Also, a 2018 study of Chinese men reported that almost 65 percent of patients with diabetes suffered from erectile dysfunction (ED).[20] Finally, diabetes is strongly associated with the risk and severity of depression. Depression is present in about 25 percent of people with type 2 diabetes.[21]

All in all, these complications pose a rather gloomy reality for anyone progressing down the very slippery slope of diabetes. Fortunately, all these conditions can be dramatically diminished, halted in their tracks, or even reversed with appropriate diet and lifestyle changes.

THE MAKING OF A METABOLIC MONSTER

The hallmark of our modern type 2 diabetes epidemic is insulin resistance. Even when adequate insulin is produced by the beta cells of the pancreas, the body cells (regardless of whether they're in muscle, liver, or fat tissue) do not respond to the insulin as they should. This can happen when there's a problem with insulin receptors or a glitch in the mechanisms that work together to move glucose into cells. Even with plenty of insulin in the bloodstream, glucose can't get into the cells to be used for energy. This means that sugar accumulates in the bloodstream, causing high blood sugar (hyperglycemia). The pancreas responds to this surge in blood sugar by supplying even more insulin. This chronic excess of insulin circulating in the bloodstream is known as hyperinsulinemia.

To be clear, insulin is an extremely important hormone in the body, helping to regulate many body systems. However, like all hormones, there's an optimal level of insulin that's needed to maintain health. When insulin in the bloodstream is persistently elevated and the body is resistant to that insulin, a metabolic mess ensues. Chronically high insulin levels can lead to weight gain, high triglyceride and uric acid levels, arteriosclerosis (hardening of the arteries), hypertension, and endothelial dysfunction (which impairs blood flow). However, as you may recall, Diane lost five pounds (2.3 kg) just prior to her type 2 diabetes diagnosis. Why would she lose weight when she had high insulin levels due to insulin resistance? In Diane's case (and for many others with a new type 2 diabetes diagnosis), her body had become so insulin resistant that she couldn't use the sugar from her food. Her blood glucose soared, and she began to dump sugar in her urine. Her body turned to its fat and muscle stores for energy, so she lost weight.

What Causes Insulin Resistance?

The vast majority of insulin resistance is a function of overweight and underactivity. While it's true that genes can be responsible for ineffective insulin receptor sites or can adversely affect the cascade of events necessary for glucose to enter cells, excess body weight, especially visceral fat (see the box on page 9), is the chief culprit.

According to the International Diabetes Federation, a waist measurement of 37 inches (94 cm) or more in Caucasian men, 35.5 inches (90 cm) or more in Asian men, and 31.5 inches (80 cm) or more in women increases risk.[22] Underactivity contributes to being overweight and to metabolic changes that further promote insulin resistance.

With unhealthy eating patterns, chronic overeating, and underactivity (and the overweight or obesity that results), metabolic mayhem ensues. This, in turn, incites five major drivers of insulin resistance and diabetes: inflammation, oxidative stress, lipotoxicity, glycotoxicity, and dysbiosis. If these terms make your head spin, just think of them as the arms that feed this metabolic monster. Let's delve a little deeper into the mechanisms behind each of these five drivers.

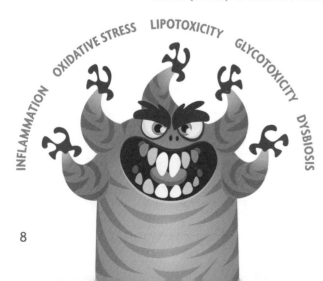

Inflammation

We're all familiar with the heat, redness, swelling, and pain associated with an injury or a sore throat; this is the result of inflammation. Inflammation is the body's way of getting rid of damaged cells and initiating tissue repair. However, there's a type of inflammation associated with many chronic diseases (including type 2 diabetes) that can't be seen or felt. It can be fueled by an unhealthy diet, food sensitivities, dysbiosis (overpopulation of bad bacteria; see page 12), alcohol, and overweight. Excess body fat, especially visceral fat, causes the release of cell-signaling proteins called cytokines that can trigger inflammation. This inflammation reduces insulin's ability to send messages to the cell to open the glucose gates. Body cells become less responsive to insulin, ultimately increasing insulin resistance. Insulin resistance itself causes inflammation, so a positive feedback loop is reinforced.[23,24,25,26]

Oxidative Stress

Oxidative stress, or oxidation, is an imbalance between substances called pro-oxidants (such as free radicals) and antioxidants. Free radicals are unstable molecules that have an electron that is unpaired (see figure 1.1, page 10). They try to stabilize by stealing electrons from other molecules. When they succeed, they turn their victim into a free radical, setting off a destructive chain reaction that creates more free radicals. Antioxidants are heroes that block the chain of destruction by offering the free radical an electron without becoming free radicals themselves (see figure 1.2, page 10).

Increased oxidative stress has been shown to promote insulin resistance and malfunction of the pancreatic cells that produce insulin. When you eat too much and exercise too little, you end up with an overload of sugar and fat. Excess sugar can bind to proteins, forming advanced glycation end products (AGEs),

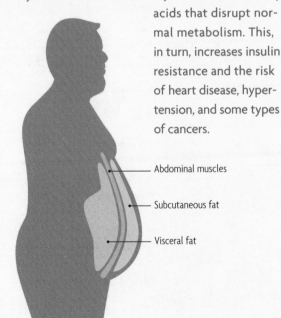

WHAT IS VISCERAL FAT?

When fat is stored just below the surface of the skin, it's called subcutaneous fat. When it's found deep within the body, in and around vital organs, it's called visceral fat. Generally, people with an apple shape (more fat in their abdomen) have more visceral fat, and those who are pear shaped (more fat in the extremities, such as hips and thighs) have more subcutaneous fat. However, even among individuals who are apple shaped, there are significant differences in the distribution of visceral versus subcutaneous fat. People with soft bellies tend to have more subcutaneous fat, while those with big, hard bellies have more visceral fat.

While all types of excess fat can adversely affect health, visceral fat is by far the most concerning. This is because it's much more biologically active than subcutaneous fat, pumping out an inflammatory set of hormones called cytokines and free fatty acids that disrupt normal metabolism. This, in turn, increases insulin resistance and the risk of heart disease, hypertension, and some types of cancers.

Abdominal muscles

Subcutaneous fat

Visceral fat

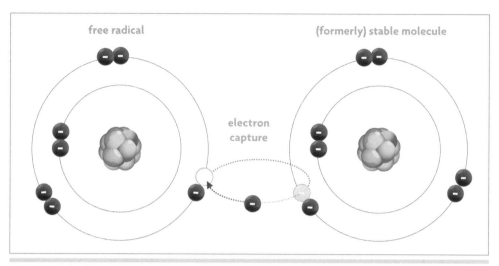

FIGURE 1.1 The free radical captures its missing electrons from stable molecules, thereby creating new free radicals.

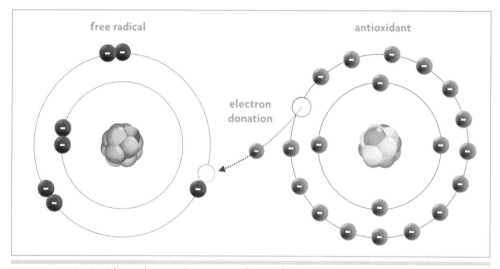

FIGURE 1.2 Antioxidants donate electrons to free radicals without becoming free radicals themselves.

which accelerate the production of free radicals. AGEs alter cell function, disrupt insulin receptors, increase insulin resistance, and promote inflammation.[27,28]

Lipotoxicity

Lipotoxicity is a condition caused by the accumulation of fatty acids in parts of the body that weren't designed to store them, such as vital organs and muscles. The human body has specialized cells called adipocytes that have an enormous capacity to store excess body fat. However, when calorie intake chronically exceeds expenditure, the storage process can back up; excess fatty acids will be stored directly in the liver or be shuttled to the pancreas, heart, or muscle tissue. Overaccumulation of fatty acids disrupts the normal workings of these cells, often leading to cell damage or cell death.

Vital organs are especially vulnerable because they're highly specialized systems that can't tolerate a significant infiltration of fatty acids. When fat is stored in the liver, it becomes less sensitive to insulin, promoting insulin resistance throughout the body. The pancreas has a particularly low tolerance for fat, so even a small exposure can cause beta cell failure. Affected beta cells can no longer secrete the expected amount of insulin in response to rising glucose. As a result, blood glucose levels sharply rise, and the diagnosis of diabetes is made. Muscle cells are also at risk, as the buildup of fatty acids inside muscle cells strongly promotes insulin resistance. These fatty acids are stored as intramyocellular lipids (intra = inside, myo = muscles, cellular = cells), or IMCL. Although IMCL is an important energy source for active muscles, an excess can be toxic to cells. Muscle insulin resistance increases the risk for diabetes, while the accumulation of fat in the liver and pancreas triggers beta cell destruction or dysfunction and full-blown diabetes.

Insulin resistance compounds the problem because one of insulin's vital roles is to promote the storage of fat and prevent the breakdown and release of fatty acids from adipocytes. In other words, insulin helps make sure fatty acids stay where they should be. When insulin resistance occurs, insulin can't perform as efficiently and fatty acids are more easily released into the bloodstream, increasing the risk of lipotoxicity. Visceral fat cells (see page 9) are already more insulin resistant than other fat cells, so people with a lot of visceral fat are at higher risk for lipotoxicity.[5,29,30,31]

Glucotoxicity

Chronically elevated blood sugar keeps the body constantly awash in a syrupy fluid that sticks to proteins and accumulates on body tissues, interfering with normal cell functions. This process is known as glucotoxicity. The price tag associated with glucotoxicity is steep. It is intrinsically linked to beta cell dysfunction and insulin resistance. Overconsumption of sugars and starches can activate enzymes that speed their conversion to fatty acids and other lipids, such as ceramides, that can be toxic to the liver.

Glucotoxicity also damages large blood vessels, leading to diseases such as atherosclerosis (plaque buildup), arteriosclerosis (hardening of the arteries), heart attacks, and strokes. Blood flow to the legs is reduced, resulting in peripheral artery disease, diabetic foot syndrome, and amputations. Muscles begin wasting away due to poor blood flow. This sea of sugar also injures small blood vessels. The lenses of the eyes become less flexible, resulting in retinopathy and possible blindness. The kidneys lose their ability to efficiently filter blood, eventually leading to nephropathy and dialysis. Nerves begin to degenerate, causing neuropathy and decreased sensation. Brain function begins to decline, increasing the risk of dementia and Alzheimer's disease. In men, the blood vessels leading to the penis are damaged, provoking erectile dysfunction. High sugar levels also cripple the immune system cells, which are usually vigilant defenders against viruses and other invaders. Glucotoxicity diminishes their ability to fight infection, and the body's capacity to heal slows to a snail's pace.[32,33,34]

Dysbiosis

The bacteria, viruses, fungi, and other single-celled organisms harbored by humans are collectively known as microbiota. The largest collection of microbes in the body is found in the gut, although the mouth, skin, and genitals are also common habitats. Each individual is host to between ten and one hundred trillion symbiotic microbes, containing a mix of communities whose balance has remarkable consequences for health. Some of these organisms promote and protect the host and are commonly referred to as "good bacteria." Those considered "bad bacteria" can harm the host and contribute to various disease processes. A normal, healthy gut is brimming with beneficial bacteria, while less desirable inhabitants are present in smaller numbers. When the balance of bacteria shifts in favor of bad bacteria, the result is a condition known as dysbiosis. Research linking dysbiosis to the epidemic of chronic disease is rapidly mounting. Correlations have been made between dysbiosis and heart disease, cancers, allergic disorders, inflammatory bowel diseases, brain diseases, liver diseases, and, not surprisingly, insulin resistance and diabetes.

Studies suggest that the gut microbiota of individuals with type 2 diabetes are altered in ways that can fuel insulin resistance. Following are some of the key mechanisms of action:

1. *Increased gut permeability.* Dysbiosis increases gut permeability, allowing intact proteins to get into the bloodstream, triggering inflammation and insulin resistance.

2. *Increased production of pro-inflammatory proteins called cytokines.* Cytokines impair insulin sensitivity by causing inflammation and by altering the inner workings of genes.

3. *Metabolic endotoxemia.* When certain types of bacteria die, their outer cell membranes release toxins that can cross the gut lining and create the inflammatory response associated with insulin resistance. While these toxins (called endotoxins) are present in low concentrations in healthy individuals, amounts can double or triple in obese individuals, resulting in a condition called metabolic endotoxemia.[35,36,37]

WHY DOESN'T EVERY OBESE PERSON DEVELOP INSULIN RESISTANCE?

You may be wondering how anyone who's very overweight or obese can manage to effectively dodge diabetes. The answer lies in the inherent differences in individual constitutions. Some people have a lot of beta cells and pump out more insulin than other people. Others have very resilient insulin receptors and highly efficient insulin signaling and are protected even when they're overweight or obese. People who manufacture fewer inflammatory cytokines may also be at reduced risk. Individuals with a high tolerance for fatty acids in their liver and pancreas will be afforded protection, while people with a lower tolerance may develop diabetes even if they're only slightly above their ideal weight. Regardless, it's important to realize that anyone who is overweight or obese will experience metabolic malfunctions that increase their risk of chronic diseases, such as heart disease and cancer, even if they don't develop diabetes. The takeaway message is that there are many reasons to keep the body's fat stores in check.

WHY ME?

If you receive a diagnosis of type 2 diabetes, you will no doubt wonder, Why me? You may, unfortunately, be saddled with genes that maximize your risk. Your genes may promote abundant adipose tissue storage, poor insulin production, weak insulin receptor sites, or reduced insulin signaling. However, if genes were the predominant perpetrator, we would expect that type 2 diabetes rates would have been relatively static over the past hundred years. Yet, a hundred years ago, type 2 diabetes was a rare occurrence; today it's a raging global epidemic. What scientists have discovered is that when it comes to chronic disease, genes act as a loaded gun. It's almost always diet and lifestyle that pull the trigger. The global culture has become one of overindulgence and underactivity. The predictable result is a rise in overweight and obesity, which dramatically increase the risk of insulin resistance, prediabetes, and type 2 diabetes.

How did this happen? Humans are hardwired to be attracted to the tastes of fat, sugar, and salt. Found in low concentrations in nature, these flavors have historically assured us that the food we're about to eat is safe and nourishing. When these substances are concentrated and used as principal ingredients in processed foods, our innate ability to control the appetite becomes unhinged. This is no mere coincidence. Foods that are hyperconcentrated in sugar, fat, and salt can, in some circumstances, stimulate pleasure centers in the brain the way that heroin, nicotine, and alcohol do, although to a lesser extent. Essentially, they can provide such pleasure that they trigger cravings. To further challenge the senses, portion sizes keep expanding. According to the Centers for Disease Control and Prevention (CDC), the average restaurant meal is four times larger than it was in the 1950s. Not surprisingly, evidence confirms that as portion sizes increase, people eat more. For anyone trying to make a living selling food, addictive flavors and larger portions mean return customers and rising sales.[38,39,40,41,42]

To add insult to injury, the level of physical activity in today's world has dwindled dramatically since the 1950s. Every possible convenience has been developed to help reduce energy expenditure. Even if people wanted to increase their activity, many neighborhoods lack sidewalks and safe places for exercise.

It's little wonder that in the United States being overweight or obese is now the new normal, with over 70 percent of the population being affected. In this environment, staying slim seems a greater mystery than becoming overweight or obese. The good news is that this dark cloud has a silver lining. By carefully controlling your environment (that is, your diet and lifestyle), you can change the expression of your genes, essentially taking your finger off the trigger. The upcoming chapters will serve as your support system, helping to guide you through this process one step at a time.[43]

Vanquishing the Monster

Diane sat in her first diabetes education session, resigned to her new reality. Her doctor was very clear that diabetes was a progressive, irreversible disease that would always be with her. It could be managed but not cured. The doctor's goal was to reduce or delay the onset of complications by tightly controlling Diane's blood sugar. The best way to do this, the doctor assured her, was to take medications as prescribed, make simple changes in diet and lifestyle, and closely monitor blood sugar levels. The diabetes education classes that were recommended were meant to give her the necessary tools to succeed in these tasks. She was apprehensive but liked the idea of group classes and the thought of making friends with people she could relate to. Dedicating an hour and a half every Tuesday evening for two months seemed a small price to pay for avoiding amputations, blindness, and dialysis.

Diane became a model patient, never missing a session. She took her medications faithfully and monitored her blood sugar several times a day. She cut back on portion sizes; swapped sugar-sweetened beverages, yogurts, and treats for sugar-free alternatives; and started eating more vegetables. Diane doubled the time she walked her dog from fifteen minutes to the recommended half hour each day. She lost two pounds (0.9 kg) in two months and kept her blood sugar close to the target goal. Although her progress was encouraging to both her and her doctor, she couldn't help but wonder if there was anything available that could more dramatically alter the course of this disease.

IS DIABETES IRREVERSIBLE?

The theory that diabetes is a progressive, irreversible disease is taught in medical schools and in diabetes educator courses. It's also embraced by many national and international diabetes and health organizations. Based on this belief, it makes perfect sense that the current conventional treatment aims to improve control over blood glucose levels rather than cure the disease. Unfortunately, some of the medications that are most effective in controlling blood sugar contribute to weight gain and inadvertently foster insulin resistance and disease progression. Both insulin injections and oral medications that increase insulin production from the pancreas promote fat storage.[1,2] This is because one of insulin's many jobs is helping to store excess calories as fat—whether those calories come from sugar, fat, or protein. Other medications commonly used in people with diabetes can boost appetite, slow metabolism, cause fluid retention, and reduce energy (leading to less physical activity). In addition, conventional diabetes diets are designed to stabilize blood glucose levels, not to fight insulin resistance or enhance beta cell function. So it's entirely understandable that reversal is not on the radar of most medical practitioners.

However, in the scientific literature it's been well established that diabetes is a reversible disease. In 2009, a consensus statement from the American Diabetes Association (ADA) published in the prestigious journal *Diabetes Care* and titled "How Do We Define Cure of Diabetes?" set standards for remission or reversal of the disease.[3] A summary of consensus definitions is provided in table 2.1, below.

In other words, there are specific criteria that determine whether a person who was diagnosed with diabetes is cured. There are three requirements for complete remission or reversal of the disease:

1. The patient is off all diabetes medications.
2. The patient has normal glycemic measures (e.g., normal HbA1c, normal fasting blood glucose).
3. Both of the above are maintained for at least one year.

There is strong and consistent evidence that many people who are motivated to kick diabetes can succeed in this task. The initial scientific data came from studies

TABLE 2.1. Summary of Consensus Definitions

PARTIAL REMISSION	COMPLETE REMISSION	PROLONGED REMISSION
Hyperglycemia below diagnostic thresholds for diabetes	Normal glycemic measures	
At least one year's duration	At least one year's duration	Complete remission of at least five years' duration
No active pharmacologic therapy or ongoing procedures	No active pharmacologic therapy or ongoing procedures	

of people who had undergone bariatric surgery. Following surgery, normal glucose metabolism is rapidly restored in the majority of patients. Liver fat declines within days, normalizing fasting blood glucose, and pancreas fat drops within weeks, restoring insulin secretion and beta cell function.[4,5] Diabetes reversal is a product of the degree of weight loss over time. People who lose the greatest amount of weight over time experience the highest success rates.[5]

The second line of evidence comes from studies of significant diet and lifestyle changes made by patients with diabetes. Several studies have established the reversal of diabetes using energy (calorie) restriction. Studies using very low-calorie diets mirror the results of bariatric surgery. For example, in 2011, one research team reported that after just one week of energy restriction (600 kcal/day), fasting glucose normalized.[6] Liver fat diminished, as did liver glucose production. By eight weeks, insulin response was superior to the nondiabetic controls and pancreatic fat declined significantly. The authors concluded that normalization of both beta cell function and liver insulin sensitivity was achieved by dietary energy restriction alone. A 2017 study reported that a twelve-week, low-calorie diet (about 1,000 kcal/day) produced normal blood glucose in 50 percent of the cohort, despite stopping all diabetes medications.[7]

In 2018, the Diabetes Remission Clinical Trial (DIRECT) released results of a clinical trial that randomized patients to a weight-management program using a total diet replacement formula (825–853 kcal/day) or a control group using best-practice care guidelines.[8] The formula provided 59 percent carbohydrate, 2 percent fiber, 13 percent fat, and 26 percent protein. It was used for three to five months, followed by a structured food-reintroduction program. At twelve months, a weight loss of at least thirty-three pounds (15 kg) was reported in 24 percent of the participants in the intervention group, but no weight loss was shown in participants in the control group. Diabetes remission was achieved in 46 percent of the intervention-group participants and 4 percent of participants in the control group. Remission rates increased with weight loss.

- 0–11 pounds (0–5 kg) weight loss = 7 percent remission rate
- 11–22 pounds (5–10 kg) weight loss = 34 percent remission rate
- 22–33 pounds (10–15 kg) weight loss = 57 percent remission rate
- 33 pounds (15 kg) or greater weight loss = 86 percent remission rate

A more gradual reversal of insulin resistance has also been demonstrated using diets that are less calorically restrictive, along with appropriate lifestyle changes. In such cases, liver and pancreas fat decline more gradually, insulin sensitivity is more slowly restored, and a healthy metabolism is reestablished. A 2012 pilot study of thirteen adults with diabetes reported impressive changes in a number of measurements (see table 2.2, page 18).[9] Sixty-two percent of participants achieved normal blood glucose levels.

TABLE 2.2. High Nutrient Density (HND) Diet: Lab Changes in Seven Months (Mean)

LAB MEASURE	BASELINE	7 MONTHS ON HND DIET
HbA1c	8.2%	5.8%
Body weight	217 lbs (98.6 kg)	173 lbs (78.6 kg)
Blood pressure	148/87	121/74
Triglycerides	171 mg/dL (1.9 mmol/L)	103 mg/dL (1.2 mmol/L)
LDL cholesterol	135 mg/dL (3.5 mmol/L)	113 mg/dL (2.9 mmol/L)
HDL cholesterol	48.3 mg/dL (1.3 mmol/L)	54.6 mg/dL (1.4 mmol/L)

A diet that was plant-rich with a high nutrient density (HND) was used in this study, incorporating foods with significant micronutrient content per calorie. Greens and other nonstarchy vegetables—such as onions, mushrooms, eggplants, peppers, tomatoes, and cauliflower—were emphasized and consumed in unlimited amounts. Foods with a high glycemic index were reduced, while carbohydrate-rich, high-fiber foods with a low glycemic index—such as beans, peas, squash, and intact grains— were included. Nuts and seeds were the primary sources of fat. Animal products were limited to no more than 10 percent of calories. The dietary protocol was as follows:

- At least one large green salad a day, with the inclusion of a salad dressing derived from nuts or seeds
- One bowl of vegetable-bean soup daily
- One to two ounces (30–60 g) of raw seeds and nuts daily (usually in a salad dressing)
- Approximately three or four servings of fresh fruits per day
- One large serving of steamed or stewed greens, with mushrooms, onions, and other low-starch veggies
- Only one serving daily (½ cup/125 ml) of starchy foods exclusive of legumes, such as squash, steel-cut oats, or brown or wild rice
- Exclusion of white flour, sweets, and oils
- Animal products, if used, limited to not more than 12 ounces (340 g) per week

We can expect to see more studies using various plant-based diets in the near future. One research group (E4 Diabetes Solutions) achieved normalization of HbA1c in 67 percent of their participants using a totally plant-based diet, although this is yet unpublished.[10] There are multiple case reports of complete remission in individuals who make the necessary diet and lifestyle changes. Each individual who has been diagnosed with diabetes but no longer meets the criteria for this diagnosis sends a powerful message to health-care providers and diabetes sufferers.

There are two main camps claiming success with diabetes reversal: the plant-based camp and the low-carb camp. Let's examine the research that speaks to each of these diet therapies.

THE PLANT-BASED CAMP

Between 1976 and 1991, a pioneering research team headed by James W. Anderson, MD, published numerous studies demonstrating that high-fiber, high-carbohydrate, plant-based diets are beneficial for people with diabetes.[11,12,13,14,15,16,17] His team compared participants consuming a plant-based, high-carbohydrate, high-fiber (HCF) diet (carbohydrates at 70 percent of calories and fiber at 35–40 g per 1,000 calories) with those consuming the conventional diabetes diet (43 percent carbohydrate) recommended by the American Diabetes Association (ADA). Participants on the HCF diet had consistently more favorable plasma glucose values, glucose tolerance, insulin sensitivity, and blood lipids than those on the ADA diet. In addition, the majority of patients on the HCF diet were able to discontinue or dramatically reduce their oral medications and insulin. Even when participants shifted to a maintenance diet providing fewer carbohydrates (55–60 percent of calories) and less fiber (25 g per 1,000 calories), most were able to sustain favorable changes in lab measurements after an average of fifteen months, while staying off medications and insulin. These studies suggest that diets rich in fiber and unprocessed carbohydrates result in lower insulin requirements than higher-fat conventional diabetes diets. The practical implications of these findings are impressive.

1. A diet providing 70 percent of energy from carbohydrate and containing 35–40 g of fiber per 1,000 calories can rapidly reduce the plasma glucose level and the requirement for insulin or oral hypoglycemic agents in patients with diabetes. It can also lower serum cholesterol and elevated triglyceride levels.

2. Improvements can be maintained long term in patients following a modified high-carbohydrate, high-fiber diet providing 55–60 percent of energy from carbohydrate, 15–20 percent from protein, and 20–30 percent from fat, with 25 g of plant fiber per 1,000 calories.

From 1992 to 1995, Dr. Anderson's team released results of another series of studies that examined the impact of very low-calorie diets (VLCD) in obese individuals with diabetes. Diets providing 400–800 calories per day resulted in an average weight loss of forty-six pounds (21 kg) in sixteen weeks. In addition, significant reductions in blood glucose, HbA1c, total cholesterol, LDL cholesterol, triglycerides, and blood pressure were reported.[18,19,20] Further, between 1999 and 2013, the team reported favorable changes in glucose and lipid levels with the intake of specific plant foods, including beans, psyllium, whole grains, and raisins,[21,22,23,24,25] and in renal function with the intake of soy protein.[26,27]

David Jenkins, MD, the architect of the glycemic index (see page 94), or GI, coauthored numerous articles demonstrating favorable metabolic consequences of consuming plant-based diets or specific plant-based foods, such as whole grains, nuts, and legumes.[28,29,30,31,32,33,34,35,36,37] In 2018, his team released a systematic review and meta-analysis of nine randomized controlled trials assessing the effect of vegetarian diets on individuals with diabetes. Specifically, researchers assessed the risk of developing heart disease or stroke and changes in glycemic control. Vegetarian diets significantly reduced HbA1c, fasting glucose, body weight, waist circumference, LDL cholesterol, and non-HDL cholesterol.[38]

Neal Barnard, MD, and his team at the Physicians Committee for Responsible Medicine (PCRM) published the results of several studies comparing the effects of 100 percent plant-based (vegan) diets versus conventional American Diabetes Association (ADA) diets for the treatment of diabetes. In the initial pilot study, eleven participants were randomized to a low-fat vegan diet or a low-fat conventional diet.[39] Participants who received the vegan diet had a 28 percent reduction in fasting glucose compared to a 12 percent reduction in those consuming the conventional ADA diet. In the vegan group, oral diabetes medications were discontinued in one participant and reduced in three participants, while no changes in medications were made in the ADA diet group. The participants in the vegan group also experienced significantly greater drops in body weight.

In 2006, Barnard's team published the results of a larger twenty-two-week randomized clinical trial (RCT) comparing ninety-nine participants with diabetes who were assigned a low-fat vegan diet with those assigned a control diet that met the ADA guidelines.[40] In the vegan group, 43 percent of the participants were able to reduce diabetes medications compared to 26 percent in the ADA group. Body weight fell by 14.3 pounds (6.5 kg) in the vegan group and 6.8 pounds (3.1 kg) in the ADA group. HbA1c was cut by 0.96 percentage point in the vegan group and 0.56 percentage point in the ADA group. When data excluded those who changed medications, HbA1c dropped 1.23 percentage points in the vegan group and 0.38 percentage point in the ADA group. Among those who did not change lipid-lowering medications, LDL cholesterol was down 21.2 percent in the vegan group and 10.7 percent in the ADA group.

In 2009, Barnard's group published seventy-four-week results in this cohort.[41] Weight loss was 9.7 pounds (4.4 kg) in the vegan group and 6.6 pounds (3.0 kg) in the ADA group. HbA1c declined 0.34 point in the vegan group and 0.14 point in the ADA group. Before any changes in lipid-lowering medications, total cholesterol decreased by 20.4 mg/dL (0.53 mmol/L) in the vegan group and 6.8 mg/dL (0.18 mmol/L) in the ADA group, and LDL cholesterol decreased by 13.5 mg/dL (0.35 mmol/L) and 3.4 mg/dL (0.09 mmol/L) in the vegan and conventional groups respectively. Interestingly, the study participants rated the vegan and ADA diets as being equally acceptable.[42]

Several additional reports from the PCRM team were released between 2014 and 2018. In 2014, a systematic review and meta-analysis of vegetarian diets and glycemic control in diabetes showed vegetarian diets produced a significant 0.39 point reduction in HbA1c and a nonsignificant reduction in fasting blood glucose of 0.36 mmol/L (6.5 mg/dL).[43] A 2015 twenty-week pilot study reported significant improvements in diabetic neuropathy with a low-fat vegan diet.[44] In 2018, significant improvements in beta cell function and insulin sensitivity were reported in overweight adults with no history of diabetes.[45]

Prior to joining the PCRM team as director of clinical research, the lead author of this study, Hana Kahleova, MD, conducted a number of trials using plant-based diets in the treatment of diabetes in the Czech Republic. The first, a 2011 study, randomized seventy-four participants with diabetes to a vegetarian diet or a conventional diabetic control diet with the same number of calories.[46] The vegetarian diet contained about 60 percent of energy from carbohydrate, 15 percent protein, and 25 percent fat, while the conventional diabetic diet provided about 50 percent carbohydrate, 20 percent protein, and 30 percent fat (7 percent or less saturated fat and less than 200 mg cholesterol a day). One portion of low-fat yogurt was the only animal product permitted in the diet.

In the intervention group, 43 percent of participants reduced diabetes medications compared to 5 percent in the control group. Intervention participants dropped 13.6 pounds (6.2 kg) compared to 7 pounds (3.2 kg) in the control group and had greater losses in visceral fat. The vegetarian group also had better improvements in insulin sensitivity, markers of inflammation, oxidative stress, and blood lipids.

In 2013, Kahleova's team reported improved quality of life, mood, and eating behavior with a vegetarian diet.[47] A 2014 trial comparing vegan meals with meat-rich meals containing the same calories found that the meat meal was accompanied by an impaired gastrointestinal hormone response and increased oxidative stress.[48]

A novel 2016 study compared the effects of low-calorie vegetarian versus conventional diabetes diets on physical fitness in people with diabetes.[49] Maximal oxygen consumption (VO$_2$ max) increased by 12 percent in the vegetarian group, whereas no significant change was observed in the conventional diet group. Maximal performance (watt max) increased by 21 percent in the vegetarian group but was unchanged in the conventional diet group.

A second novel trial released in 2017 examined the effects of low-calorie vegetarian versus conventional diabetes diets on thigh adipose (fat) tissue distribution in participants with diabetes. Greater reduction was observed in total leg area and in intramuscular fat in participants consuming the vegetarian diet. Only those consuming the vegetarian diet experienced a significant reduction in subfascial fat (the type of fat that lines our muscles). Participants on the vegetarian diet also had more favorable changes in HbA1c, fasting plasma glucose, and beta cell insulin sensitivity.[50] In 2019, a study involving sixty men (twenty with diabetes, twenty obese, and twenty healthy) reported favorable effects on gut hormones and satiety in those eating a vegan meal with tofu compared with a meat-and-cheese-based meal matched for energy and macronutrients.[51]

A Korean research team measured glycemic control in patients with diabetes on a carbohydrate-rich vegan diet compared with a control group on a conventional diabetic diet.[52] The vegan diet consisted of whole grains (predominantly brown rice), vegetables, fruits, and legumes, along with a selection of foods that don't spike blood sugar levels (green vegetables and seaweed). The conventional mixed diabetic diet provided 50–60 percent carbohydrate, 15–20 percent protein, less than 25 percent fat, less than 7 percent saturated fat, minimal trans-fat intake, and 200 milligrams or less per day of cholesterol.

HbA1c levels decreased by 0.5 percentage point in the vegan group compared with 0.2 percentage point in the conventional group. When the analysis was restricted to participants who were highly adherent to their respective diets, HbA1c dropped 0.9 percentage point in the vegan group and 0.3 percentage point in the conventional diet group. The inclusion of individuals older than age sixty in this trial, and in the majority of vegetarian trials mentioned in the meta-analysis above, supports recommending plant-based diets to all age groups with diabetes, including older adults. The authors concluded that both diets led to reductions in HbA1c levels; however, glycemic control was better with the vegan diet than with the conventional diet. They recommended that dietary guidelines for patients with type 2 diabetes should include a vegan diet for better management and treatment.

A 2016 review published in *Canadian Journal of Diabetes* reported that plant-based diets are best for people with diabetes.[53] Researchers reviewed thirteen studies that explored the efficacy and acceptability of plant-based diets as treatment for diabetes. Diabetes patients who followed a plant-based diet improved their insulin sensitivity, reduced their diabetes medications, and lowered their intakes of saturated fat and cholesterol. Results also showed high acceptance rates and, as a result of decreased meat consumption, lower disease prevalence among those who followed a plant-based diet. The research team called on clinicians to provide more frequent and standardized nutrition education and support for plant-based diets as diabetes treatment.

In 2017, an American review of plant-based diets in the prevention and treatment of diabetes was published. In this report, plant-based diets are defined as eating patterns that emphasize legumes, whole grains, vegetables, fruits, nuts, and seeds and discourage most or all animal products.[54] The authors provide evidence from observational and interventional studies demonstrating the benefits of plant-based diets in treating and reducing key diabetes-related macrovascular and microvascular complications. They suggest that the focus of the diet should be on overall eating patterns while including unrefined versus refined carbohydrates, monounsaturated and polyunsaturated versus saturated and trans fats, and plant rather than animal protein. They also thought the best way to highlight the advantages of a plant-based diet would be to underscore its benefits: the promotion of a healthy body weight, increased intake of fiber and phytonutrients, improved food–microbiome interactions, and decreased intake of saturated fat, advanced glycation end products (see page 76), nitrosamines (a possible carcinogen), and heme iron (a form of iron associated with heart disease).

Three reviews that looked at plant-based diets in the prevention and treatment of diabetes were released in 2018.[55,56,57] The first review, from the United States, concludes that health-care providers should feel confident in recommending a vegetarian diet to patients who have prediabetes or diabetes.[55] However, they clearly distinguish between healthful and unhealthful plant-based diets. The use of diets rich in whole grains, fruits, vegetables, nuts, legumes, and unsaturated fats are advised, while the use of diets containing higher amounts of refined grains, added sugars, and saturated fats are cautioned against. The authors add that there is evidence that a healthful vegan diet has the greatest therapeutic value, especially for reducing fasting blood glucose levels and reducing the risk of complications, such as cardiovascular disease.

The second review, from Indonesia, concludes that in patients with diabetes, HbA1c reduction is greater in those consuming plant-based diets compared with patients consuming a conventional diet.[56] The third review was a meta-analysis of eleven studies and 433 participants with diabetes.[57] Eight of the trials reported on vegan diets and three on vegetarian diets. In six of the studies, patients reduced or discontinued medications used to treat diabetes or symptoms of diabetes. Participants reported improvements in blood glucose levels as well as blood cholesterol levels. They also experienced improvements in physical health and mental health. Nerve pain diminished, depression levels dropped, and overall quality of life was enhanced.

In 2006, I had the privilege of serving as the lead dietitian on a diabetes lifestyle research project in the Republic of the Marshall Islands (RMI), which lies about 2,300 miles southwest of Hawaii. The project was funded by the United States and was a joint venture of the RMI Ministry of Health and Canvasback Missions, Inc.

In several countries of the South Pacific, the prevalence of diabetes among adults is in the range of 25–33 percent. The RMI has the highest prevalence of diabetes in the world, with 32.9 percent of all adults being affected.[58] A century ago, when people lived off the land and sea and were slim and physically active, diabetes was virtually unheard of. The Marshallese diet consisted of edible plants, such as coconut, breadfruit, taro, pandanus, bananas, and leafy greens, along with fish and other seafood. In the 1950s, only three people in the RMI were known to have the disease. By the 1990s, the prevalence had reached 30 percent, and now more than half of all hospital admissions in the capital city of Majuro are due to diabetes and its complications.

Today, the majority of Marshallese are sedentary and live predominantly on imported, processed foods. A typical adult's breakfast consists of cake donuts or sweet pancakes and coffee, while children often start the day with popsicles, chips, soda pop, sweet cereal, or dry ramen noodles with Kool-Aid powder sprinkled on top for extra flavor. Lunch and dinner feature sticky white rice with meat or fish. Favorite meats are Spam, canned corned beef, grilled chicken, and variety meats, such as turkey tails. Meals are often washed down with a sweetened beverage. It would be difficult to design a diet that could more efficiently induce diabetes than the diet that has been adopted by the Marshallese people.

Our team conducted a randomized controlled trial with five groups and a total of 169 participants. We compared an intensive diet-and-lifestyle program with conventional treatment for type 2 diabetes. One group followed a whole-foods, plant-based diet that was high in fiber, antioxidants, and phytochemicals (the protective substances in plants). They also received daily education about nutrition and lifestyle, including shopping tours, cooking classes, and instruction in growing vegetables to keep food costs down. Participants took part in one-hour fitness classes at least four times a week, walked after each meal, and were encouraged to do strength and flexibility exercises at home.

As early as two weeks into the program, success was remarkable. Blood glucose dropped an average of 71 mg/dl (3.9 mmol/l). A measure of inflammation known as hsCRP went down almost 40 percent. A measure of insulin resistance (HOMA-IR) fell over 40 percent. Participants reported dramatic reductions or complete disappearance of pain in their legs, arms, and joints, and walking became much easier. Almost everyone reported increased energy and greatly improved regularity. Weight loss averaged about five pounds (2.25 kg). Almost 90 percent of the participants stopped taking oral medications, both for diabetes and other diabetes-related issues.

After twelve weeks, average weight loss was approximately ten pounds (4.5 kg) per person. Blood sugars were still down about 48 mg/dl (2.7 mmol/l) from baseline, and HbA1c was down an average of nearly two points. Every percentage point drop in HbA1c can reduce the risk of complications in the small blood vessels of the eyes, kidneys, and nerves by 40 percent, so a two-point drop is extraordinary. For many participants, these changes seemed nothing short of a miracle.

These pioneers of the Pacific provided hope amid a deep sense of hopelessness. They overcame seemingly insurmountable mountains of Spam, doughnuts, ramen noodles, and cola. They managed despite the high cost of fresh produce and the lack of fitness facilities or walking trails.

Some people ask if this type of program could work at home. The answer is simple: If there is hope in the Marshall Islands, considering the enormous barriers they face, there is hope at home. But that hope rests on the integration of lifestyle medicine into our health-care systems. It must be offered as a treatment option, and preferably as the first line of treatment. If you do find such a program in your area, get on board! The added support from a like-minded community will help guide you and keep you on the road to recovery. Additional support can also be found online with one of many whole-food, plant-based programs that have reported success in treating, and often reversing, type 2 diabetes. Their websites, along with excellent general informational websites, are listed in the resources on page 231.

Anecdotal evidence does not provide scientific proof; however, it often provides the inspiration and information needed to affect change in individuals. My favorite testimony from my own personal clinical experience is the story of Carlos. These are his words:

CARLOS'S STORY

I was diagnosed with type 2 diabetes when I was fifty. For the next twenty years, I was injecting between 35 and 40 units of insulin (both L and N) per day. I was also on other diabetic medications, including DiaBeta and metformin. In total, I was taking seventeen pills a day. I had coronary artery disease and had already had one heart attack. I also had high blood pressure, early signs of kidney failure, peripheral artery disease, and chronic gout, among other ailments. I believed that my conditions were irreversible and progressive. With respect to my diabetes in particular, based on what my doctors told me and on the widely distributed literature about diabetes, I "knew" that diabetes was an irreversible disease. Then, my oldest son was diagnosed with cancer, and he decided to adopt a whole-foods, plant-based diet. To support him, my wife and I changed our diets as well.

I was being treated at UC San Francisco, so I was confident that I needed the medication I was taking and that my conditions could be managed to some extent but not reversed. What happened after I changed my diet was unbelievable to me. Within weeks I had cut my medication significantly, lost weight, and started feeling a fundamental change in my body. Today, after about a year and a half on a whole-foods, plant-based diet, I'm taking zero insulin and zero pills. My fasting glucose is now between 80 and 87 on a daily basis and my A1c is normal. My average blood pressure is now 115/70. (Even with all the medication, my blood pressure was high and never reached an average normal range.) My arteries have opened up, and I needed no procedures or surgeries. The scar tissue resulting from my heart attack has shrunk, indicating potential tissue regeneration. My kidney function is now perfectly normal, and I'm no longer taking the medication I had been prescribed for this problem. I averted (and possibly reversed) peripheral artery disease. In short, I reversed all the conditions that I "knew" were progressive and irreversible. Today I had to go to the DMV to renew my driver's license. I could not believe that I answered no to the question "Do you have diabetes?" I am no longer diabetic. This all may sound incredible, but it's true. My story is supported by medical exams and records that reflect my conditions before and after I changed my diet.

It's been over seven years since Carlos began this healing journey. He remains free of the chronic diseases that nearly took his life, and his son Andres is still in remission from his cancer.

THE LOW-CARB CAMP

Low-carbohydrate (commonly referred to as low-carb) and very low-carbohydrate or ketogenic diets have recently gained tremendous favor as treatments for people with diabetes. The basic premise is that if someone can lower carbohydrate intake sufficiently, their blood sugar will also naturally stay low because there is less available glucose. As a result, the body will have to use an alternative fuel called ketone bodies (or ketones). In theory, the need for insulin or diabetes medications will plummet, and diabetes will be reversed.

Ketone bodies, or ketones, are formed during starvation or fasting, when the body's primary fuel source, glucose, is not available. When blood glucose drops and no source of carbohydrate is consumed, the body uses up its stored glucose (glycogen stores). When glycogen stores are depleted (usually within twenty-four hours of carbohydrate deprivation), the body generates glucose through a process called gluconeogenesis (literally, "the making of new sugar") that utilizes amino acids (from muscle stores), lactate (a by-product of glucose metabolism), and glycerol (the backbone of triglycerides from fat stores).

Gluconeogenesis is necessary for survival because only cells with mitochondria can use fatty acids as an energy source; red blood cells, which do not have mitochondria, must use glucose. However, gluconeogenisis does not produce enough glucose for the whole body, so the body is forced to rely more heavily on ketones. Ketones are a by-product of fatty acid breakdown that can be used as fuel by muscle and other body tissues, including the brain and central nervous system. As with episodes of fasting or starvation, low-carbohydrate diets also trigger the production of ketones because sources of dietary glucose are not consumed. Not surprisingly, prolonged strenuous physical activity will also induce ketone formation if glucose is not replenished.

When the levels of ketones in the body are high, it is referred to as ketosis. In a person who does not have diabetes, ketosis is a normal adaptation to starvation. However, in someone with type 1 diabetes, or in someone with sudden intractable insulin resistance (perhaps from an infection or steroid use), the levels of ketones in the body can get so high that a life-threatening condition called diabetic ketoacidosis (DKA) can emerge. DKA is generally the product of severe hyperglycemia (high blood glucose levels) in the absence of insulin. The body begins burning fatty acids at a very high rate, and ketone production goes through the roof. Ketosis is *not* the same as ketoacidosis, which is much more dangerous.

Going into ketosis using a modified fast or very low-calorie diet (see chapter 4) can be a powerful way to force your body to use up some of its stored energy. It can induce some impressive physiological adaptations, including the reduction of inflammation and elimination of damaged cells.[3] It can also help to significantly reduce lipotoxicity.[4] So there can be a place for these diets in a diabetes treatment regimen, but they do require careful medical monitoring and should be plant-based. Going into ketosis using a fast or a plant-based modified fast is far safer than going into ketosis using a long-term, very low-carbohydrate, high-animal-fat diet. Let's dive a little deeper into the latter.

How Are Low-Carb Diets Defined?

Low-carb diets are those that restrict the intake of carbohydrates to varying degrees. In typical low-carb diets, the percent of calories from macronutrients generally ranges from 5–25 percent carbohydrate, 10–30 percent protein, and 50–85 percent fat. At one end of the spectrum are the strictest low-carb diets known as ketogenic (or keto) diets. These diets generally allow no more than 20–30 grams of carbohydrate or 5 percent (or less) carbohydrate. Another popular option is the low-carb, high-fat diet (LCHF), which limits carbohydrates to under 100 grams per day and focuses on unprocessed foods, such as meat, seafood, eggs, dairy products, nuts, healthy fats, and nonstarchy vegetables. This diet would allow up to 20 percent of calories from carbohydrates. Still another well-known low-carb plan is the Atkins diet. There are four phases, beginning with an induction phase, which allows no more than 20 grams of carbohydrate per day, up to a phase-4 maintenance level that allows up to 100 grams of carbohydrate per day. More moderate low-carb diets allow 100–130 grams of carbohydrate or about 25 percent of total calories. It is important to understand that all categories of whole plant foods, with the exception of very high-fat foods (such as nuts, seeds, coconut, and avocado), provide an average of 58–92 percent of calories from carbohydrate. Even nonstarchy vegetables contain close to 60 percent of calories from carbohydrates (see figure 2.1, page 28).

Low-carb diets generally contain few plant-based foods. Grains, legumes, starchy vegetables, and fruit are restricted, and in more rigid programs they are completely eliminated (with the exception of a few berries). The plant foods permitted are nonstarchy vegetables and high-fat plant foods, such as nuts, seeds, coconut, and avocado. Even though nonstarchy vegetables contain close to 60 percent carbohydrate, they are so low in calories that total carbohydrate content is generally quite low.

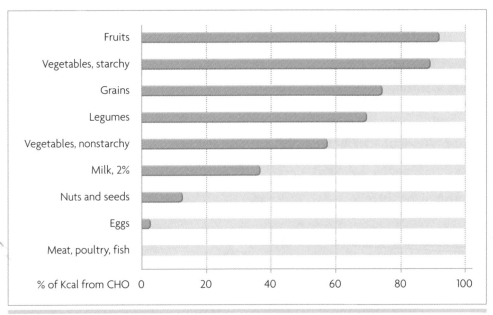

FIGURE 2.1 Average percentage of calories from carbohydrates in common foods.

Source: USDA Nutrient Database.

Some people are under the impression that if you follow a low-carb diet, you can eat unlimited amounts of nonstarchy vegetables. This is not the case. For example, if someone following a keto diet with a limit of 20 grams of carbohydrate wanted to meet the recommended nine to ten servings of vegetables and fruits per day (without including any fruits), that person could eat about six cups (1.5 L) of greens (6 g carbs), one cup (250 ml) of raw broccoli (6 g carbs), and a total of two cups (500 ml) of a combination of salad vegetables, such as cucumber, radishes, celery, and peppers (8 g carbs). Table 2.3 (opposite page) provides the carbohydrate content of common nonstarchy vegetables. As you can see, at a limit of 20 grams total carbohydrate, even nonstarchy vegetables would have to be restricted. For comparison, the carbohydrate content of one cup (250 ml) of whole grains (such as oatmeal, quinoa, or rice), starchy vegetables (potato or corn), or legumes ranges from 30–50 grams. A large banana, apple, or pear has about 30 grams of carbohydrate. See table 2.4 (opposite page) for the carbohydrate content of other foods. More moderate low-carb programs allow small amounts of these higher carbohydrate foods.

In low-carbohydrate diets, most of the calories come from fat. The predominant fat sources are meat, poultry, fish, eggs, dairy, nuts, seeds, avocados, coconut, and concentrated fats and oils, such as coconut oil (which is considered a superfood by many low-carb eaters).

TABLE 2.3. Carbohydrate Content of Nonstarchy Vegetables

FOOD, SERVING SIZE	CARB CONTENT (g)
Artichoke hearts, cooked, 1 medium	14
Brussels sprouts, cooked, 1 cup (250 ml)	11
Broccoli, cooked, 1 cup (250 ml)	10
Green beans, cooked, 1 cup (250 ml)	10
Eggplant, cooked, 1 cup (250 ml), cubed	9
Turnips, cooked, 1 cup (250 ml), cubed	8
Asparagus, cooked, 1 cup (250 ml)	7
Carrots, raw, 1 large	7
Tomato, raw, 1 large	7
Broccoli, raw, 1 cup (250 ml), chopped	6
Peppers, 1 cup (250 ml), sliced	6
Cauliflower, cooked, 1 cup (250 ml)	5
Cabbage, raw, 1 cup (250 ml)	4
Cucumber, 1 cup (250 ml), sliced	4
Radish, 1 cup (250 ml), sliced	4
Mushrooms, raw, 1 cup (250 ml)	3
Peas in pods, 10	3
Celery, 1 large stalk	2
Sprouts, raw, 1 cup (250 ml)	1-6
Greens, raw, 1 cup (250 ml)	1

Source: USDA National Nutrient Database for Standard Reference 1 Release, April 2018.

TABLE 2.4. Carbohydrate Content of Other Foods

FOOD, SERVING SIZE	CARB CONTENT (g)
Granola, 1 cup (250 ml)	66
Bagel, 1 medium	56
Rice, brown, cooked, 1 cup (250 ml)	52
Barley, cooked, 1 cup (250 ml)	44
Instant oatmeal, raisin spice, 1 cup (250 ml)	43
Beans/lentils, cooked, 1 cup (250 ml)	40
Quinoa, cooked, 1 cup (250 ml)	40
Potato, 1 medium	37
Pasta, cooked, 1 cup (250 ml)	36
Corn, cooked, 1 cup (250 ml)	31
Apple, 1 medium	30
Banana, 1 medium	27
Mango, raw, 1 cup (250 ml)	25
Bran flakes, 1 cup (250 ml)	24
Blueberries, 1 cup (250 ml)	21
Squash, winter, cooked, 1 cup (250 ml), cubed	15
Whole wheat bread, 1 slice	15
Strawberries, 1 cup (250 ml)	13
Milk, whole, 1 cup (250 ml)	11
Cream, light, 1 cup (250 ml)	9
Cream cheese, 2 Tbsp (30 ml)	1.5
Sour cream, 2 Tbsp (30 ml)	1
Cheese, 1 oz (30 g)	1
Butter, lard, oil	0
Meat, chicken, fish, eggs	0

Source: USDA National Nutrient Database for Standard Reference 1 Release, April 2018.

A typical keto menu looks something like this:

Breakfast: a three-egg omelet with sausage, spinach, and cheese, cooked in oil

Lunch: salad greens, meat, cheese, avocado, celery, tomatoes, and oily dressing

Dinner: pork chops (cooked in oil) with mushroom sauce (made with heavy whipping cream and butter) and asparagus with cheese sauce

Snacks: meat or fish jerky, cubed cheese, nuts and seeds, pork rinds, avocados, veggies with a cream cheese or sour cream dip.

How Low-Carb Diets Measure Up

How do low-carbohydrate eaters do when it comes to diabetes and related health issues? Five comprehensive reports (systematic reviews and meta-analyses), including four from 2018 and one from 2017, address this question. The most recent report, out of Norway, assessed the results of twenty-three studies.[59] Although reductions in HbA1c and triglycerides were slightly greater using a low-carbohydrate diet compared with a higher-carbohydrate diet, there were no differences in changes in body weight; total, LDL, and HDL cholesterol; or blood pressure. The HbA1c advantage disappeared within six months. The authors concluded that the proportion of daily energy provided by carbohydrate is not an important determinant of response to dietary management, especially when longer-term trials are factored in.

The second 2018 meta-analysis came from a research team in Australia. The effects of carbohydrate-restricted diets (less than 45 percent of energy coming from carbs) were compared with those of higher-carbohydrate diets (more than 45 percent of energy from carbs) on glycemic control in adults with diabetes.[60] Low-carbohydrate diets (less than 26 percent carbohydrates) produced greater reductions in HbA1c at three months (-0.47 percentage points) than higher-carbohydrate diets, although there were no significant differences at twelve or twenty-four months.

A third 2018 report, from a research team in the Netherlands, included thirty-six trials comparing low-carbohydrate diets (some with less-strict carb restriction—up to 40 percent of calories) with conventional (not plant-based) low-fat diets (30 percent fat or less) in patients with type 2 diabetes.[61] In short-term studies (up to eight weeks), HbA1c declined more in the low-carb eaters than in the low-fat eaters (the mean difference was -1.38 percentage point in the low-carb group and -0.36 percentage point in the low-fat group). However, differences diminished over time, and after two years there was no significant reduction in HbA1c and no difference between the two groups. It was noted that the low-carb group did have better results for fasting glucose, triglycerides, and HDL cholesterol concentrations. There was little to no difference between the two groups in LDL cholesterol, body weight, waist circumference, blood pressure, or quality of life. The authors concluded that the current available data show with low to moderate certainty that a diet that restricts carbohydrates to a maximum of 40 percent of calories yields slightly better metabolic control than reduction in fat to a maximum of 30 percent in people with type 2 diabetes.

A fourth 2018 meta-analysis, from a research team in the UK, reported on outcomes of eighteen interventions using low-carbohydrate diets versus traditional high-carbohydrate, low-fat diets in the management of diabetes.[62] The low-carbohydrate diets promoted more favorable changes in HbA1c, triglycerides, and HDL cholesterol and reduced requirements for diabetes medication. Seven studies provided data after one year. In these studies, the low-carb diet resulted in a drop in HbA1c of 0.28 percentage point, an HDL cholesterol increase of 2.3 mg/dL (0.06 mmol/L), a triglyceride reduction of 21.26 mg/dL (-0.24 mmol/L), and a systolic blood pressure reduction of 2.74 mmHg. Body weight, total cholesterol, LDL cholesterol, and diastolic blood pressure did not differ significantly between intervention groups. The authors concluded that a very low-carbohydrate diet (less than 50 grams per day) seems unrealistic for many individuals; however, a low-carbohydrate diet (less than 130 grams per day) appears to be achievable.

The fifth meta-analysis, from China, was released in 2017. This report included nine studies comparing low-carbohydrate diets with normal or high-carbohydrate diets in patients with type 2 diabetes. Findings were favorable for HbA1c (with a mean difference of -0.44 percentage point), triglycerides, and increased HDL cholesterol. No benefits were found for total or LDL cholesterol or long-term weight loss. The authors concluded that low-carbohydrate diets provided effective management of type 2 diabetes.[63]

In summary, there are benefits associated with low-carbohydrate diets, particularly in the short term. These diets are associated with weight loss, improved blood glucose levels, decreased triglycerides, and increased HDL cholesterol (although this may or may not be an advantage). On the other hand, there are known disadvantages, particularly when carbohydrate intakes are below 50 grams a day. Reports suggest that there are short-term detrimental impacts on LDL cholesterol, kidney function, kidney stones, glucose tolerance, gut microflora, bone health, nutritional status, markers of inflammation, and athletic performance.[64,65,66,67] Individuals on very low-carbohydrate diets also often complain of constipation, headaches, bad breath, and muscle weakness.[64] In the long term, low-carbohydrate diets have been associated with increased mortality, increased exposure to persistent organic pollutants (POPs), reduced bone density, impaired artery function, and increased risk of cardiovascular disease, birth defects, and possibly colon cancer (with high meat intakes).[64,68,69,70,71,72,73,74]

A 2018 study from an American research team reported on mortality from all causes in over fifteen thousand people eating various amounts of carbohydrate.[68] After adjusting for any variables that might influence the outcome, the study found that people consuming moderate amounts of carbohydrate (50–55 percent of calories) fared best. Those eating the fewest carbohydrates (less than 40 percent of calories) had the highest rates of mortality, followed by those eating the most carbohydrates (more than 70 percent of calories). However, results varied according to the sources of the macronutrients. Mortality increased by 18 percent when carbohydrates were exchanged for animal-derived fat or protein and decreased by 18 percent when the substitutions were plant-based (a difference of 36 percent). In this trial, very high-carbohydrate diets (more than 70 percent of calories) were associated with economically disadvantaged areas where refined carbohydrates, such as white rice and white flour products, are dietary staples. These types of diets reflect poor food quality and confer a chronically high glycemic load (see page 94).

WHY CHOOSE PLANT-BASED OVER LOW-CARB?

Low-carb diets, particularly ketogenic diets, do reduce the need for insulin and do lower and stabilize blood glucose. However, they *do not* reverse insulin resistance. In fact, if people who eat a low-carb diet are challenged with a load of carbohydrate (such as a bowl of oatmeal), they tend to have huge spikes in blood glucose because they remain so insulin resistant. This is because low-carb diets are relatively ineffective at reducing many of the drivers of insulin resistance. Of course, any strategy that produces sufficient weight loss will improve markers of diabetes. However, weight loss can be achieved by eating almost any combination of foods, just as long as an adequate caloric deficit is produced.

So although there are wildly divergent methods of producing weight loss and improving glycemic control, it makes sense to opt for the way that will best minimize health risks over the long term. It seems wise to select a pattern of eating that reduces the chances of developing heart disease, cancer, intestinal disorders, hypertension, and other lifestyle-induced diseases. Plant-based diets are associated with the greatest longevity and the lowest rates of chronic diseases of all dietary patterns. They maximize the most protective dietary components and minimize those that are the most pathogenic. Table 2.5 (pages 34–35) and table 2.6 (pages 36–37) explain some of the most vital differences between plant-based and low-carb dietary patterns.

In summary, plant-based diets outpower low-carb diets when it comes to diabetes reversal or almost any other desirable health outcome. David Katz, MD, one of the most recognized voices in health and nutrition (he's the founding director of Yale University's Prevention Research Center, past president of the American College of Lifestyle Medicine, and author of over two hundred scientific articles and fifteen books), provides a compelling argument against ketogenic or very low-carbohydrate diets in the following intriguing opinion piece:[75]

There is, for starters, no evidence that ketogenic diets are conducive to, or even compatible with, human health across the lifespan, or longevity. There is, instead, bountiful evidence that the very foods such diets exclude are associated with less diabetes, cancer, heart disease, dementia, and premature death in general. There is as well the experience of free-living populations. To date, every population group around the world found to experience remarkable vitality and longevity has a dietary pattern in which whole, nutrient-rich plant foods predominate, the very opposite of ketogenic. Vitality and longevity even in the last of the planet's hunter-gatherers, or foragers, is similarly linked to a plant-predominant, high-carbohydrate diet.

So, OK, ketogenic diets might help people live long and prosper, but there are, to date, no such people. Admittedly, the Inuit, for want of choice, have a very low-carbohydrate diet which may at times be ketogenic, but they do not experience enviable health or longevity.

There is, as well, the inconvenience factor of being on a "diet" for the rest of one's life. The argument for ketogenic diets reeks of fad because, like all fad diets, the benefits derive from eliminating most of the foods most people around the world like to eat. If ever there was a case of "fool me once, shame on you, fool me ten thousand times, shame on me," the marketing of the next diet fad is surely it.

Arguments for ketogenesis as anything other than the next batch of Kool-Aid brewed specially for suckers need to navigate past all such impediments. There is more, however. While such diets are likely to be harmful to the health of people, they are certain to be devastating for the fate of the planet. The clamor for ketogenic diets is at odds with every trend necessary to preserve our aquifers, wild places, biodiversity, and climate.

So maybe a diet low in vegetables, fruits, whole grains, beans, lentils, nuts and seeds— a diet low in antioxidants and phytonutrients and devoid of fiber—could be good for you in spite of it all. If you are reaching for your credit card accordingly, you should understand you are paying for the privilege of making a leap of faith. Time will tell about the landing.

DIETARY PATTERNS AND RISK

Overall dietary patterns have been carefully examined by researchers. Those patterns that are more plant-based consistently come out as being the most highly protective against both prediabetes and type 2 diabetes.

In 2011, a research group from Spain released an extensive review of diabetes and dietary patterns.[76] The study authors concluded that along with the maintenance of ideal body weight, the promotion of a prudent diet (characterized by a higher intake of plant-based foods and a lower intake of red meat, meat products, sweets, high-fat dairy products, and refined grains) or a Mediterranean dietary pattern rich in olive oil, fruits, and vegetables, including whole grains, pulses (legumes), nuts, and low-fat dairy products and allowing moderate alcohol consumption (mainly red wine) appears to be the best strategy for decreasing diabetes risk. The observational studies

TABLE 2.5. Protective Effects of Plant-Based vs Low-Carb Diets

PROTECTIVE DIETARY FACTORS	HEALTH EFFECTS	PRESENCE IN PLANT-BASED DIETS	PRESENCE IN LOW-CARB DIETS
Fiber	Improves gut microbiome; prevents constipation and other GI disorders; reduces risk of colorectal cancer, gallstones, cardiovascular disease, diabetes, and overweight.	High. Plants are the only sources. Legumes and grains are the most concentrated sources.	Low. The only sources are the limited plant foods included. Richest dietary sources (legumes and grains) are excluded.
Phytochemicals	Antioxidant and anti-inflammatory action. Block tumor formation; reduce inflammation; eradicate carcinogens; fight viruses, bacteria, and fungi; and protect blood vessels.	High. Plant foods are the only sources.	Low to moderate, depending on degree of carbohydrate restriction.
Plant enzymes	Help turn certain phytochemicals into their active forms; may aid digestion.	High. Concentrated in raw and sprouted plant foods.	Variable, depending on degree of carbohydrate restriction and inclusion of raw and sprouted foods.
Antioxidants	Protect against free radicals and oxidative stress; potentially reduce risk of artery damage, cancers, arthritis, cataracts, stroke, and other diseases.	High. Most whole plant foods are rich sources, so almost everything consumed will contribute to overall intake.	Variable. Intake depends on inclusion of plant foods, herbs and spices, coffee, cocoa, and tea. Animal products contain smaller amounts.
Pre- and probiotics	Support a healthy gut microbiome, protect against pathogens, boost nutritional status, reduce cancer risk, keep the intestinal wall healthy, support immune function, reduce inflammation, promote healthy body weight, and support brain function.	Probiotics: variable, depending on use of fermented and cultured foods. Prebiotics: high. Prebiotics come exclusively from plant foods, such as beans, whole grains, and some vegetables and fruits.	Probiotics: variable, depending on use of fermented and cultured foods. Prebiotics: low to moderate, as the only sources (plants) are restricted.
Plant sterols and stanols	Reduce cholesterol absorption from the gut, lowering total and LDL cholesterol. Blunt inflammation pathways.	Variable. Depending on intake of high-fat plant foods (such as nuts, seeds, avocados, wheat germ, and vegetable oils) and other plant foods, such as sprouts.	Variable. Depending on intake of high-fat plant foods (such as nuts, seeds, avocados, wheat germ, and vegetable oils) and other plant foods, such as sprouts.
Macronutrients (carbohydrate, protein, and fat)	Provide energy, help with building and rebuilding of body tissues, and provide structure and function.	Variable. Whole-food, plant-based diets provide a healthful balance of macronutrients. Plant-based protein is associated with disease risk reduction. Carbohydrates from whole plant foods are consistently protective to health. Unprocessed plant-based fats are associated with disease risk reduction. Omega-3 fats must be included.	Low-carb diets provide an unhealthy balance of macronutrients. In practice, animal-protein intake often exceeds healthful limits. Unrefined carbohydrate and fiber is too low. Intake of healthy fats is generally more than adequate; disproportionately high in saturated fat.

PROTECTIVE DIETARY FACTORS	HEALTH EFFECTS	PRESENCE IN PLANT-BASED DIETS	PRESENCE IN LOW-CARB DIETS
Micronutrients	Vitamins and minerals perform hundreds of roles. They support tissue and bone growth and repair, heal wounds, boost immune function, convert food into energy, and participate in essential chemical reactions. One measure of nutritional adequacy is nutrient density—the amount of vitamins and minerals (and sometimes other protective factors, such as fiber) in a food.	High. The most nutrient-dense foods are green leafy vegetables, followed by other vegetables, fruits, legumes, fish, nuts and seeds, and grains.	Low to moderate. One of the concerns about low-carb diets is nutritional deficiencies. The food with the lowest nutrient density is concentrated fat (which is almost devoid of vitamins and minerals). Fried foods, cheese, meat, and eggs also have low nutrient density.

reviewed in this report found two categories of foods clearly associated with elevated diabetes risk: animal products and processed foods. This includes red meat, processed meat, high-fat dairy products, packaged foods containing trans fats, fried foods, soft drinks, and foods high in refined carbohydrates (such as white flour and sugar). The dietary factors most strongly associated with decreased risk were plant-based foods or food components, such as vegetables, fruits, whole grains, and fiber.

In 2014, a team of experts from the Harvard School of Public Health released a comprehensive review that examined the evidence surrounding the prevention and management of diabetes.[77] Dietary factors associated with increased risk were excessive energy intakes leading to overweight or obesity, higher intake of saturated and animal fat, carbohydrate-rich foods with a high glycemic index and load, refined grains, sugar-sweetened beverages, high iron stores, and low vitamin D status. Frequent consumption of red meats, especially processed red meats (such as bacon, sausages, and hot dogs), was strongly associated with higher diabetes risk, while fish and seafood intake had no significant association. Intake of green leafy vegetables lowered risk, as did intake of whole fruits (such as apples, blueberries, and grapes). Dairy product intake was associated with a moderately lower diabetes risk, with yogurt intake being more beneficial than other dairy products. Consumption of nuts, especially walnuts, was associated with reduced diabetes risk. Alcohol intake in small amounts (22–24 g per day—about ¾ ounce) appeared to lower risk but became harmful in larger amounts (50–60 g per day, or about 2 ounces). Coffee intake was associated with lower risk. The authors concluded that the most healthful dietary patterns for diabetes prevention and management are typically rich in whole grains, fruits, vegetables, nuts, and legumes; are moderate in alcohol; and are lower in refined grains, red and processed meats, and sugar-sweetened beverages.

TABLE 2.6. Pathogenic Effects of Plant-Based vs Low-Carb Diets

PATHOGENIC DIETARY FACTORS	HEALTH EFFECTS	PRESENCE IN PLANT-BASED DIETS	PRESENCE IN LOW-CARB DIETS
Trans-fatty acids	Increase risk of cardiovascular disease, diabetes, and other chronic diseases. They are the most damaging fats of all.	Zero or low. Plant-based diets minimize processed foods that contain manufactured trans-fatty acids and eliminate animal products, which may contain natural trans-fatty acids.	Low to moderate. Although foods containing manufactured trans-fatty acids are minimized or excluded, fatty animal products with natural trans fats are generously consumed. Although less harmful than manufactured trans fats, both impair insulin sensitivity and increase oxidative stress.
Excessive saturated fat	Increases total and LDL cholesterol and risk of cardiovascular disease; impairs insulin sensitivity.	Low. Plant-based diets are generally the only diets that meet the recommended limit of 5–6 percent saturated fat to reduce heart disease risk.	Very high. Saturated fat varies from 20–50 percent of total calories. The upper limit for saturated fat in a 2,000 kcal diet is about 22 grams based on the upper limit of 10 percent set for the general population. A typical low-carb diet providing 70 percent of calories from fat could easily contain over 90 grams of saturated fat.
Refined carbohydrates	Increase risk of overeating and obesity, promote fatty liver, increase insulin resistance and diabetes risk, and adversely affect blood lipids and cardiovascular disease risk.	Low to moderate. Most plant-based diets promoted for disease risk reduction dramatically reduce refined carbohydrates and rely on whole plant foods. However, some permit the use of white rice and some white flour products.	Zero to very low. As carbohydrates are limited primarily to vegetables, refined carbohydrate foods are eliminated.
Excessive animal protein	Consistently linked to increases in all causes of mortality and increased risk of heart disease, diabetes, and several cancers.	Zero to very low. Most plant-based diets exclude animal protein, although some allow 5–10 percent. Excessive intake is not an issue.	High. Low-carbohydrate diets are generally high animal-protein diets. Many contain 20–25 percent of calories from protein, which has been associated with increased mortality and disease risk in many scientific studies.
Excessive sodium	Increases risk of hypertension and cardiovascular disease, osteoporosis, and some cancers. People with diabetes who have poor blood glucose control are at very high risk for cardiovascular disease with high sodium intakes.	Variable, depending on sodium added to foods and use of condiments and processed foods.	Variable, depending mostly on sodium added to foods and use of condiments, as well as use of processed meat and cheese.

PATHOGENIC DIETARY FACTORS	HEALTH EFFECTS	PRESENCE IN PLANT-BASED DIETS	PRESENCE IN LOW-CARB DIETS
Chemical contaminants	Increase oxidative stress, fuel inflammation, disrupt hormones (obesogenic), damage vital organs, damage DNA and the central nervous system, and increase risk of diabetes and other chronic diseases.	Low to moderate. Pesticide residues from conventional produce can be contributors. Organic foods contain much less. Very low in heavy metals (except for arsenic in rice), drugs given to animals, and persistent organic pollutants (POPs), such as PCBs, DDT, and dioxins.	Moderate to high. POPs become more concentrated as they are moved up the food chain, with the most in fish and meat. Heavy metals are highest in fish, shellfish, meat, and dairy products. Heavy metals are concentrated in fish and chicken. Hormones, antibiotics, and antimicrobial agents come mainly from meat, poultry, dairy, and fish.
Products of high-temperature cooking	Increase risk of cancer, diabetes, Alzheimer's disease, and other chronic conditions. Promote oxidative stress and inflammation.	No heterocyclic amines. Presence of polycyclic aromatic hydrocarbons varies with cooking methods: higher with dry heat and high temperatures. Acrylamides vary with use of potato products (especially when cooked with dry heat or fried). AGEs vary but are generally low.	Heterocyclic amines are generally high, formed with high-temperature cooking of meat, poultry, and eggs. Polycyclic aromatic hydrocarbons vary; higher with dry heat and high temperatures, especially frying. Acrylamides are generally low, as most of the concentrated sources are potato products. AGEs are generally high, most concentrated in processed meats.
Heme iron	Oxidative stress. Increases risk of insulin resistance, metabolic syndrome, diabetes, cardiovascular disease, and some cancers.	Zero to very low. Only present in diets containing meat.	High.
Neu5Gc	Induces inflammation and diseases triggered by inflammation.	Zero to very low. Only present in diets containing meat.	Variable. Increases as red meat increases.
TMAO	Induces inflammation, contributes to plaque formation and kidney disease.	Zero to very low. Only formed with meat consumption or intake of fish.	High. Formed with meat consumption or direct intake from fish.
Endotoxins	Associated with inflammation, insulin resistance, diabetes, and obesity.	Low. Animal products are the primary sources.	Moderate to high. Found in the outer cell membranes of gram-negative bacteria. Come from the breakdown of gut bacteria or food bacteria (meat, poultry, and dairy products).

The 2018 Clinical Practice Guidelines for Nutrition Therapy (Diabetes Canada) reviewed the scientific literature on dietary patterns and diabetes risk.[78] The patterns most consistently associated with reduced risk were Mediterranean diets, vegetarian diets, DASH diets, the Portfolio Diet, and the Nordic diet (a combination of Mediterranean, DASH, and National Cholesterol Education Program dietary patterns). In all of these diets, emphasis is placed on whole plant foods: vegetables, fruits, legumes, whole grains, and nuts and seeds. Some recommend moderate amounts of low-fat dairy products and fish; some suggest the addition of olive oil. Others suggest the use of vegetable protein rather than animal-protein sources. All advocate for low intakes of meat, especially red and processed meats, refined carbohydrates, and sugar-sweetened beverages.

In 2016, an innovative Harvard study that looked at specific plant-based dietary patterns and risk was published.[79] In this report, researchers examined different types of plant-based diets to ascertain which would be most protective. They used data from the Nurses' Health Study and the Health Professionals Follow-Up Study, including over 130,000 individuals. They created a healthful plant-based diet index (hPDI), in which nutritious plant foods (whole grains, fruits, vegetables, nuts, legumes, vegetable oils, tea, and coffee) received positive scores, while less-nutritious plant foods (fruit juices, sweetened beverages, refined grains, potatoes, sweets, and desserts) and animal products received negative scores. They also created an unhealthful plant-based diet index (uPDI) by assigning positive scores to less healthy plant foods and negative scores to healthy plant foods and animal products. The hPDI was associated with a 45 percent reduction in diabetes risk, although this dropped to 34 percent when adjusted for body mass index (BMI), a measure of body fatness (see page 58). The uPDI was associated with a 16 percent increase in diabetes risk, even after BMI adjustment.

The take-home message is that plant-based diets are well recognized by scientists as being the dietary patterns associated with the greatest reduction in type 2 diabetes risk. The plant-based diets that are most protective are those that rely on whole plant foods as their foundation.

ARE PEOPLE EATING PLANT-BASED DIETS AT LOWER RISK FOR DIABETES?

There is no controversy: People who eat mainly plants suffer less type 2 diabetes. The most impressive evidence to date comes from the Adventist Health Study-2 (AHS-2) and the Taiwanese Buddhist studies.

In the AHS-2, compared to health-conscious nonvegetarians, vegans had the lowest odds of having diabetes, followed by lacto-ovo vegetarians, pesco-vegetarians (who occasionally eat fish), and semi-vegetarians (who occasionally add meat).[80] Data was adjusted for all confounding variables except body mass index (BMI). However, when

TABLE 2.7. Risk Reduction for Plant-Based Eaters Compared to Health-Conscious Meat Eaters

RISK REDUCTION	VEGAN	LACTO-OVO VEGETARIAN	PESCO VEGETARIAN	SEMI-VEGETARIAN
Adjusted for all confounders, EXCLUDING BMI	68%	57%	44%	31%
Adjusted for all confounders, INCLUDING BMI	49%	46%	30%	24%

BMI was also adjusted for, the differences were still remarkable. When the participants who did not have diabetes were followed for two years, the odds of developing diabetes (when adjusted for all factors, including BMI) was lowest among vegans. See the table above for the findings.

In 2014, a research group from Taiwan published findings that compared diabetes rates in health-conscious Taiwanese Buddhist volunteers who consumed vegetarian (near-vegan) or omnivorous diets.[81] After adjustments for age, BMI, education, family history of diabetes, physical activity, smoking, and alcohol consumption, vegetarian (near-vegan) diets lowered risk by 51 percent in men, by 74 percent in premenopausal women, and by 75 percent in postmenopausal women.

In 2018, almost three thousand Taiwanese Buddhists who were free of diabetes were followed for a median of five years to see who would develop diabetes.[5] Consistent intake of vegetarian diets was associated with a risk reduction of 35 percent, while converting from a nonvegetarian to a vegetarian pattern was associated with a risk reduction of 53 percent.[82]

In 2008, an AHS-2 study reported that participants who consumed meat weekly were 29 percent more likely to develop diabetes. Participants who consumed any amount of processed meat were 38 percent more likely to develop diabetes, and those who had long-term adherence to a diet that included at least weekly meat intake was associated with an increase in risk of 74 percent. Even after controlling for weight (body fatness) and weight change, weekly meat intake increased diabetes risk by 38 percent.[83]

CAN EVERYONE KICK DIABETES?

The majority of people can kick diabetes, though not everyone. If someone has sustained too much damage to their pancreas to produce sufficient insulin, their diabetes may be chronic regardless of which dietary pattern they follow. They may overcome insulin resistance, reduce lipotoxicity, overcome inflammation and oxidative stress, and reestablish a healthy gut microbiome, yet their blood sugars won't completely normalize. Preliminary evidence suggests that in the face of huge insulin demands, beta cells can become overwhelmed and go into a dormant or resting state. They go on strike, if you will. In most cases, it appears that these cells can be turned back on when insulin sensitivity is restored and insulin demands are diminished. This means that in many people with diabetes, beta cell function can be recovered. Generally, the degree of achieved weight loss is the main determinant of remission. However, the longer a person has the disease, the more challenging complete reversal becomes. In people who have had the disease for a long time, a greater degree of weight loss appears to be necessary for reversal than is needed in people who have developed the disease more recently.[5]

It can be devastating to make sufficient lifestyle changes to reverse insulin resistance only to discover that your pancreas is too damaged to reverse your diabetes. No matter how brilliantly your diet is designed and how physically active you become, if you're in this group, you'll require injected insulin for the rest of your life because your pancreas function can no longer meet your body's insulin needs. However, regardless of your insulin production, take heart that overcoming insulin resistance itself will dramatically improve your health and quality of life. Restoring your body's insulin sensitivity reduces your risk for many conditions, including heart disease, hypertension, certain types of cancer, and dementia. Overcoming insulin resistance also means that you'll need the lowest possible insulin doses, which effectively reduces your risk for the most dreaded complications of diabetes.

WHY ARE VEGAN FOODS SO PROTECTIVE?

Research points convincingly to the success of vegan diets in helping people kick diabetes, but why? Are all plant foods beneficial, or are some better than others? What specific factors in these foods make them so effective for overcoming insulin resistance?

The answers lie not only in what vegan diets contain but also in what they eliminate. In the next chapter we'll explore the research that provides these answers.

Chapter 3

Diet Smarts and Lessons to Live By

When Elaine asked Diane if she would be willing to watch a new documentary film called *Eating You Alive,* Diane said yes, just to please her. The DVD sat on Diane's kitchen counter for over a week before Elaine asked her if she had a chance to watch it. She responded honestly but promised Elaine that she would watch it that night—and a promise is a promise. As Diane popped in the DVD, she thought about the many more important things she could be doing and felt a tinge of resentment. Within the first five minutes, however, her mood began to shift. Could the claims they were making be true?

If so, for Diane this message was no less than earth-shattering. She listened to story after story of healing from diseases that she was so certain were incurable. She heard expert after expert building a case for lifestyle medicine that was far too compelling to ignore. The take-home message was ridiculously simple: If what we eat is the problem, perhaps what we eat is also the solution. The film provided Diane with her first glimmer of hope that a lifetime of diabetes is not a foregone conclusion. She vowed on the spot that she would dig as deep as she could to uncover the truth. She discovered a wealth of resources—DVDs, books, websites, and even research articles—that confirmed the basic premise of the original film. (For such a list, see page 231.) Then Diane made a decision that would change the course of her life. If diabetes can be reversed, then she would do whatever it takes to reverse it.

She went online and started searching for more information about plant-based diets and diabetes. That's how she found the online plant-based support program that turned her life right-side up. It was a program that offered live audio and video conferences, one-on-one support, group support, cooking instruction, and comprehensive lab testing. Diane knew in an instant that she had arrived at exactly where she needed to be, and she has never looked back. The information in this chapter provides a glimpse of the evidence that suggests Diane's decision to go plant-based was a wise one.

Research has clearly demonstrated that healthful lifestyle choices can change the expression of our genes, turning off disease-promoting genes and turning on disease-preventing genes.[1] With the appropriate choices, experts estimate that we could prevent 90 percent of type 2 diabetes, and there is strong consensus that diet is the kingpin.[2] Adopting healthy diet and lifestyle choices after the onset of type 2 diabetes can change the course of the disease and, in some cases, reverse it altogether.[3,4,5]

So what is it about eating plants that gives people an advantage? There are two factors that are crucial: (1) plant-based diets maximize the dietary components proven to be protective to human health, and (2) plant-based diets minimize the dietary components that are known to be harmful. Let's delve a little deeper into each of these.

PLANT-BASED PROTECTION: THE FRIENDS IN FOODS

Part of the reason people eating plant-based diets are protected is because they are less likely to be overweight or obese.[7,8] However, it's the inherent nutritional profile of plants that affords the lion's share of the protection. The dietary components that are most strongly tied to risk reduction are concentrated in plants. These dietary components help protect against obesity, insulin resistance, inflammation, oxidative stress, lipotoxicity, glucotoxicity, and dysbiosis. They essentially disable the key drivers of the disease. Consequently, they not only protect but also improve outcomes and increase the chances of recovery. There are a number of these protective dietary components that are particularly notable.

Fiber

This indigestible part of plants helps control blood sugar, lowers blood cholesterol, keeps the gastrointestinal system healthy, encourages a health-supportive mix of gut bacteria, and aids with weight loss by staving off hunger. All whole plant foods contain fiber; it provides their shape and structure. Animal flesh foods, dairy products, sugar, and oil provide none.

Multiple studies have demonstrated an inverse relationship between fiber intake and diabetes risk—the more fiber you eat, the lower your risk.[9,10,11,12,13] One recent meta-analysis of seventeen studies, including almost five hundred thousand participants and over nineteen thousand incident cases of type 2 diabetes, reported a 6 percent decrease in diabetes risk for every 2 grams of fiber consumed.[9] Diabetes risk was reduced as follows:

15 grams fiber/day → 2 percent

20 grams fiber/day → 3 percent

25 grams fiber/day → 11 percent

30 grams fiber/day → 24 percent

35 grams fiber/day → 34 percent

Although data wasn't provided for people who consumed higher amounts, we can do the math. A person eating a whole-foods, plant-based diet would easily consume 50 grams of fiber per day. If we assume a 34 percent risk reduction for 35 grams, this would mean adding an extra 15 grams of fiber. Based on the general estimate of 6 percent per 2-gram increase, risk reduction would be about 79 percent (34 + 15/2 x 6). This figure is very similar to the actual risk reduction reported in people who eat a 100 percent plant-based diet.

Higher fiber intakes have also been associated with better outcomes for people who have diabetes—weight loss, improved glycemic control, better insulin sensitivity, and a healthier gut microbiome.[13,14,15,16]

Phytochemicals

Thousands of protective phytochemicals (plant chemicals) cut the risk of type 2 diabetes and enhance the potential for effective dietary treatment. Phytochemicals accomplish these tasks by reducing inflammation and oxidative stress, improving the balance of gut microbiota, improving fasting blood glucose and insulin sensitivity, preventing weight gain, slowing or reducing carbohydrate absorption, stimulating insulin secretion from the pancreas, activating insulin receptors, and promoting insulin signaling.[17,18,19,20,21,22,23]

Phytochemicals also add glorious color and flavor to plant foods. Like fiber, phytochemicals are plentiful in plants but absent from animal products. Examples of phytochemicals known to afford protection are curcumin in turmeric, capsaicin in hot chiles, gingerol in ginger, catechin in tea, resveratrol in grapes and berries, genistein in soy, and quercetin in onions.[24,25]

A review of curcumin and diabetes reported improvements in inflammation, oxidative stress, hyperglycemia, insulin sensitivity, hyperlipidemia (high blood lipids), and beta cell dysfunction or death. In addition, curcumin ameliorates many of the complications of diabetes, including neuropathy, nephropathy (kidney damage), and vascular disease.[25] Capsaicin has been reported to suppress inflammation, improve insulin resistance and glucose tolerance, and improve blood lipids.[26] A meta-analysis of ten studies reported a significant beneficial effect of ginger on blood glucose control and insulin sensitivity in people with type 2 diabetes.[27] Reports suggest beneficial effects of tea due to its antioxidant and antidiabetic properties and its ability to target risk factors, such as obesity, high cholesterol, and hypertension.[28,29] Resveratrol may improve glucose control, decrease insulin resistance, protect pancreatic beta cells, improve insulin secretion, and reduce oxidative stress and inflammation.[30,31] Genistein, derived from soy, has been shown to protect pancreatic beta cells and reduce obesity-related low-grade inflammation.[32] Quercetin, a key phytochemical in onions, berries, apples, and other vegetables and fruits, exhibits positive effects on gene expression, fat metabolism, and inflammation and reduces the risk of obesity. It has also been shown to stimulate glucose uptake and reduce glucose production in the liver. In human studies, quercetin decreases the signs and symptoms of neuropathy.[33]

Plant Enzymes

Raw plant foods contain enzymes that help to convert specific phytochemicals into their active forms. The most plentiful sources of these important plant enzymes are raw cruciferous and *Allium* vegetables.[34] For example, an enzyme called myrosinase in cruciferous vegetables (such as arugula, broccoli, Brussels sprouts, cabbage, cauliflower, collards, kale, kohlrabi, radishes, turnips, and watercress) helps to convert a group of phytochemicals called glucosinolates into an active form called isothiocyanates. The active compounds help us process and eliminate harmful substances. Another enzyme called alliinase in *Allium* vegetables (such as chives, garlic, leeks, and onions) converts a phytochemical called alliin to allicin, its active form. Allicin has antimicrobial, antiviral, and antifungal properties. It lowers cholesterol and fights inflammation. The enzymes myrosinase and alliinase are released in plants when the food is chopped, mashed, blended, or chewed. Once released, the conversion of phytochemicals into their active forms begins. Cooking foods destroys some or all of these enzymes, depending on how long they are cooked and the temperature used. Although we have not yet identified enzymes in other plant foods that serve in this capacity, this is a relatively new area of research, so we can expect others may soon be discovered.

Antioxidants

Common antioxidants that protect from free radicals and oxidative stress (see page 9) are vitamins C and E, selenium, carotenoids, and flavonoids. The most concentrated sources of antioxidants are colorful vegetables, fruits, herbs, spices, legumes, whole grains, nuts, and seeds.

One recent review reported that carotenoids enhance insulin sensitivity and protect the body from long-term complications of diabetes, including nephropathy and nervous system and eye abnormalities.[35] Another review reported that insufficient dietary antioxidants, such as beta-carotene, vitamin C, and vitamin E, can induce oxidative stress and inflammation, especially in people who are obese.[36] Oxidative stress, in turn, induces beta cell dysfunction, insulin resistance, and complications of diabetes.

Pre- and Probiotics

Prebiotics are food for beneficial bacteria, stimulating their growth and activity. The best sources are plants with indigestible sugars, such as asparagus, bananas, chicory, garlic, Jerusalem artichokes, leeks, onions, and sweet potatoes. Probiotics are beneficial bacteria that come in foods or supplements. The richest plant sources are sauerkraut, tempeh, miso, certain fermented beverages (kombucha), naturally fermented vegetables, nondairy yogurts, and nut cheeses. Probiotics also can be taken as supplements. Prebiotics and probiotics can improve your community of gut microbes, which can reduce chronic inflammation, improve insulin sensitivity and insulin signaling, and control blood sugar. Eating foods with plenty of polyphenols can increase the population of good bacteria and reduce some particularly nasty bugs. Great sources include grapes, blueberries, cocoa, broccoli, almonds, onions, and green tea.[37,38,39]

Omega-3 Fatty Acids

Omega-3 fatty acids, particularly the long-chain omega-3 fatty acid EPA (and DHA to a lesser extent), have impressive anti-inflammatory action.[40,41] Alpha-linolenic acid (ALA) appears to have antiobesity effects, and all three omega-3s appear to improve insulin secretion and insulin sensitivity.[42] These fatty acids are produced by microalgae (which is cultured for supplements) and are found in fish or produced internally from plant omega-3s in chia seeds, flaxseeds, hemp seeds, and walnuts.

Plant Sterols

With favorable effects on health, plant sterols are most concentrated in nuts and seeds (and their oils), avocados, and legumes (especially adzuki beans, chickpeas, kidney beans, lentils, peas, and soybeans). Lesser amounts are found in vegetables (especially cruciferous vegetables, such as Brussels sprouts, broccoli, and cauliflower, as well as corn, dill, and parsley), fruits (especially apricots, figs, oranges, and passion fruit), and whole grains. Although research is limited and often done using supplements rather than foods, plant sterols and stanols may reduce blood lipids, markers of oxidative stress and inflammation, and improve endothelial function.[43,44,45]

Commonsense Conclusions

As you go down the list of beneficial food components, the critical role of plant foods in the prevention and reversal of diabetes becomes clear. Almost every protective dietary component is found either exclusively or predominantly in plant foods. These food factors work together to turn off disease-promoting genes, reduce inflammation, boost immune function, balance hormones, enhance detoxification systems, maintain blood glucose levels, and keep blood pressure and blood cholesterol levels in check. The bottom line is that any dietary arsenal powerful enough to kick diabetes must be loaded with whole plant foods.

PLANT FOODS: FORTIFYING THE EVIDENCE

ot surprisingly, intakes of specific plant foods are consistently associated with reduced diabetes risk. Let's explore the most recent evidence.

Vegetables and Fruits

Studies consistently demonstrate that higher intakes of vegetables and fruits are associated with lower rates of type 2 diabetes. In the EPIC-Norfolk study, compared with participants in the bottom 25 percent (quartile) of intake, risk was reduced by 81 percent for those in the highest quartile, 66 percent for those in the second highest quartile, and 30 percent for those in the second lowest quartile.[46] In a recent study from China, compared to the lowest quartile of fruit and vegetable intake, the risk of type 2 diabetes in women was 34 percent lower in the highest quartile of intake, 50 percent lower in the second highest quartile, and 9 percent lower in the second lowest quartile of intake.[47] A meta-analysis of ten studies reported that for every serving of vegetables consumed per day, type 2 diabetes risk was reduced by 10 percent, and for every serving of fruit, type 2 diabetes risk was reduced by 7 percent. For every 0.2 serving of green leafy vegetables per day (equivalent of ⅓ cup or 50 ml), risk was reduced 13 percent.[48] Finally, a meta-analysis of thirteen studies reported a minor risk reduction for type 2 diabetes of 2 percent with vegetable intake, although risk dropped 9 percent when vegetable intake rose to 10.5 ounces (300 g).[49] The same study reported a 7 percent risk reduction for the highest versus lowest fruit consumers, and risk fell by 10 percent when intakes reached 7–10.5 ounces (200–300 g).

Legumes

Not only are legumes the richest dietary sources of fiber, but these protein powerhouses also have a very low glycemic index and are sources of a wide variety of bioactive compounds, such as phytochemicals and plant sterols. Studies consistently show that soybeans and other legumes improve insulin sensitivity and produce significant reductions in HOMA-IR (a measure of insulin resistance). One comprehensive review detailed the mechanisms of action, including antioxidant activities, increased glucose transporter levels, inhibition of adipogenesis (fat deposits), and improved gut microbiota.[50]

One study of legume intake in over 150,000 participants in India reported that daily legume intake resulted in a 54 percent reduction in risk of type 2 diabetes in women and a 38 percent risk reduction in men (although the finding in men was not statistically significant). Weekly legume intake was associated with a 49 percent risk reduction in both men and women (all figures were adjusted for confounding variables, including BMI).[51] In the Shanghai Women's Health Study, risk of developing type 2 diabetes was 38 percent lower in those with the highest quintile of legume intake and 47 percent lower in those with the highest quintile of soy intake.[52] A large meta-analysis reported a 13 percent risk reduction for the highest versus lowest soy consumers and a 26 percent risk reduction in women.[53]

Whole Grains

While refined grains are commonly associated with increased risk of type 2 diabetes, whole grains are consistently associated with reduced risk. In a meta-analysis of sixteen studies, every three servings of whole grains per day was associated with a 34 percent risk reduction.[54] In a second meta-analysis of sixty-six studies, participants consuming three to five servings of whole grains per day had a 26 percent lower risk of type 2 diabetes than those who rarely or never consumed whole grains.[55] In a third meta-analysis of thirteen studies, a 23 percent risk reduction was reported in the highest versus lowest whole-grain consumers. Each serving of whole grains resulted in a 13 percent risk reduction.[49] A recent Danish study reported that for every whole-grain serving, type 2 diabetes risk was reduced by 11 percent for men and 7 percent for women.[56]

Nuts

A recent study from the Middle East of almost two thousand participants reported that people consuming at least four servings, each serving being 1 ounce (30 g), of nuts per week had a 53 percent lower risk of diabetes than those consuming less than one serving per week, when the data was fully adjusted for confounding variables.[57] In a meta-analysis of eighteen studies, each serving per day of nuts reduced the risk of type 2 diabetes by 20 percent, although this effect was reduced when adjusted for BMI.[58]

Seeds

Although there are few studies looking at the association between seed consumption and type 2 diabetes, it makes sense that there would be more impressive findings with seeds than with nuts based on their nutrient profile (more fiber, essential fatty acids, and trace minerals than nuts). A 2017 study reported that 1 ounce of chia or flaxseeds favorably affected blood glucose response, with chia being slightly more effective than flax.[59]

WESTERN DIET WOES: THE FIENDS IN FOOD

Just as there are dietary components that are protective against diabetes, there are components that can be pathogenic, increasing risk or accelerating the disease and its complications. There are a number of specific "fiends" in foods that are associated with both promotion and progression of diabetes.

Refined Carbohydrates

Although carbohydrates have been vilified in the popular press, the amount of carbohydrate in someone's diet does not appreciably influence diabetes risk.[60] Rather, it is the quality of carbohydrates that determines health outcomes. Refined carbohydrates with a high glycemic index and glycemic load (see page 94) are particularly problematic, while carbohydrates intrinsic to whole plant foods are protective. Refined carbohydrates have been stripped of fiber and other protective components. They are consumed as sugars (such as white or brown sugar or syrups) or as sugars that are a major component of sweet items (such as beverages, candies, jams, jellies, and gelatin-based desserts), starches (such as white flour used in breads and crackers), or both sugar and starches together (such as sugar and white flour in cakes, pies, and cookies). Refined carbohydrates promote overeating and obesity, fuel inflammation, impair immunity, promote insulin resistance, increase blood sugar levels and triglycerides, and contribute to nonalcoholic fatty liver disease (NAFLD).[61,62,63,64,65,66,67]

Trans-Fatty Acids

Trans fats are the most damaging fats in the diet. They're formed when fats are turned from liquid oils to solids during hydrogenation (adding hydrogen under pressure). A 2018 study of US adults reported that those with the highest intakes of trans-fatty acids (from all sources) had more than double the risk of type 2 diabetes compared with those eating the least.[68] Trans fats increase insulin resistance, adversely affect glucose metabolism, boost LDL (bad cholesterol) and triglycerides, and decrease HDL (good cholesterol).[69,70,71,72] The main sources are shortenings and processed and deep-fried foods containing partially hydrogenated oils.

Saturated Fat

Although saturated fat is present in all whole foods, it is most concentrated in animal products and tropical oils. Generally, the more solid a fat is at room temperature, the greater the percent of the total fat that is saturated. Approximately 11 percent of the calories in most American diets come from saturated fat, with low-carbohydrate diets often containing 20 percent or more. The US Dietary Guidelines recommend that saturated fat account for less than 10 percent of total calories. Only 29 percent of Americans achieve that goal.[73] According to the American College of Cardiology and the American Heart Association, people who are at high risk for heart disease (such as individuals with type 2 diabetes) are advised to limit saturated fat to not more than 5–6 percent of total calories.[74] Saturated fat is associated with insulin resistance, inflammation, reduced insulin secretion from the pancreas, and increased blood cholesterol levels.[74,75,76,77,78]

Food sources that contribute the highest amounts of saturated fat in the US are dairy cheeses and desserts, pizza, processed meats, grain-based desserts (made with ingredients such as butter, eggs, and coconut oil), burgers, cow's milk, eggs, butter, and potato chips.[73] Although tropical oils contain a higher percentage of calories from saturated fat than animal products, total intake from these oils has traditionally been much smaller. This is beginning to change with the rise in popularity of coconut products and tropical oils used in place of partially hydrogenated fats in processed foods. Fifty to 87 percent of the fat in tropical oils is saturated, with coconut oil being at the highest end of this range. This compares to over 60 percent in dairy, about 40 percent in meat, 30 percent in chicken, and 20–30 percent in fish. The fat in plant foods (with the exception of tropical oils) ranges from 10–20 percent saturated.[79]

Environmental Contaminants

Hazardous materials that enter the food chain unintentionally can fuel inflammation, cause oxidative stress, disrupt hormones, induce dysbiosis, increase blood pressure, and damage vital organs, DNA, and the central nervous system. Environmental contaminants also contribute to beta-cell malfunction, insulin resistance, and the development and progression of diabetes.[80] Many chemicals can alter the normal function of the endocrine system. These chemicals are known as endocrine disrupting chemicals (EDCs), or simply endocrine disruptors. EDCs include industrial pollutants, heavy metals, food packaging materials, and agrochemicals.[80]

Industrial pollutants (also called persistent organic pollutants, or POPs), such as PCBs, dioxins, and TCDD (an herbicide), can result in significant damage during gestation and lactation, causing glucose intolerance in offspring. TCDD has been shown to reduce glucose uptake in adipose tissue, the pancreas, and the liver; increase the production of inflammatory cytokines; and decrease insulin secretion, potentially contributing to the onset of type 2 diabetes.[80] The main source of POPs is animal fat, which contributes about 95 percent of total intake.[81]

Heavy metals, such as mercury, arsenic, and cadmium, have been linked with the progression of impaired insulin secretion and decreased insulin sensitivity. Mercury is most concentrated in fish and seafood; arsenic is present in rice, rice products, chicken, seaweed, and fruit juices; and cadmium is derived mainly from cigarette smoke, grains, fish, seafood, organ meats, seaweed, root vegetables, and cocoa powder.[80,82]

Food packaging materials, such as bisphenol A (BPA), can act as chemicals that mimic estrogen (xenoestrogens). They can cause insulin resistance, insulin oversecretion, and beta cell exhaustion, contributing to the development and progression of type 2 diabetes.[80]

Agrochemicals, such as pesticides, can contribute to oxidative stress, induce pancreatitis and beta cell damage, and impair glucose uptake and insulin secretion.[80] A systematic review and meta-analysis reported that those in the top tertile (one-third) of participants who had exposure to any pesticides had a 61 percent higher risk of developing type 2 diabetes than those in the bottom tertile.[83]

Products of High-Temperature Cooking

Cooking at high temperatures can generate products of oxidation that are damaging to human health. These substances contribute to oxidative stress and inflammation and can contribute to the development and progression of disease, including diabetes. The most notorious are heterocyclic amines (HCAs), polycyclic aromatic hydrocarbons (PAHs), and advanced glycation end products (AGEs).

HCAs are chemicals that are formed when meat, poultry, and fish are subjected to high temperatures, particularly with grilling, frying, or cooking with dry heat. They're not present in plant foods because the formation of HCAs requires the presence of the amino acids creatine or creatinine, and these compounds are found only in animal tissue. HCAs have been linked to increased diabetes risk, whether the source is red meat or chicken. In a recent study of over 138,000 individuals, the risk of developing type 2 diabetes was 28 percent higher in those eating meat cooked with an open flame or at high temperatures more than fifteen times a month compared with those eating it less than four times a month.[84]

PAHs are a group of several hundred chemically related compounds that are formed by the incomplete burning of organic substances, including foods that are heated to temperatures above 350 degrees F (176 degrees C). The most concentrated dietary sources are grilled or charred meat, poultry, or fish; grain products; fats and oils; and sweets. Although grain products cooked with dry heat or grilling can contain relatively high levels, whole grains that are soaked, sprouted, boiled, or steamed are negligible sources. In a recent study of over 8,600 participants, the risk of developing type 2 diabetes was 73 percent higher in those with the highest quintile of exposure (top quarter of the participants) compared with those in the lowest quintile of exposure (bottom quarter of the participants).[85,86]

AGEs are harmful end products of fat oxidation or the Maillard reaction (browning of foods that occurs when sugars combine with amino acids). They are also produced within the body during sustained hyperglycemia (elevated blood glucose). AGEs are associated with oxidative stress, decreased glucose-stimulated insulin secretion, insulin resistance, and beta cell damage. The main sources are broiled, seared, or fried meats, especially processed meats; other grilled or fried foods; butter; margarine; and roasted nuts. Fructose forms AGEs at a more rapid rate than glucose.[80,87,88]

TMAO

Trimethylamine N-oxide (TMAO) is an inflammatory compound that is formed in the body during the metabolism of primarily carnitine (red meat being the main source) or choline (eggs are the main source). Trimethylamine (TMA) is first produced by gut bacteria and then delivered to the liver, where enzymes convert it to TMAO. TMA and TMAO can also be consumed directly from fish. High-protein or high-fat diets increase TMAO production, as do Western diets. Some vegetables (especially cruciferous vegetables, such as broccoli) and pistachios appear to reduce TMAO production. In addition, people eating plant-based diets appear to have far lower amounts of TMA-producing bacteria in their guts than people eating omnivorous diets.

TMAO has been linked to the prevalence of and poor prognosis in cardiovascular disease. It promotes vascular inflammation, plaque formation, and endothelial dysfunction. People with type 2 diabetes or chronic kidney disease have higher levels of TMA-producing bacteria. TMAO may also exacerbate impaired glucose tolerance and inhibit insulin signaling in the liver, thereby increasing risk or complications associated with the disease.[89,90]

Neu5Gc

This particular sugar molecule is produced in most mammals and found on their cell surfaces. Humans are an exception, completely lacking the ability to produce Neu5Gc, but it can be incorporated into human cells through the consumption of muscle meats, organ meats, and some dairy products. Neu5Gc has been associated with inflammation and cancer, and preliminary evidence suggests it may negatively affect endothelial function and aggravate atherosclerosis.[91,92] As people with diabetes are at increased risk for these diseases, limiting or avoiding Neu5Gc may prove beneficial.

Endotoxins

Although the evidence is limited, endotoxins may induce obesity and insulin resistance through an inflammation pathway. Endotoxins are complex molecules composed of fats and sugars (lipopolysaccharides) that are found in the outer membranes of particular types of bacteria (gram-negative), such as *E. coli*. They can come from gut bacteria or from dead bacteria in food. The most significant dietary sources are ground meat (such as hamburger), dairy products (such as yogurt, cheese, and ice cream), and chocolate.[93,94,95]

Heme Iron

Heme iron is a highly absorbable form of iron that is present in animal products, such as meat, poultry, and fish. A recent review of the scientific literature reported a positive association between dietary heme iron, serum ferritin (iron stores), and risk of type 2 diabetes. A meta-analysis of nine studies reported a 73 percent increased risk for serum ferritin in participants with the highest versus lowest (top versus bottom fifth) intake. Three recent meta-analyses reported a 28–33 percent increased diabetes risk in people consuming the highest amounts of heme iron versus those with low intakes.[96]

Excessive Sodium

An estimated 50–75 percent of people with type 2 diabetes have hypertension, with rates highest among obese adults. Diabetes and hypertension are a lethal combination, dramatically increasing the risk for heart attack or stroke and the chances of developing kidney or eye diseases. Sodium intake is positively associated with hypertension risk. Although no direct link between sodium intake and diabetes risk has been established, one study reported an almost twofold increase in diabetes risk for those who regularly add salt to meals compared with those who never add salt.[97] A Japanese study of over 1,500 participants reported that in individuals with type 2 diabetes, those eating the greatest amount of sodium had over double the risk of developing cardiovascular disease (CVD) compared with people eating the least. In addition, those with an HbA1c of 9 percent or above had an almost tenfold increase in CVD.[98] The American Heart Association recommends that people at risk for cardiovascular disease, including everyone with diabetes, limit sodium intake to 1,500 milligrams per day. The most concentrated sources of sodium are processed foods, which contribute about 75 percent of average intakes.[99,100]

Artificial Sweeteners

Although artificial sweeteners are often considered allies for people with type 2 diabetes, research suggests that they may have significant adverse health effects.[101] In a large meta-analysis including seventeen studies, people who always or almost always used artificial sweeteners had an 83 percent increased risk of type 2 diabetes compared with those who never or rarely consumed them. When results were adjusted for BMI (body fatness), there was still a 33 percent increase in risk.[102] Artificial sweeteners have been shown to induce glucose intolerance through changes to the gut microbiota, so their use in people with diabetes is not advised.[103]

Commonsense Conclusions

As you go down the list of pathogenic dietary components, you will quickly notice that they are concentrated into two categories of foods: highly processed foods and animal products. These pathogenic factors have been linked to insulin resistance, inflammation, oxidative stress, dysbiosis, hormonal imbalances, high blood cholesterol levels, and hypertension. By minimizing or avoiding these components, you will maximize your disease-fighting capacity. Chapter 8 (page 125) will guide you step by step to a diet blueprint that will help you to heal your body.

ANIMAL PRODUCTS AND PROCESSED FOODS: FORTIFYING THE EVIDENCE

Not surprisingly, intakes of specific animal products and processed foods are consistently associated with increased diabetes risk. Let's review the most recent evidence.

Red Meat

In a review of fifteen studies, red meat was associated with a 21 percent increased risk in the highest versus lowest consumers. Each 3.5-ounce (100-g) portion increased risk by 17 percent.[49] Another review of thirteen studies was associated with a 22 percent increased risk in the highest versus lowest consumers.[53]

Processed Meat

Processed meat is strongly and consistently associated with an increased risk of type 2 diabetes, as well as an increased risk of heart disease, cancer, and mortality. A review of eleven studies reported a 39 percent increase in diabetes risk for high versus low consumption of processed meat.[53] Another review of fourteen studies reported a 27 percent increased type 2 diabetes risk for highest versus lowest consumers. For each 1.75-ounce (50-g) serving, risk was increased by 37 percent.[49]

Poultry

Studies regarding poultry intake are less consistent than those for red or processed meat. A recent study from Singapore reported a 15 percent higher risk for participants in the highest versus lowest intake quartiles. It is interesting to note that this association disappeared when it was adjusted for heme iron intake, which suggests that heme iron was largely responsible for its adverse effects.[104] One study reported a 22 percent increase in type 2 diabetes risk for the highest quartile of consumers of chicken that had been cooked with an open flame or at high temperatures.[84] Another study reported an 81 percent increase in risk of gestational diabetes in women consuming more than one serving of fried chicken per month.[105]

Fish

In a review of nine studies, fish intake was associated with a 3 percent increase in type 2 diabetes risk in the highest versus lowest amount of fish consumption.[51] In another meta-analysis of sixteen studies, the risk increased to 4 percent for the highest versus lowest fish consumption and to 9 percent for each additional daily 3.5 ounces (100 g) of intake, but the findings were not statistically significant.[47] Generally, a strong positive association was reported for fish intake and risk of type 2 diabetes in American studies, while an inverse association was reported in Asian studies. It is possible this could be explained by differences in methods of preparation or the type of fish consumed. For example, in China, stewing, braising, steaming, and quick stir-frying are the usual cooking methods, while grilling, barbecuing, broiling, pan-frying, and roasting are more widely practiced in Western countries.[84] One study reported a 68 percent higher risk of gestational diabetes in women consuming at least one serving of fried fish per month compared to those consuming none.[105] Fish with higher mercury content may also increase diabetes risk and adversely affect beta cells.[106]

Dairy Products

Although research on the consumption of dairy products and diabetes has been mixed, a few studies have examined the risk associated with specific dairy subgroups. A study of more than 112,000 adults with prediabetes or recently diagnosed diabetes reported a 2 percent decrease in risk of prediabetes for every 100-gram serving of skimmed or fermented dairy products, such as low-fat yogurt and cheese. However, the risk of newly diagnosed type 2 diabetes was increased by 16 percent for participants in the highest tertile (highest third) of full-fat dairy product consumption, by 8 percent for every 5-ounce (150-g) serving of milk, and by 5 percent for every 3.5-ounce (100-g) serving of nonfermented dairy.[107] An earlier large, systematic review examined the evidence for the association of dairy consumption to the risk of cardiovascular-related outcomes, including type 2 diabetes. Low-fat dairy products and yogurt were associated with a reduced risk of type 2 diabetes, while high-fat milk and its products and fermented dairy had a neutral association.[108] Another large review and meta-analysis of twenty-one studies reported a 9 percent reduction in type 2 diabetes risk in the highest versus lowest dairy consumers. For every 7-ounce (200-g) serving, risk fell 3 percent. However, the risk reduction was only observed in Asian and Australian studies, not in American or European studies.[49]

Eggs

In an analysis of five studies, high versus low egg consumption was associated with a 3 percent increased risk of type 2 diabetes. It is interesting to note that the results varied wildly in different populations. For example, a study group from Finland showed a 38 percent reduced risk in the highest versus lowest egg consumers.[109] Another team in the United States reported a 58 percent higher risk in men consuming seven or more eggs per week and a 77 percent higher risk in women consuming seven or more eggs per week. The same research team reported a 52 percent increased risk in African Americans who consumed five or more eggs per week.[110] More recently, a Korean team reported that participants with the highest versus lowest egg intakes had 2.8 times the increased risk of cardiovascular disease.[111]

Refined Grains

A meta-analysis and review of fifteen studies reported a 6–14 percent increased risk of type 2 diabetes in participants consuming 7–14 ounces (220–400 g) of refined grains per day, although the risk was not increased with lower intakes.[49] In a meta-analysis of four studies, the pooled diabetes risk was 55 percent higher in Asian populations consuming the highest versus lowest amounts of white rice and 12 percent higher among Western populations consuming the highest versus lowest intakes. It is important to note that in Asian populations, consumption is three to four servings (1.5–2 cups/375–500 ml) per day, while Western intakes are one to two servings (0.5–1 cups/125–250 ml) per week. In the total population, type 2 diabetes risk increased by 11 percent for each serving of white rice consumed per day.[112] In a study of 1,776 Chinese adults, intake of bread and noodles (not including rice noodles) was associated with almost 2.5 times the increased risk of diabetes, while the intake of coarse grains resulted in a 73 percent risk reduction.[113] In a study examining the quality of carbohydrates consumed, higher carbohydrate intakes were not associated with diabetes risk. However, the highest versus lowest quintiles of starch (refined grains) intakes were associated with a 23 percent increased risk, while the highest versus lowest quintile of fiber intake was associated with a 20 percent risk reduction. Participants with the highest starch to cereal-fiber ratio (such as refined versus whole grains) had a 39 percent increased diabetes risk.[114]

Sugar-Sweetened Beverages

A review of ten studies reported a 30 percent increase of type 2 diabetes risk for the highest versus lowest consumers of sugar-sweetened beverages. Each serving of 1 cup (250 ml) increased risk by 21 percent.[49] A second review of eleven studies reported a 26 percent increased risk of developing type 2 diabetes in the highest versus lowest consumers of sugar-sweetened beverages (most often one to two servings per day in the highest consumers).[115]

Fast Foods and Fried Foods

Western dietary patterns rich in fast foods and fried foods are consistently associated with increased risk of chronic disease, including type 2 diabetes.[116,117] In a study of Western-style fast-food consumption in Singapore, participants with the most frequent intake of fast foods (two or more servings per week) had a 27 percent higher risk of developing diabetes and a 56 percent higher risk of dying of coronary heart disease.[118] Another study from Sweden reporting on food environments and diabetes risk in over four million individuals found that relative to individuals whose access to whole foods did not change, those who moved into areas that had more health-harming food outlets (such as fast-food restaurants) developed almost a fourfold increase in risk of developing type 2 diabetes. Among those who did not move, living in an area that increased access to health-harming food outlets was associated with a 72 percent increased risk of diabetes.[119] In a large study of over fifteen thousand women, those who consumed fried foods more than seven times a week were at more than twice the risk of developing gestational diabetes than women who did not consume them. Consuming fried foods one to three times a week was associated with a 13 percent increased risk, and consuming them four to six times a week was associated with an increased risk of 31 percent.[120]

Chapter 4

Get Lean

Diane started dieting when she was thirteen years old. It wasn't that she was fat; it was just that she wasn't thin. And she knew for a fact that she didn't stand a chance with Tyler Morgan unless she was as thin as Amy Jones, the most popular girl in eighth grade. So Diane said no to fries, soda, ice cream, and her favorite chocolate bars. She got thin enough that the popular girls began paying attention to her . . . and so did Tyler Morgan. That was the year that marked the beginning of Diane's weight-loss roller coaster—up and down all through high school and college. It was the birth of her first child that brought the roller coaster to a grinding halt. The downhill rush was over, and the slow, steady climb began in earnest, culminating with her diabetes diagnosis. Diets didn't work for Diane, and to be perfectly honest, she felt as though she had been on enough diets to last the rest of her life. What she learned about weight loss in her diabetes program changed everything. For the first time in years, the scale began to move in the right direction.

Approximately 90 percent of people with diabetes are overweight or obese.[1] Shedding just 5–10 percent of initial body weight can improve insulin sensitivity, glycemic control, blood pressure, and blood lipids in people with type 2 diabetes.[2,3] Depleting fat stores is a prerequisite for reversing diabetes, but even relatively small decreases in fat stores, especially visceral fat stores, will help to improve insulin sensitivity. People eating 100 percent plant-based or vegan diets have the lowest rates of overweight and obesity of all dietary categories.[4,5]

Overweight and obesity are defined as excessive fat accumulation, resulting in weight that is higher than the healthy range for any given height. There is no one ideal weight for a person of a particular height because healthy weight depends on bone structure, muscle mass, body fat, and body build. However, there are tools that can help you determine if you're carrying excess weight. The most accurate method is to determine how much of your body weight is fat. Body fat of more than 17 percent in men and 27 percent in women indicates overweight, while a body fat of greater than 25 percent in men and 31 percent in women indicates obesity. Unfortunately, getting accurate body-fat measurements can be inconvenient and costly. More commonly, a simple tool called Body Mass Index (BMI) is used to estimate total body fatness. While BMI can be calculated with a simple formula that divides weight in kilograms (1 kilogram = 2.2 pounds) by the square of height in meters (1 meter = 39.4 inches), BMI calculators are widely available online. Once your BMI is determined, see table 4.1, opposite page, for your predicted weight category.

It is important to note that BMI is not a diagnostic tool, as it doesn't always accurately predict fat mass. However, BMI is strongly correlated with adverse health outcomes, so it does serve as a useful tool. The key limitation to BMI is that it doesn't take into account differences in body composition between genders, racial and ethnic groups, or age groups.[6] BMI may be most accurate for Caucasian women and small-boned men. For men with more muscle mass or larger bone structure, and for black people of either gender who have denser, more muscular builds (note that this does not apply to all black people), it is less reliable.[7] Thus, for many men and some women, a BMI of 25–27 could be very healthy. For such individuals, shifting the cutoffs up by two points could improve accuracy. Likewise, for individuals with smaller bone structures and muscle mass, the BMI range may need to be adjusted down a couple of points. This is especially true for Asians, who are commonly at increased risk of disease when they are within, but closer to the top, of the healthy BMI range (23–24.9).[8,9,10]

Given the option, very few of us would choose to be overweight or obese. So why are over 70 percent of Americans overweight and almost 40 percent of Americans obese?[11] There is no question, if you eat more than you need, you gain weight; if you eat less than you need, you lose weight. While it seems a clear matter of energy balance, overweight and obesity are the products of a highly complex interplay of physical, environmental, and emotional factors.

From a physiological perspective, we are all unique. Some people are metabolically efficient—they are designed to survive famine. Unfortunately, those who are best able to survive famine are the least able to survive excess. For these individuals, moderate food intake and vigorous physical activity are necessary to avoid weight gain. Less commonly, overweight and obesity are triggered by hypothyroidism or the use of medications that can slow metabolism, increase appetite, or cause water retention.

It doesn't help that our environment is becoming increasingly obesogenic—likely to cause obesity. Hyperpalatable foods infused with sugar, fat, and salt beckon us at every turn. These flavors once gave us the assurance that our food supply was safe

TABLE 4.1. Body Mass Index (BMI)

Weight (lb)	Height (in)																
	60	61	62	63	64	65	66	67	68	69	70	71	72	73	74	75	76
100	20	19	18	18	17	17	16	16	15	15	14	14	14	13	13	12	12
105	21	20	19	19	18	17	17	16	16	16	15	15	14	14	13	13	13
110	21	21	20	19	19	18	18	17	17	16	16	15	15	15	14	14	13
115	22	22	21	20	20	19	19	18	17	17	17	16	16	15	15	14	14
120	23	23	22	21	21	20	19	19	18	18	17	17	16	16	15	15	15
125	24	24	23	22	21	21	20	20	19	18	18	17	17	16	16	16	15
130	25	25	24	23	22	22	21	20	20	19	19	18	18	17	17	16	16
135	26	26	25	24	23	22	22	21	21	20	19	19	18	18	17	17	16
140	27	26	26	25	24	23	23	22	21	21	20	20	19	18	18	17	17
145	28	27	27	26	25	24	23	23	22	21	21	20	20	19	19	18	18
150	29	28	27	27	26	25	24	23	23	22	22	21	20	20	19	19	18
155	30	29	28	27	27	26	25	24	24	23	22	22	21	20	20	19	19
160	31	30	29	28	27	27	26	25	24	24	23	22	22	21	21	20	19
165	32	31	30	29	28	27	27	26	25	24	24	23	22	22	21	21	20
170	33	32	31	30	29	28	27	27	26	25	24	24	23	22	22	21	21
175	34	33	32	31	30	29	28	27	27	26	25	24	24	23	22	22	21
180	35	34	33	32	31	30	29	28	27	27	26	25	24	24	23	22	22
185	36	35	34	33	32	31	30	29	28	27	27	26	25	24	24	23	23
190	37	36	35	34	33	32	31	30	29	28	27	26	26	25	24	24	23
195	38	37	36	35	34	33	32	31	30	29	28	28	27	26	25	24	24
200	39	38	37	35	34	33	32	31	31	30	29	28	27	26	26	25	24
205	40	39	37	36	35	34	33	32	31	30	29	29	28	27	26	26	25
210	41	40	38	37	36	35	34	33	32	31	30	29	28	28	27	26	26
215	42	41	39	38	37	36	35	34	33	32	31	30	29	28	28	27	26
220	43	42	40	39	38	37	36	35	34	33	32	31	30	29	28	27	27
225	44	43	41	40	39	37	36	35	34	33	32	31	31	30	29	28	27
230	45	43	42	41	39	38	37	36	35	34	33	32	31	30	30	29	28
235	46	44	43	42	40	39	38	37	36	35	34	33	32	31	31	29	29
240	47	45	44	43	41	40	39	38	36	35	34	33	33	31	31	30	29
245	48	46	45	43	42	41	40	39	37	36	35	34	33	32	32	30	30
250	49	47	46	44	43	42	40	39	38	37	36	35	34	33	32	31	30

UNDERSTANDING BMI	
BMI ‹ 16: indicates severe underweight	BMI 25–29.9: indicates overweight
BMI 16–16.9: indicates moderate underweight	BMI 30–34.9: indicates class 1 obesity
BMI 17–18.49: indicates mild underweight	BMI 35–39.9: indicates class 2 or severe obesity
BMI 18.5–24.9: indicates healthy weight for most people	BMI ≥ 40: indicates class 3 or extreme obesity

and nourishing, but they're only present in small amounts in nature. When concentrated and used as principal ingredients in processed foods, our innate ability to control appetite becomes unhinged. This is no mere coincidence. These food components are purposefully concentrated in processed foods to keep us coming back for more.[12,13,14] Environmental chemicals (both natural and synthetic) may also act as obesogens.[15,16] These compounds can mimic hormones in the body, adversely affecting the metabolic pathways involved in fat storage, fat cell function, energy metabolism, hunger, and appetite regulation.[17,18]

For many individuals, overweight has more to do with emotions than physical hunger. Not only do we celebrate joy, excitement, success, victory, good news, and special occasions with food, we numb the pain of difficult interactions, disappointment, embarrassment, stress, boredom, and overwork with food. Emotional eating, in its most severe form, can lead to eating disorders, such as compulsive overeating or binge eating, the most common types of eating disorders in America.[19,20]

A PERMANENT SOLUTION

Diets are generally designed to produce a calorie deficit or to ensure that you take in fewer calories than you burn so you will lose weight. Most diets succeed in this task. All sorts of creative food combinations can work, as long as they leave you with a caloric deficit. If most diets succeed in producing weight loss, why do the vast majority fail for the long term? The answer is simple: they end. If there is no plan for lifelong lifestyle change, old habits return, as does the weight. So while some more-extreme diets, such as modified fasting regimens, can and do work to rid the body of stored fat and restore insulin sensitivity, they need to be carefully paired with permanent diet and lifestyle changes in order to get permanent results.

People with type 2 diabetes are insulin resistant. The insulin resistance is a function of the drivers of insulin resistance discussed in chapter one—inflammation, oxidative stress, lipotoxicity, glucotoxicity, and dysbiosis—all of which are fueled by excess body fat. So it makes perfect sense to force the body to use up fat stores by eating significantly fewer calories than what the body requires for weight maintenance. You can do this by cutting 500–1,000 calories per day, which typically means a very slow, steady loss of about one to two pounds (0.45–0.9 kg) per week. The higher your current caloric intake, the more calories you can afford to remove without risking nutritional shortfalls. Gradual weight loss is predictably accompanied by gradual improvements in insulin sensitivity. A second option is to kick-start your weight loss by using one of the more extreme regimens that promote rapid reduction of lipotoxicity and insulin resistance. This is worth serious consideration, as results are rapid and encouraging for most individuals. There are two distinct options: a very low-calorie diet used over a limited period of time (one week to one month) or either fasting or modified fasting.

VERY LOW-CALORIE DIETS

Very low-calorie diets have shown to be effective in helping to improve insulin sensitivity and, in some cases, reversing type 2 diabetes (see pages 26–27).[21,22,23] In chapter 10, a very low-calorie menu is provided to kick-start your healing. It is designed to be used for seven to fourteen days, depending on your preference and how much weight you have to lose. The diet is somewhat flexible, offering 600–1,000 calories per day, depending on your current energy needs. It is carefully constructed to reduce inflammation and lipotoxicity (see pages 10–11). Following the initial one to two weeks, you'll graduate to a moderate-calorie, high-fiber, therapeutic plant-based diet.

FASTING AND MODIFIED FASTING DIETS

Humans have a remarkable ability to survive the absence of food through a series of physiological adaptations. When the body is deprived of nutrition, it turns to its body stores. Within twenty-four to forty-eight hours, its very limited stores of glucose (glycogen) are used up. It is absolutely critical that blood glucose levels are maintained, as some body tissues (such as red blood cells and liver cells) can use only glucose as a fuel, so the body turns to stores of protein and fat, transforming them into glucose through a mechanism called gluconeogenesis (meaning "generation of new sugar"). Although some of the newly manufactured glucose is made from amino acids (muscle tissue) and lactate (a glucose breakdown product), most comes from fat stores.

Fat is used preferentially because it contains concentrated energy reserves and is expendable. Fats are stored mainly as triglycerides, which are composed of three fatty acids attached to a glycerol backbone. It is the glycerol part of the molecule that is used to make glucose. Long-chain fatty acids can't be used as direct energy sources, so they are converted into short-chain fatty acids and ketones, which can be used for energy by the brain, muscle, and other body tissues.

One of the key adaptations of food deprivation is reduced inflammation and atrophy of body tissues and organs to reduce energy expenditure. In addition, the body attempts to rid itself of damaged or deranged cells. Upon refeeding, stem-cell-based regeneration of a portion of these cells takes place. Some evidence suggests that this process can result in the regeneration of pancreatic beta cells, which is exciting news for anyone who has a reduced ability to make insulin.[24,25]

For individuals with type 2 diabetes, any type of fasting program requires close medical supervision, particularly if the individual is on insulin or other medications. Because true fasting or water fasting eliminates all foods, it should only be carried out in a treatment facility with medical monitoring, especially when the fast is extended for more than a few days. Modified fasts that allow some caloric beverages or food are generally safer choices. However, these regimens are not nutritionally adequate long term, so if they are used, they need to be carefully controlled. A comprehensive weight-loss strategy needs to be included, as well as ongoing support.[26] There are three popular variations on fasting or modified fasting:

Time-Restricted Feeding (TRF)

This method of modified fasting restricts food intake to a limited window of time in a twenty-four-hour period.[25,27,28,29] Regimens restrict eating for fourteen to twenty-two hours each day, allowing a range of two to ten hours for eating. With fourteen hours of fasting, you would stop eating after dinner (say at 6:00 or 7:00 p.m.) and not begin eating again until 8:00 or 9:00 a.m. the next morning. With a sixteen-hour fast, you would eat only two meals a day. The first could be at 10:00 or 11:00 a.m. and the second at 5:00 or 6:00 p.m. With a twenty- to twenty-two-hour fast, you would consume just one meal a day. Of course, your meals would be healthy, high in fiber, and plant-based.

Intermittent Fasting (IF) or Intermittent Energy Restriction (IER)

This is a type of modified fast that involves full-day food abstinence or restriction, but only on specified days of the week.[29,30] So, for example, you might do a fast or modified fast one day a week or eat normally for five days and then fast for two consecutive days; this is called a 5:2 regimen. Some intermittent fasts involve a fast or modified fast every other day. Intermittent fasting may be done using water fasts, juice fasts (with fresh vegetable juices), or very low-calorie diets.

Periodic Fasting

This type of fasting is based on extended periods of food abstinence or restriction, such as four to five days at a time.[31] Periodic fasting can be done using water-only fasts under supervision, juice fasts, or very low-calorie diets. One of the most popular periodic fasts is what is commonly referred to as a fasting-mimicking diet. Originally developed by Valter Longo, PhD, a longevity expert from the University of Southern California, the plan is vegan, but it does rely more heavily on high-fat plant foods. Even though the percentage of calories from carbohydrates is higher than it is on keto-genic weight-loss diets (about 30 percent of calories compared to 5 percent), it still produces ketosis because total calories are very low (about 1,100 calories on day one and 800 calories for the next four days). Participants follow a modified fast for five days, then eat a high-fiber, plant-based diet for twenty-five days. For someone with diabetes, at least three fasting cycles are recommended or as many as are needed to achieve the desired results.

GETTING TO YOUR GOAL WEIGHT ONE DAY AT A TIME

T he first and most critical step to permanently overcoming overweight or obesity is to redirect your focus from thinness to health. Restoring health must be your top priority. Remember that every single cell of your body is the product of the food that you put into your mouth—your food serves as your basic structural material. Resist the urge to select foods on the basis of their caloric content or perceived effectiveness as diet foods. Instead, select foods on the basis of their ability to nourish and protect your body. Before you bite into a sugar-free "diet" cookie, ask yourself whether white flour, processed vegetable oil, and artificial sweeteners are the best materials with which to rebuild your brain cells.

There is no question that weight loss requires a decrease in energy input and an increase in energy output; in other words, you must eat less (fewer calories) and move more. But this is only one prerequisite. It's also important to reestablish an environment that will effectively reset metabolic machinery. One of the greatest challenges in the quest for wellness is to break old, destructive habits and replace them with habits that truly support and promote health. For example, if you descend into an abyss of junk food while watching television after dinner, consider the possibility of filling your evenings with dancing, walking, bird-watching, pottery classes, or whatever else tickles your fancy. The plan must involve creating a new routine and following that routine robotically for a set period of time—one month is a good goal. If you set a time frame for yourself, it will make sticking to the routine a little easier. Once you've repeated a behavior for a month, you'll be well on your way to turning it into a good habit for life. To make your plan foolproof, be sure to surround yourself with a strong support system.

Think positively. It is more important to be on the right path, inching your way to your goal, than to worry about how far along you are on that path. Listen carefully to your body, as it communicates with you constantly, honestly, and openly. Let it guide you as you gradually reclaim your health. On this journey there are no interviews, no exams, and no reprisals. There is nothing to fear. Take on only what you are able and ready to take on. Be prepared for stumbling blocks and resistance. Don't beat yourself up when things don't go according to plan. Instead, use each disappointment as a valuable lesson about what works and what doesn't.

Get on the Road to Recovery

Shedding excess pounds and reclaiming your health may feel like the most challenging journey of your life, but it is equally rewarding. Set goals and focus on those that will get you to your destination—improving your fitness level; increasing your fiber intake; eating more leafy greens and beans; stabilizing blood glucose levels; reducing blood pressure, blood cholesterol, or triglycerides; managing stress; improving energy; curtailing mood swings; overcoming addictions; and getting enough rest. Get rid of the foods and other items that tempt you, and restock your pantry with foods that are consistent with your health goals. If you've been a junk-food or fast-food eater, join a whole-foods, plant-based cooking class.

Reclaim Your Health

Trust in your body's innate ability to heal itself. Lifestyle-induced diseases respond to lifestyle changes. No one can eat for you, exercise for you, or manage stress for you. You are at the helm of that ship, and you have everything at your disposal to steer that ship in the direction of health and healing. Begin by working to overcome common roadblocks.

1. **Overcome food addictions and cravings.** Ultraprocessed fat-, sugar-, and salt-laden foods can be physically addictive. Food cravings work much like an itch—the more you scratch them, the worse they become. Breaking the addiction means replacing these harmful foods with healthful choices. For many people, success is dependent on keeping blood sugar levels in check. Eat meals containing a balance of carbohydrate, protein, and fat. For example, if you eat cooked grains for breakfast, throw in some lentils. Top your breakfast bowl with nuts or seeds, and be sure your nondairy milk is unsweetened. Avoid caloric beverages, sugar, and artificial sweeteners.

2. **Control inflammation.** Inflammation is one of the key driving forces behind overweight, obesity, insulin resistance, and diabetes. There are many ways dietary factors can generate inflammation. Overeating, leading to overweight and obesity, can itself trigger inflammation. Healthy fat cells produce a balance of pro-inflammatory and anti-inflammatory hormones. When fat cells become bloated or overfilled with fat, production of pro-inflammatory hormones increases while production of anti-inflammatory hormones decreases. This imbalance promotes insulin resistance.[32,33] Food sensitivities and allergies, environmental contaminants, and deficiencies of certain nutrients, such as vitamin D and omega-3 fatty acids, can also promote inflammation. Anti-inflammatory compounds from vegetables, fruits, legumes, whole grains, nuts, seeds, herbs, and spices are your best defense.

3. **Repair your leaky gut.** "Leaky gut" is a popular term used to describe increased intestinal permeability, which has been shown to be a contributing factor to obesity.[34,35,36] The major driving forces are thought to be dysbiosis, an unhealthy diet, micronutrient deficiencies, and food sensitivities and allergies. Foods that may be especially problematic are fried foods and other high-fat foods, foods cooked

at very high temperatures, refined sugars, alcohol, and food allergens (such as gluten or dairy products for some individuals). High-fiber, whole plant foods, anti-inflammatory compounds (such as curcumin in turmeric), and foods rich in omega-3 fatty acids may help to promote gut healing.[37,38,39,40,41,42]

4. **Reinforce detoxification systems.** There is growing evidence that suggests a link between environmental contaminants—such as BPA, heavy metals, persistent organic pollutants, and pesticides—and body-fat accumulation.[43,44] While we can't completely eliminate our exposure to these compounds, we can minimize them and reinforce the body systems that help us to excrete these compounds. Animal products, including fish, are significant sources of environmental toxins. Cruciferous vegetables, rich in phytochemicals, support the detoxification processes. Choose organic, when possible. Numerous vitamins, minerals, amino acids, phytochemicals, and antioxidants play a role in this process, so good nutritional status is important.

5. **Enhance nutritional status.** Even if you feel as though you're doing everything right, you can easily fall short on nutrients when calories are restricted. Take care to include adequate protein, iron, and zinc in your diet, as well as good sources of calcium, magnesium, and selenium. Be sure to include reliable sources of vitamin B_{12}, vitamin D, and iodine as well. When curtailing calories, there is little room for foods with *high energy density* (a lot of calories per gram). Focus instead on foods with *high nutrient density* (a lot of nutrients per calorie). The best choices are vegetables (especially leafy greens), legumes, fruits, nuts, seeds, and intact whole grains (rather than grains that have been ground into flour). When the body is fueled with high-quality, organic whole plant foods, the genetic switches that promote overweight and obesity are turned off.

6. **Balance hormones.** Optimal health and metabolism are highly dependent on the production and release of hormones, including thyroid, stress, and sex hormones. Thyroid hormones control metabolism and can have a significant effect on body weight. Consuming too much or too little iodine can have a profound effect on the production of thyroid hormones. Insufficient selenium and vitamin D can also adversely affect thyroid function, particularly in people who have autoimmune thyroid conditions.[45] Environmental contaminants can also disrupt thyroid function.[46] Under conditions of chronic stress, levels of the stress hormone cortisol rise and fat is shuttled into visceral fat deposits in the abdomen (see page 9). Elevated cortisol levels are also associated with increased appetite and cravings of foods rich in fat and sugar.[47,48] The best way to balance hormones and boost metabolism is by adopting a whole-foods, low-glycemic-load, nutrient-dense, plant-based diet; removing food allergens (particularly gluten); adding supplements (if needed); reducing stress; and increasing physical activity.

FINE-TUNING FOOD CHOICES FOR
HEALTHY BODIES AND HEALTHY WEIGHTS

Here's a bucket list of things you can do to shed excess pounds and, more importantly, sustain the weight loss for a lifetime. Once you make them part of your daily routine, following this list will become a healthy habit.

Emphasize Foods with a Low Caloric Density

Foods with a low caloric density are those that take up a lot of space on your plate and in your stomach but pack few calories per bite. Foods with the lowest caloric density are nonstarchy vegetables, which provide about 100 calories per pound (0.45 kg). Eat them liberally. Foods with moderate caloric density should be included to ensure that you feel well fed and are well nourished. This includes fruits, which provide about 300 calories per pound (0.45 kg), as well as legumes, starchy vegetables, and whole grains, which provide 400–600 calories per pound (0.45 kg). Calorically dense healthy whole foods, such as avocados, nuts, and seeds, should also be included but in small amounts. Calorically dense unhealthy refined foods, such as sugars, processed flour products, and fried foods, are what need to go. Concentrated fats and oils provide about 4,000 calories per pound (0.45 kg) and are also best excluded. The only foods with lower nutrient density are sugars.

Emphasize Foods with a High Nutrient Density

Foods with a high nutrient density are those that provide the greatest amount of nutrients per calorie. Some nutrient density indexes, such as the Aggregate Nutrient Density Index (ANDI) by Joel Fuhrman, MD, also factor in fiber, plant sterols, phytochemicals, and antioxidants.[49] Using the ANDI score, nothing compares to green leafy vegetables (see table 4.2, at left). All whole plant foods are nutrient-dense choices—vegetables, fruits, legumes, whole grains, nuts, and seeds. Foods with the lowest nutrient density, such as sweet beverages, oils, and deep-fried foods, will work against your quest for health and are best avoided.

TABLE 4.2. Aggregate Nutrient Density Index (ANDI)*

FOOD	NUTRIENTS/CALORIES (AVERAGE)
Green leafy vegetables	500–1000
Other nonstarchy vegetables	100–500
Fruit	50–200
Starchy vegetables	30–180
Legumes and tofu	50–100
Nuts and seeds	25–100
Fish	30–50
Whole grains	25–40
Milk, yogurt	20–35
Meat, poultry, eggs	10–30
Cheddar cheese	11
Olive oil	10
Cola	1

Source: Summary of the ANDI index by Joel Fuhrman, MD, providing ranges of ANDI scores for various food groups.

Focus on Fiber at Every Meal

Fiber keeps you full, maintains regularity, feeds your gut bacteria, and moderates your blood glucose. The foods highest in fiber are legumes. Other fiber-rich choices are whole grains, vegetables, fruits, nuts, and seeds. Include these foods at every meal. (See pages 87–94 for more fiber guidelines.)

Fill Your Plate with Whole Plant Foods

Whole plant foods don't come with an ingredient list. What you see is what you get. Aim for at least seven servings of nonstarchy vegetables, three servings of legumes, and three servings of fruits each day. Eat moderate portions of grains and starchy vegetables based on your energy (calorie) needs. For weight loss, intakes may be as low as two or three servings a day. Nuts and seeds are very high in calories, so use small portions—one to two servings per day. Eat these foods as they're grown—unprocessed.

Eliminate Ultraprocessed Foods

Ultraprocessed foods are made entirely or predominantly from non-nutritive substances extracted from foods—starch, oil, sugar, additives, colors, flavors, and preservatives. Most are based on refined carbohydrates and refined fats. These foods are subjected to many layers of commercial preparation. For example, the wheat used in making an apple Danish pastry will be ground into flour and then refined to remove the bran and germ. The apple used in the filling will have its peel removed. Sugar, salt, starch additives, colors, and preservatives will be added to enhance the final product. Finally, the sweet treat is deep-fried and coated in sugar.

Not all processed foods are off-limits. Minimally processed foods, such as frozen herbs, shelled frozen edamame, some sprouted breads, washed and packaged greens, canned beans, and some jarred tomato sauces can make food prep a little easier. Read the ingredient list!

Minimize Your Use of Concentrated Sweeteners and Avoid Artificial Sweeteners

Humans are naturally attracted to sweet tastes. Whether the sugar comes from high-fructose corn syrup or organic dehydrated cane juice matters less than the amount of sugar you ingest. Regardless of the source, sugar is sugar, and it indicates empty calories with little or no other nutrients. If you're using a packaged food, read the label. Avoid artificial sweeteners; they provide no real assistance in your quest for health and may negatively affect metabolism, microbiota, and appetite control. If you do use a sweetener, monk fruit and stevia derivatives would be the best options. (For more information, see pages 85–87. Table 5.4, page 84, provides a list of sugar in common foods.)

Minimize Concentrated Fats and Oils and Avoid Solid Fats

Fats and oils are extracted from whole foods. During this process, fat-soluble vitamins, minerals, phytochemicals, and fiber are left behind. Extracted fats and oils are to the world of fats what sugars and white flour are to the universe of carbohydrates. Both are highly processed foods with most of their nutrients removed, and it's best to minimize their use. Fats and oils contain about 120 calories per tablespoon (15 ml), which is about two and one-half times more than pure protein or carbohydrate. Avoid solid fats, such as margarines and coconut oil, as they are particularly high in saturated fat.

Make the Most of Herbs and Spices

Herbs and spices are the most recently hailed health heroes. They not only make foods taste better, but they also do so without adding sodium or fat. Several herbs and spices have shown some promise as weight-loss allies due to their ability to boost metabolism, calm inflammation, or balance blood glucose levels. Among the spicy superstars are black pepper, cardamom, cayenne, cumin, cloves, cinnamon, ginger, ginseng, mustard seeds, oregano, rosemary, and turmeric. Grow your own herbs on your windowsill; they are hardy plants that can be enjoyed year-round. Herbs can be frozen or dehydrated for later use.

Drink Water, Not Sugar

Sweet beverages are loaded with calories. A 12-ounce (375 ml) serving of lemonade, fruit punch, or soda contains 120–150 calories. A 12-ounce (375 ml) beer provides 110–170 calories; distilled spirits, about 110 calories per 1.5 ounces (45 ml); liqueurs, 150–190 calories per 1.5 ounces (45 ml); and wine, about 80 calories per 4 ounces (120 ml). Water is our best thirst quencher and is calorie-free. Herbal teas are also good choices. It is best to avoid getting calories from beverages, as they don't provide satiety the way that solid foods do.

The one exception is fresh-pressed green vegetable juice, which has a unique value as an antioxidant booster. If you consume nondairy milks, select those that are unsweetened. If you include smoothies, be very selective with ingredients, and use them as meal replacements (not as snacks) no more than once a day. (See the recipe for Green Smoothie on page 194.) Avoid calorie-free beverages containing artificial sweeteners. These beverages seem to confuse our appetite control center and metabolic hormones and are of no value to health.

Rule Out Food Allergies and Sensitivities

Eating foods you are sensitive to can cause inflammation, which triggers insulin resistance and may contribute to weight gain. Consider doing a modified elimination diet by removing foods that you think you might be sensitive to for three to four weeks. The most common culprits are dairy, wheat (sometimes gluten), shellfish, fish, eggs, corn, peanuts, and soy.

FINE-TUNING FOOD BEHAVIORS FOR HEALTHY BODIES AND HEALTHY WEIGHTS

There are also some smart practices you can adopt to augment your good eating habits. Learn to pace your meals, then check out the following tips for creating an environment that helps support a healthy body and a healthy weight for the long term:

Listen to Your Body

Your food choices should be a reflection of the powerful connection between those choices and your well-being, rather than a function of convenience or habit. Learn to respond to natural hunger signals and avoid the temptation to eat when you're not hungry or deprive yourself when you're famished. If you think you're hungry, drink a glass of water, then wait fifteen minutes before eating anything. It's easy to mistake thirst for hunger.

If you're not hungry at your regular mealtime, postpone your meal. If that's not practical, wait until your next meal to eat or eat very lightly. Stop eating when you're comfortable but not full. Remember that it takes about twenty minutes (and sometimes even longer) after you start eating for your body to register fullness. If you eat too quickly, you can easily overeat, as you haven't allowed enough time for your satiety hormones to do their job.

Eat Mindfully

Make mealtimes special. Set the table, light a candle, and play some quiet music. Eat slowly, chew your food well, and savor every bite. Put your utensils down between bites. All of this can help reduce the amount you eat and aid digestion. It can also help to reduce the amount of air you swallow and the resulting intestinal gas this air can produce. Be aware of where your food comes from and be grateful to all the individuals who had a hand in getting it on your plate.

Build Healthy Habits

1. **Eat regular, moderately sized meals.** Skipping meals can leave you so hungry that you overeat at the next meal.

2. **Eat at home or eat food prepared at home when you're out and about.** Eating at home helps promote a healthy body weight and healthy eating. It allows for complete control over the ingredients that go into meals. If you eat at work or school, bring a box lunch. Restaurant food is designed to impress the palate, which means it includes extra fat, sugar, and salt. Although eating out can fit into a healthy meal plan, it should be an occasional adventure rather than a daily affair.

3. **Keep portion sizes moderate.** The more food on your plate, the more you will eat. Using smaller cups, plates, and bowls will also help to keep portions reasonable.

4. **Forgo snacks.** For most people, snacks add calories to their day. Instead, focus on eating three good meals, and drink water or tea in between meals. Avoid eating after dinner. Eating close to bedtime drives up insulin levels, triggering fat storage.

5. **Shop smart.** Stick to a shopping list. Go shopping after a meal rather than on an empty stomach. Don't be duped into buying foods labeled low calorie, low fat, or sugar-free. While such foods may contain 10–15 percent fewer calories than the foods they are replacing, it is easy to convince yourself that you're justified in eating twice as much.

6. **Fill your plate or bowl before you get to the table.** When you serve food family-style with bowls on the table, it takes incredible willpower to stop eating. Fill your plate or bowl at the stove or counter. The exceptions are healthy foods you want to eat more of—raw vegetables, salad, and steamed vegetables.

7. **Eat your food while sitting down at the table.** Always put your food in a bowl or on a plate, and sit down to eat. Eating while standing can induce mindless overeating.

8. **Avoid eating while cooking.** You may need to suck on a cinnamon stick or chew some mint if this is a major challenge for you.

9. **Minimize distractions.** Keep your hands busy while you're watching TV to avoid snacking. If you eat while you're watching TV, you'll be less conscious of how much you're consuming. Enjoy a craft project, take up knitting, or do some stretching exercises to keep yourself otherwise occupied.

10. **Bring in reinforcements.** Share your goals with trusted family members and friends. Enlist their support. Find a buddy who has similar goals. Consider joining a support group.

11. **Consider intermittent fasting.** Wait at least twelve hours between your evening meal and breakfast. Fasting for one day a week or adopting a fasting-mimicking diet (see pages 61–62) are also considerations.

12. **Self-monitor your weight.** While experts used to advise against daily weighing, evidence is now clear that this strategy leads to improved long-term weight maintenance.[50]

Chapter 5

Getting a Grip on Carbohydrates

When Diane was diagnosed with diabetes, the internet searches began. She wanted to know if sugar caused her diabetes. She wondered which artificial sweeteners tasted the best and were the safest. She was curious to know if steering clear of carbohydrates could help her get off her medications. She even thought about a keto diet—it sure did the trick for Ken, a treasured colleague who taught high school science right across the hall from her. She was disheartened by the inconsistency of the information from reputable health-care providers. She wasn't sure who or what to believe. For the most part, carbohydrates seemed guilty as charged. Her perspective shifted entirely when she embraced a plant-based diet. In her diabetes program, she learned why carbohydrates have such a bad reputation. She also learned that she had been listening to only one side of the carbohydrate story.

Carbohydrate-rich foods are the most important sources of food energy in the world. Across the globe, intakes range from 40–80 percent of calories, with people in developing countries tending toward the higher end and those in Western nations falling near the lower end of the range.[1] So why are carbohydrates commonly viewed as villains by popular nutrition authorities and consumers? The answer lies in the quality of the carbohydrates. Because the vast majority of carbohydrates consumed by populations in which obesity and diabetes are prevalent have been refined, all high-carbohydrate foods are considered suspect. This is a mistake. By minimizing carbohydrates, you reduce the intake of beneficial components associated with whole plant foods: fiber, phytochemicals, antioxidants, plant sterols, pre- and probiotics, vitamins, minerals, and essential fatty acids. People who rely on whole plant foods for most of their carbohydrates are consistently protected against obesity and diabetes. It's not carbohydrates per se that are the problem. Rather, it's refined carbohydrates.

Refined carbohydrates are extracted from plant foods and have been stripped of most of their beneficial components by food-processing techniques. There are two main categories of refined carbohydrates: starches and sugars. When starches and sugars are separated from plants, many substances of value to human health are left behind. For example, during the process of refining wheat to produce white flour, two of the three parts of the wheat kernel are removed: the germ and the bran. The germ is the kernel's nutrient storehouse; it concentrates essential fatty acids, vitamins, minerals, and phytochemicals in order to support the life and growth of a new plant. The bran is the outer husk, which protects the contents of the grain. Although the bran provides nutrients and phytochemicals, its main claim to fame is fiber. What is left after the germ and bran are removed is called the endosperm, which is mainly starch, some protein, and a miniscule amount of vitamins and minerals. In the process of turning wheat kernels into white flour, 70–90 percent of the vitamins, minerals, and fiber are lost. To add insult to injury, a two-hundredfold to three-hundredfold loss in phytochemicals occurs.[2] Figure 5.1 (below) shows the amount of fiber and key nutrients that remain when wheat berries are processed into white flour.

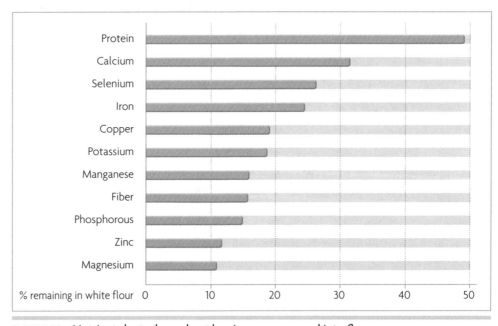

FIGURE 5.1   Nutrients lost when wheat berries are processed into flour.

Source: USDA Nutrient Database. *Note:* Calculations based on 72 percent extraction (138 pounds of wheat produces 100 pounds of white flour, according to Prairie Grains 2003).

Granted, some nutrients may be added back. For example, when wheat or rice is refined into flour, it is often enriched with four B vitamins (thiamin, riboflavin, niacin, and folic acid) and the mineral iron. However, other vitamins and minerals (such as vitamin B_6, pantothenic acid, vitamin E, selenium, magnesium, zinc, potassium, manganese, and boron) are not added back, nor are the phytochemicals or fiber. And, of course, no one eats a bowl of plain white flour. Varying amounts of sugar, salt, fat, colors, flavors, and preservatives are added to enhance the palatability and appearance of the final product, which is then consumed as bread, cake, cereal, cookies, crackers, pasta, pastries, pretzels, pancakes, or other flour products. So not only are the most protective parts of the plant removed, but also a number of potentially harmful ingredients are added. This is a risky trade-off for human health.

To prevent or reverse diabetes, rely on high-quality carbohydrates, such as unrefined whole plant foods (vegetables, fruits, legumes, whole grains, nuts, and seeds). Minimize or avoid low-quality carbohydrates, such as refined starches (white flour products and concentrated starches, such as cornstarch) and refined sugars and syrups. When carbohydrate-rich foods are refined, the fiber that slows the absorption of carbohydrates into the bloodstream is removed and their glycemic index rises. In addition, the nutrients needed to metabolize those carbohydrates are shaved away, so the body is less able to deal with the fast influx of these energy-giving nutrients.

WHAT ARE REFINED CARBOHYDRATES?

Refined carbohydrates are made from processed grains (such as white flour), other processed starchy foods (such as peeled potatoes), or processed sweeteners (such as white or brown sugar). In other words, these are low-quality carbohydrate sources. Examples of foods rich in refined starches are breads or pastas made with white flour. Examples of foods rich in refined sugars are sodas, candies, and sugar-sweetened jams or jellies.

WHAT ARE UNREFINED CARBOHYDRATES?

Unrefined carbohydrates are naturally present in whole plant foods, such as vegetables, fruits, legumes, whole grains, nuts, and seeds. In other words, these are high-quality carbohydrate sources. Examples of foods rich in unrefined starches are barley, quinoa, sweet potatoes, and beans. Examples of unrefined foods with natural sugars are fruits, dried fruits, and nonstarchy vegetables, such as broccoli, cucumbers, leafy greens, peppers, and tomatoes.

Eliminate processed foods with added refined flours and sugars, shift away from packaged foods, and leave the skin on the starchy vegetables you eat. Choose black, red, or brown rice instead of white rice and intact whole grains instead of flour products. To fine-tune your diet even further, select lower GI foods within each food category (see pages 94–100).

In addition to the quality of the carbohydrates you eat, there's also the issue of quantity. Important considerations include the percentage of total calories as carbohydrate, the amount or grams of carbohydrates consumed each day, and the spacing or regularity of carbohydrate intake. If most of your food provides high-quality, unrefined carbohydrates, the range of intake that will support and promote health is quite wide. Established diabetes guidelines recommend 45–60 percent of calories from carbohydrates.[3] The upper limit can be successfully extended to 70 percent (or slightly higher) with very high-fiber diets. On the other hand, if you eat mostly poor-quality, refined carbohydrates, you may see health benefits from cutting carbs, especially if fat and protein sources are carefully selected. However, a healthier approach would be to swap the low-quality refined carbohydrates for high-quality unrefined carbohydrates. Dipping below the 45 percent mark is not recommended, as low carbohydrate intakes are associated with escalating intakes of saturated fat and animal protein.

Your total carbohydrate intake and the spacing and regularity of intake can impact body weight and blood glucose control. If your goal is weight loss, portion sizes of carbohydrate-rich foods will need to be controlled. If you're consuming a whole-foods, plant-based, weight-loss diet of 1,400–1,800 calories, your upper limit for carbohydrate would be 245–315 g (based on 70 percent of calories from carbohydrates). This amounts to 80–100 grams of carbohydrate per meal. To put this into perspective, 1 cup (250 ml) of beans or whole grains has about 40 grams; one large apple, about 30 grams; 1 cup (250 ml) of blueberries, about 20 grams; and 1 cup (250 ml) of broccoli, about 10 grams. Refer back to tables 2.3 and 2.4 (page 29) for the carbohydrate content of other common foods. Although carbohydrate counting is not necessary, keeping track of your intake for a week or two can help you become more familiar with the carbohydrate content of specific foods.

The quantity of carbohydrates you consume will affect your blood glucose levels, even when those carbohydrates come from whole plant foods. You'll want to space your intake throughout the day to help keep blood glucose levels relatively stable and avoid extreme highs and lows. To accomplish this, eat regular, balanced meals. Although distributing carbohydrate intake throughout the day is most important for individuals who take insulin, it can also be helpful for anyone who is trying to improve blood glucose control. One simple way of doing this is to include one or two servings of carbohydrate-rich foods per meal, depending on your caloric needs (see chapter 10 for specific guidelines). Most meals will include a whole grain or starchy vegetable. For more aggressive weight-loss regimens, sufficient carbohydrates can be obtained from legumes and nonstarchy vegetables or fruits.

PUT A LID ON SUGAR

Humans have a soft spot for sweets. We were born that way, and for good reason. In nature, sweetness generally signals safety, while bitterness serves as a warning flag. It would be difficult to consume excessive sugar when eating foods in the form in which they are grown. Yet when sugars are extracted and concentrated, then added to ultraprocessed foods, our hardwiring for sweets works against us. Our appetite control center becomes unhinged, and satiety signals fail to protect us from overconsumption.

In 1700, annual per capita sugar consumption averaged 4 pounds (1.8 kg) per person per year in the UK. It was not until the mid 1800s that sugar became a common part of everyday diets.[4] Since 2015, total added sugar intakes have hovered around 15 percent of calories in the US, down from 18 percent in 1999.[5] The average American adult now consumes about 19 teaspoons (80 g) per day. The US Dietary Guidelines Advisory Committee recommends limiting added sugars to not more than 10 percent of total calories (12 teaspoons/50 g in a 2,000-calorie diet).[6] The World Health Organization concurs but adds that greater health benefits would be achieved by lowering intake to not more than 5 percent of calories (6 teaspoons/25 g in a 2,000-calorie diet). Actual intakes exceed all of these recommendations.

How damaging is sugar to health? Sugar itself is not inherently harmful. In fact, when it is naturally present in the matrix of a whole food, it's the preferred fuel for the human body, and we are well equipped to handle it. It's excess sugar that's the issue, particularly when it comes from concentrated sweeteners. While it's the dose that makes the poison, whenever concentrated sugars are involved, it is best to minimize their intake or avoid them completely.

The adverse effects of sugar are most pronounced when there is a surplus of calories. It is particularly problematic when consumed in the absence of fiber, as is the case with beverages and many ultraprocessed foods. Diets containing a high proportion of calories as concentrated sugars (and, in most instances, other refined carbohydrates) are associated with a laundry list of adverse health consequences:

Poor nutrition. Sugar, which provides significant calories but insignificant nutrients, can crowd out more nutrient-dense foods. This may result in an overall reduction in micronutrient intakes and potentially shortfalls.[4]

Hypertension. There is growing evidence that excessive sugar intake may raise blood pressure.[4] A meta-analysis reported an 8 percent increase in risk for every serving of sugar-sweetened beverage consumed.[7]

High triglycerides. High-sugar diets increase triglycerides, especially when simple sugars exceed 20 percent of energy. Fructose has the most profound impact of all sugars. The effect appears to be even greater in men, in sedentary and overweight individuals, and in people with metabolic syndrome or diabetes. High triglycerides can increase the risk for cardiovascular disease. [4, 8,9,10]

Decreased HDL cholesterol. Most but not all studies show reductions in beneficial HDL cholesterol with increasing sugar intake. Fructose appears more potent than sucrose in reducing HDL cholesterol levels.[8,10]

Insulin resistance and type 2 diabetes. Chronic, excessive sugar intake can result in sustained, elevated blood glucose levels, increased insulin output, and insulin resistance.

This means that the body fails to respond properly to insulin, and blood glucose is not efficiently cleared. There is increased risk for metabolic syndrome, prediabetes, and type 2 diabetes. Fructose is associated with increased levels of visceral fat (fat in and around vital organs), further increasing insulin resistance.[11,12]

Increased cancer risk. There is limited evidence that high intakes of sucrose increase risk of colorectal cancer.[13,14,15] One study reported a greater than twofold increase in the incidence of breast cancer in postmenopausal women who were regular consumers of sugar-sweetened beverages compared to women who seldom or never consume them.[16]

Overconsumption, overweight, and obesity. Increasing added sugars, especially from beverages, can result in an increase in total energy consumption, leading to overweight, obesity, and a higher risk of chronic disease.[17,18,19]

Poor dental health. High sugar intakes are strongly associated with dental caries and reduced dental health.[8]

Nonalcoholic fatty liver disease (NAFLD). NAFLD is a key driver of insulin resistance, metabolic syndrome, type 2 diabetes, and cardiovascular disease. The prevalence is approximately 43 percent in people with impaired glucose tolerance and 62 percent in those with newly diagnosed type 2 diabetes.[20] Excessive sugar intake has been associated with NAFLD, with excessive fructose intake being especially problematic.[21,22,23,24]

Gout. Excess sugar intake, particularly from sugar-sweetened beverages, is positively associated with increased uric acid levels and gout. Fructose appears to be especially effective at driving up uric acid levels.[25,26]

Inflammation. Sugar excesses have been shown to increase inflammation, especially in insulin-sensitive tissues. Proinflammatory molecules may rise with elevated blood glucose levels.[27,28,29]

Increased formation of advanced glycation end products (AGEs). Limited research suggests that fructose is linked to AGE formation within body cells and is approximately eight times more likely to form these compounds than glucose. AGEs contribute to numerous disease processes and accelerate aging.[30,31]

EXPLAINING FRUCTOSE

Excess fructose appears to be even more damaging than excess glucose. When it is consumed in excess, it promotes nonalcoholic fatty liver disease, elevated triglycerides, increased LDL cholesterol, insulin resistance, elevated blood pressure, visceral fat accumulation, and the formation of advanced glycation end products more sharply than glucose.[4,30,31]

Understanding the metabolic fate of fructose helps to explain this phenomenon. For many years scientists believed that fructose was metabolized exclusively by the liver. More recent evidence suggests that much of the fructose we consume is converted into glucose and other metabolites in the intestines.[32] However, if fructose intake is very high, the intestines can't keep up and the excess is either shuttled to the liver for processing or it passes into the colon where it feeds harmful bacteria. Every cell in the human body can use glucose for energy, while fructose, once in the bloodstream, is metabolized almost exclusively by liver cells. In the liver, the preferred fate of fructose is to replenish glycogen stores. In fact, fructose is a better substrate for making glycogen than glucose. Once liver glycogen is replenished, any additional fructose is converted into triglycerides or fatty acids and stored in fat cells, muscles, or vital organs. As you may recall, when excess fat is stored in the muscles or vital organs, lipotoxicity, a major driver of insulin resistance, can result (see pages 10–11).

On a positive note, there is a rapid response to fructose restriction. In a study of children with features of metabolic syndrome, just nine days of fructose restriction (with an equal calorie substitution for complex carbohydrates) resulted in reductions in fasting glucose and insulin levels, improved glucose tolerance, and better lipid profiles.[33] Liver fat concentrations decreased by 22 percent on average. The conversion of carbohydrates to fatty acids, a process known as de novo lipogenesis, was reduced by 56 percent. Similarly, in a metabolic study of adult men, de novo lipogenesis was almost 19 percent when the men were fed a high-fructose diet (25 percent of calories from fructose) compared to 11 percent when they were eating a low-fructose diet (less than 4 percent of calories from fructose). Liver fat concentration also significantly increased when fructose intake was high.[34]

The problem is *not* fructose from fruits and vegetables. The human body is well equipped to handle the relatively small amounts of fructose naturally present in whole plant foods. However, when the diet is loaded with concentrated fructose, the body's capacity to handle it quickly becomes overwhelmed. Concentrated fructose is found not only in high-fructose corn syrup but also in agave syrup, table sugar, honey, and other common sweeteners. Particularly problematic are sweetened beverages. Even unsweetened fruit juices can pack a lot of fructose.

It's interesting to note that between 1970 and 1995, sugar intake increased by 19 percent, but the most notable change was not in the amount of sugar consumed but rather in the type of sugar consumed. While intake of sucrose (in the form of table sugar from sugarcane and beets) declined by 38 percent, the intake of high-fructose corn sweeteners increased by 387 percent.[35] By 2007, 45 percent of total added sugars came from table sugar (sucrose), 41 percent came from high-fructose corn syrup, and 14 percent came from glucose syrup, pure glucose, and honey.[36]

The fructose content of a serving of fruit is 2–12 grams, averaging about 6 grams. Fruit juices can contain higher amounts. The fructose content of a 12-ounce (375-ml) soda, regardless of whether it is sweetened by high-fructose corn syrup or sucrose, is about 20 grams or slightly more. See table 5.1 (below).

Table 5.2 (opposite page) provides a summary of the types of sugars in common sweeteners. Note that sucrose is half glucose, half fructose. Essentially, our two

TABLE 5.1. Fructose Content of Fresh Fruits and Beverages

FOOD	SERVING SIZE	FRUCTOSE CONTENT (g)	FOOD	SERVING SIZE	FRUCTOSE CONTENT (g)
FRUIT			Plums	1 (66 g)	2.0
Grapes	1 cup (250 ml)	12.4	Apricots	3 (35 g each)	1.0
Pear	1 medium	11.4	**FRUIT JUICES, UNSWEETENED**		
Apple	1 medium	10.7	Grape juice	1 cup (250 ml)	18.6
Mango, pieces	1 cup (250 ml)	7.7	Pomegranate juice	1 cup (250 ml)	15.9
Cherries	1 cup (250 ml)	7.5	Apple juice	1 cup (250 ml)	14.2
Blueberries	1 cup (250 ml)	7.4	Pineapple juice, unsweetened	1 cup (250 ml)	9.5
Banana	1 medium	7.1	Grapefruit juice	1 cup (250 ml)	8.3
Orange	1 medium	6.1	Orange juice	1 cup (250 ml)	5.6
Watermelon	1 cup (250 ml)	6.0	**SWEETENED BEVERAGES**		
Papaya, pieces	1 cup (250 ml)	5.9	Lemon-lime soda	1 can (12 oz/ 375 ml)	21.6
Peach	1 medium	5.9	Cola	1 can (12 oz/ 375 ml)	21.2
Honeydew melon, cubes	1 cup (250 ml)	5.0	Cranberry juice cocktail	1 cup (250 ml)	14.0
Figs, fresh	3	4.5	Ginger ale	1 can (12 oz/ 375 ml)	13.5
Grapefruit	1 medium	4.4	Iced green tea, sweetened	1 can 12 oz/ 375 ml	12.6
Strawberries	1 cup (250 ml)	3.8	Red Bull	1 can 12 oz/ 375 ml	6.0
Blackberries	1 cup (250 ml)	3.5			
Pineapple, chunks	1 cup (250 ml)	3.5			
Kiwi	1 medium	3.1			
Cantaloupe, cubes	1 cup (250 ml)	3.0			
Raspberries	1 cup (250 ml)	2.9			

Source: [37]

TABLE 5.2. Types of Simple Sugars in Common Sweeteners

SUGAR	FRUCTOSE	GLUCOSE	SUCROSE (GLUCOSE + FRUCTOSE)	OTHER SUGARS
White sugar	0	0	100	0
Agave syrup	75 (57–90)	20 (5–38)	0	0
Coconut sugar	3–9	3–9	70–79	—
Corn syrup	0	100	0	0
HFCS-42	42	53	0	5
HFCS-55	55	41	0	4
HFCS-90	90	5	0	5
Honey	50	44	1	5
Maple syrup	1	4	95	0
Molasses	23	21	53	3
Tapioca syrup	55	45	0	0

Source: [40]

most common sweeteners (sucrose and high-fructose corn syrup) provide roughly equal amounts of glucose and fructose. The main difference between high-fructose corn syrup and sucrose is that in sucrose the glucose and fructose are bound together and must be cleaved apart by an enzyme or acid before being absorbed.[38] In high-fructose corn syrup, the fructose is not bound to glucose; instead, both the fructose and glucose are present as single sugars (known as free monosaccharides). Preliminary evidence suggests that blood levels of fructose are higher with the consumption of high-fructose corn syrup compared with equal amounts of sucrose from beverages.[39]

TOP TIPS FOR KICKING THE SUGAR HABIT

Sugar is everywhere, and most people were introduced to it early in life, so it's normal to expect sweet flavors in your foods. The good news is that you can overcome the hold that sugar has on you.

Rewire Your Taste Buds

Sugar is addictive. It increases a brain chemical called dopamine, which is associated with the brain's reward system. This is the same system that is triggered by drugs, alcohol, and nicotine. While sugar provokes a less dramatic surge in dopamine than drugs, its effect is still quite profound, especially with large intakes. Excess sugar causes a spike in dopamine that makes you feel good, but when dopamine falls, you crave more sugar. The cycle leads to tolerance, so you need more sugar to get the same reward.

The good news is, by decreasing your sugar intake, your taste buds can readjust and your brain can be rewired to crave sugar less.[41] If you are a sugarholic, you may need to reduce intake gradually. Cut intake in half for a week, then in half again, until you are using little or none. If need be, some of the sugar can be replaced with a natural noncaloric sweetener (see pages 85–87) while your taste buds are adjusting. However, this too should be eliminated over time because your taste buds require a reduction of all things sweet in order to appreciate the natural flavors in foods. The advantage of the natural noncaloric sweetener over sugar is that it won't cause a spike in blood glucose.

Steer Clear of Beverages with Added Sugars

Nearly half of the sugar in American diets comes from sweet beverages.[42] The average 12-ounce (375-ml) serving of soda or fruit drink packs about 150 calories from sugar. That is close to 10 teaspoons (40 grams) of sugar per serving—and some drinks have even more. Consuming sugar-sweetened beverages is strongly linked to weight gain and diabetes risk.[43] If you add just one 12-ounce (375-ml) can of regular soft drink to your daily diet, you can expect to add about 15 pounds (6.9 kg) per year. While you might imagine that you would eliminate calories elsewhere, this is not always the case. When you drink your calories, your body fails to register those calories with the appetite control center the way it does when you eat solid food.

The bottom line is simple: avoid *all* sugar-sweetened beverages, including soda, energy drinks, sports beverages, sweetened coffee or tea beverages, fruit drinks, and sweet alcoholic beverages. Sugar-sweetened beverages contribute to the development of insulin resistance, prediabetes, and diabetes because these are conditions of abnormal glucose metabolism and high blood sugar. The last thing you want to do when you have these conditions is to consume highly absorbable liquid sugar.

Eat Whole Foods Instead of Packaged Foods

About 90 percent of the added sugars consumed by Americans come from packaged foods.[44] Cutting out or cutting down on these foods will dramatically reduce sugar intake. When sugar is within the matrix of a whole food that is rich in fiber, it is safe to consume.

You can't always trust your instincts when selecting packaged foods. Often products that you might assume are low in sugar are not. For example, barbecue sauce, ketchup, and many other ready-made sauces get most of their calories from sugar, as do many low-fat salad dressings. Instant oatmeal, breakfast bars, granola bars, protein bars, bottled smoothies, canned baked beans, canned fruits, and ready-to-eat breakfast cereals (even healthy-sounding ones) are often high in sugar. See table 5.4 (page 84) for the amount of sugar in common foods.

If You Eat Packaged Foods, Read the Label and Select Products with Less Added Sugar

Go to the Nutrition Facts panel and check the serving size—servings are often smaller than you might imagine. To determine the number of teaspoons of sugar per serving of food, find the total grams of sugar and divide this number by four. (The precise conversion is 4.2 grams per teaspoon; rounding down to four makes for easier calculation). So, 16 grams of sugar in a serving of food would equal about 4 teaspoons (20 ml). Remember that 1 gram of sugar has 4 calories. So, if a serving of a food has 100 calories and 10 grams of sugar, that means the food derives 40 percent of its calories from sugar (10 x 4 ÷ 100).

The total sugar listing in the Nutrition Facts panel does not distinguish between the sugars naturally present in food and added sugars. (Fortunately, in the United States, by early 2021, all food manufacturers will have to declare both total and added sugars on food labels, with added sugars appearing directly below total sugar.) On a label that does not list added sugars, it can be difficult to know how much of the total sugar comes from natural sources (such as fruit) and how much comes from added sugar. If there are no natural sugars (from fruits, vegetables, or dairy products), then the sugar listed is all added sugar. The exception to this rule is fruit juice concentrate, which is included as an added sugar.

If there are natural sugars from fruits, dried fruits, or even vegetables (such as tomatoes), then some further detective work is called for in order to figure out how much added sugar might be present. You will need to scrutinize the ingredient list, and although this will not tell you the precise division of natural and added sugars, it will provide some helpful information. Ingredients are listed in descending order according to their weight. If sugar is near the top of the list, this is a clue that added sugars are high. Some manufacturers try to push sugars lower down on the ingredient list by using smaller amounts of several different sweeteners, some of which consumers might not even recognize as sugar. Of course, you will see the usual suspects, such as beet sugar, brown sugar, cane sugar, coconut sugar, confectioner's sugar, corn sugar, date sugar, invert sugar, turbinado sugar, and other sugars. You may find a variety of syrups, such as agave syrup, brown rice syrup, corn syrup, corn syrup solids, high-fructose corn syrup, malt syrup, and maple syrup, along with other easily recognizable sugars, such as honey and molasses. However, you may also notice ingredients such as dextrin and maltodextrin or ones that end in "ose," such as dextrose, fructose, glucose, lactose, and maltose. All of these are sugars. The following tips will help you keep added sugars to a bare minimum:

- Purchase products labeled "unsweetened" or "no added sugar," such as nondairy milks, applesauce, nut butters, oatmeal, and canned fruit.
- Compare products such as tomato sauce, salad dressings, and condiments, and select a product with no added sugar or with the least added sugar.
- Don't let words such as "natural" or "organic" fool you. These words are no guarantee of low sugar.
- If you're buying a sweetened product, such as a bar or cereal, select one that uses fresh or dried fruit as the primary sweetener instead of sugars or syrups.

Don't Be Duped into Believing That There Is a Healthy Sugar

The simple truth is that the differences between various concentrated sugars are of relatively minor consequence to health. Most sugars are essentially glucose, fructose, or some combination of the two. Although a few sweeteners contain tiny amounts of nutrients, you would have to eat far more than you should to make a significant contribution to your nutritional needs (see table 5.3, opposite page).

One notable exception is blackstrap molasses, which is an impressive mineral source. For example, 2 tablespoons (30 ml) of blackstrap molasses provides 353 milligrams of calcium, 7.2 milligrams of iron, and 1,023 milligrams of potassium—more calcium than 1 cup of milk, more iron than an 8-ounce steak, and more potassium than two large bananas.[37] Date sugar is made from dried and ground dates, so it's a whole-food sugar, which is preferable to refined sugars. Coconut sugar is dried coconut nectar, and it is more nutrient dense than typical refined sugars.

Regardless, the bottom line is that sugar is sugar. Even the sugars derived from whole-food sources, such as date or coconut sugar, will have a significant impact on blood glucose and should be minimized. The best advice is to kick the sugar habit and get used to foods with less sweetness.

Make Fruit Your Go-To Sweet Treat

Fruit is an ideal sweet treat that provides significant advantages over added sugars. Fruit is rich in fiber, phytochemicals, antioxidants, and a host of vitamins and min-

TABLE 5.3. Nutrients in Sweeteners

NUTRIENTS IN 2 TBSP (30 ML)	RDA FOR FEMALES AGES 19–50	WHITE SUGAR	BROWN SUGAR	HONEY	AGAVE NECTAR	COCONUT SUGAR	MAPLE SYRUP	BLACKSTRAP MOLASSES
B₁ (mg)	1.1	0	0	0	0.05	0	0.03	0
B₂ (mg)	1.1	0.005	0	0.16	0.07	n/a	0.50	.06
B₃ (mg)	14	0	0.02	0.05	0.29	n/a	0.03	0.9
B₆ (mg)	1.3	0	0.008	0.10	0.1	n/a	0.001	0.6
Calcium (mg)	1,000	0	16	3	0	2	82	353
Iron (mg)	18	0.01	0.14	0.18	0.04	0.5	0.04	7.2
Zinc (mg)	8	0	0.01	0.09	0	0.5	1.2	0.42
Magnesium (mg)	320	0	2	1	0	7	16	88
Potassium (mg)	4,700	1	26	22	2	258	170	1,023

Source: [37]

erals. It is convenient and relatively economical. Eat fruit whole, chop it into a fruit salad, slice it and serve with a little nut butter, freeze it and blend it to the texture of ice cream or sorbet, or bake it. Step outside of your comfort zone and try fruits that are new to you. Dried fruits can be used in place of sugar in homemade cereals, baked goods, desserts, and treats. Although they are naturally high in sugar, dried fruits, when used judiciously, are healthful, high-fiber, nutrient-dense alternatives to sugar.

Take Advantage of Herbs and Spices to Flavor Foods Instead of Sugar

Use vanilla beans or vanilla extract, citrus zest, or spices, such as allspice, cardamom, cinnamon, ginger, nutmeg, and star anise to bring out the natural sweetness in foods. Not only are these seasonings sugar-free, but they also are great sources of antioxidants and phytochemicals. Add them to cereals, puddings, baked goods, and beverages. Some of them also work well in savory dishes. You can enhance the flavor of commonly sweetened savory foods, such as pasta sauce, with herbs and caramelized onion. Root vegetables, such as carrots and beets, also add sweetness to main and side dishes.

TABLE 5.4. Sugar Content of Common Packaged Foods

FOOD	SERVING SIZE	GRAMS SUGAR	TEASPOONS SUGAR (1 tsp = 4 g)
Milkshake with chocolate candies	1 regular (12 oz/375 ml)	85	21
Soda, all types	20 oz (600 ml) bottle	72	18
Large vanilla blended iced coffee	16 oz (454 g)	58	15
Ice cream, soft, chocolate	1 medium (298 g)	58	15
Superfood smoothie (commercial, bottled)	1 bottle 15.2 oz (450 ml)	51	13
Fruit cocktail, canned in heavy syrup	1 cup (250 ml)	44	11
Yogurt, low fat	1 cup (250 ml)	42	11
Chocolate bar (with caramel)	1	40	10
Applesauce, canned, sweetened	1 cup (250 ml)	36	9
Ice cream, mint chip	1 cup (250 ml)	34	8.5
Apple pie, commercial	1 slice (⅛ pie)	29	7.5
Coconut yogurt, blueberry	8 oz (250 ml)	27	7
Baked beans	1 cup (250 ml)	22	5.5
Hazelnut spread, chocolate	2 Tbsp (30 ml)	20	5
Soy ice cream	½ cup (125 ml)	20	5
Tomato sauce	1 cup (250 ml)	18	4.5
Almond milk (vanilla)	1 cup (250 ml)	14	3.5
Cereal, frosted flakes	1 cup (250 ml)	14	3.5
Cookies, chocolate chip	2	14	3.5
Chocolate bar, 70% cocoa	50 g (½ bar)	12	3
Granola	½ cup (125 ml)	12	3
Donut, glazed	1	10	2.5
Granola bar	1 bar	10	2.5
Soymilk (vanilla)	1 cup (250 ml)	8	2
Salad dressing, raspberry balsamic vinaigrette	2 Tbsp (30 ml)	8	2
Ketchup	2 Tbsp (30 ml)	8	2
Soymilk (original)	1 cup (250 ml)	6	1.5

Source: [37]

THE GOODS ON ALTERNATIVE SWEETENERS

Alternative sweeteners are divided into two categories: sugar alcohols and high-intensity sweeteners. Sugar alcohols are nutritive or caloric sweeteners (that is, they contain calories). High-intensity sweeteners are mostly non-nutritive or calorie-free.

Sugar alcohols (also known as polyols) are a distinct category of sweet carbohydrates. Part of their chemical structure resembles a carbohydrate, while another part resembles alcohol. They are resistant to digestion, so they behave a lot like fiber. The effects are similar to those of oligosaccharides; they go undigested into the large intestine and are fermented by the bacteria that reside there. When consumed in large amounts, sugar alcohols can cause gastrointestinal distress, such as abdominal pain, gas, bloating, and diarrhea.

Even though sugar alcohols exist naturally in foods such as fruits and vegetables, most are manufactured from starches and sugars and are used in processed foods. Because they provide on average about half the calories of other carbohydrates and are thought to be relatively safe, sugar alcohols are often considered excellent sugar substitutes for people with diabetes. However, in order to train your palate to prefer less-sweet tastes, it is still best to minimize their use.

The most common sugar alcohols are erythritol, maltitol, sorbitol, and xylitol. Erythritol has the fewest calories at 0.2 calories per gram, while the other sugar alcohols range from 1.6–3 calories per gram (compared to 4 calories per gram for carbohydrates).[45] Erythritol is the one sugar alcohol that tends to not have adverse digestive effects because it is mostly absorbed into the bloodstream and excreted in the urine rather than passing through into the large intestine.[46] Although sugar alcohols do affect blood glucose, their impact is significantly less than that of other carbohydrates. They are very shelf stable because they are not as likely as sugar to attract bacteria or mold. These attributes make sugar alcohols very attractive to food manufacturers. On food labels, sugar alcohol content is listed separately from other carbohydrates. If you're counting carbohydrates, you can omit sugar alcohols if the total content is 5 grams or less or if the sugar alcohol is erythritol. However, if the total is more than 5 grams, simply divide the total by two and add it to your carbohydrate count. For example, if you eat 10 grams of sugar alcohols, you would count only 5 grams.

Sugar alcohols do not promote tooth decay, so they are the sweetener of choice in many dental hygiene products, such as toothpastes and mouth rinses. They also are used in breath mints and gums and in a variety of processed foods, such as ice cream, candy, and fruit spreads. Products containing sugar alcohols are often labeled sugar-free.

The second category of alternative sweeteners is high-intensity sweeteners. Some of these are artificial or synthetically produced while others are natural. Most are non-nutritive or essentially calorie-free. High-intensity sweeteners are regulated by national governments, and not all are permitted for use in all countries. In the United States, the Food and Drug Administration (FDA) has approved the use of six high-intensity artificial sweeteners: acesulfame-K, advantame, aspartame, neotame, saccharin, and sucralose.[47] Of these six, aspartame is the only one that is considered nutritive because it contains calories. However, it is about two hundred times sweeter than sugar, so it's used in such small amounts that it's considered calorie-free.

There are two approved high-intensity natural sweeteners: steviol glycosides and luo han guo (monk fruit) extracts. Both are non-nutritive or essentially calorie-free. Steviol glycosides, such as rebaudioside A (also called reb A), stevioside, rebaudioside D, or various mixtures of these compounds, are extracted from the stevia plant. These components are two hundred to four hundred times sweeter than sugar. While these constituents of stevia have been approved for use as sweeteners in the United States, the stevia leaf and crude stevia extracts have only been approved for use as nutritional supplements and not as sweeteners. Although there is controversy about the safety and side effects of stevia, recent scientific studies have been largely favorable.[48,49,50,51]

Stevia is approved for use in several countries and has been the principal non-nutritive sweetener used in Japan for several decades. Luo han guo, or monk fruit, is a fruit from southern China that has been used in Chinese medicine to treat coughs and sore throats and as a longevity aid. Monk fruit extracts contain a compound called mogrosides, which are 100–250 times sweeter than sugar.

The safety of high-intensity sweeteners is very controversial, although most health organizations, including the American Diabetes Association, Diabetes Canada, and the Academy of Nutrition and Dietetics (formerly American Dietetic Association), approve their use.[52,53,54] One of the reasons they are thought to be safe is that most are not metabolized by the body. However, it is possible for nonmetabolized compounds to exert adverse health effects.[55] Recent findings suggest that some high-intensity sweeteners promote dysbiosis, which can in turn increase insulin resistance and blood glucose regulation.[56,57,58]

High-intensity sweeteners are used mainly to help people lose weight and gain glycemic control without sacrificing sweet flavors. Unfortunately, the results of several studies suggest that the effects of these substances are counterintuitive; that is, they don't provide the expected benefits and, in some cases, could actually increase weight gain and impair glycemic control. There are several explanations for this.[59,60,61,62] First, studies suggest that when people use sugar-free foods, they make up for the missing calories by eating more food. By eating what's perceived to be a healthy, low-calorie item, people are more likely to give themselves permission to overconsume less-healthful food.

The second possible explanation is more about physiology than psychology. When you consume high-intensity sweeteners, your brain thinks you are consuming something with calories, but you get less than what your body expects (as happens with calorie-reduced solid foods) or you get none (as with artificially sweetened beverages).

This triggers the release of hunger hormones that increase appetite, so again you eat more food. In essence, your ability to regulate the intake of normal foods is decreased when your body expects calories that never come.

Another possibility is that the intense sweeteners cause people to become desensitized to sweetness. Sweet whole foods, such as fruits, become less appealing, and you're drawn to less-nutritious foods containing powerful sweeteners; it's a slippery slope from a nutritional perspective. Some research suggests that there are sweetness receptors in fat tissue that could trigger weight gain by stimulating the development of new fat cells. Evidence is also building that weight gain may be induced by the negative impact these sweeteners have on the gut microbiome.[57]

The bottom line is that sugar alcohols and intense sweeteners are used to enhance the flavor of ultraprocessed foods and beverages. These are not foods that will help you reclaim your health. Rather, they are the kinds of foods that promote overeating and diabetes. When you stick to whole plant foods, you don't have to worry about intense sweeteners, as they are not found in whole plant foods. If you must use a sweetener during your transition to a whole-foods, plant-based diet, your safest options are derivatives of monk fruit or stevia. Use them in the tiniest amounts possible, with a goal of removing them altogether.

BULK UP ON FIBER

Fiber is what gives plants their structure, and it's not present in any animal foods. Acting as nature's broom, fiber keeps food moving smoothly and efficiently through the intestinal tract. While fiber is a type of carbohydrate, it can't be broken down into digestible sugar molecules like most other carbohydrates. Although it passes through the intestinal tract relatively intact, it has a significant and positive impact. It is well known that fiber prevents constipation, but it can also help lower blood cholesterol and blood pressure, reducing the risk of heart disease. Fiber can improve blood sugar control and insulin sensitivity, reducing the risk of diabetes, and it can diminish the risk of diverticular disease and some cancers, especially colorectal cancer.

Fiber also helps to support a healthy gut flora, which supports every body system, including optimal functioning of the brain.[63,64,65] As discussed previously (see page 12), people with type 2 diabetes are at increased risk for dysbiosis (unhealthy gut microbiota), which is a key driver of insulin resistance. The most effective way of establishing and maintaining a health-supporting microbiome is to boost the volume and variety of dietary fiber in your diet. For example, to boost volume, add beans to your breakfast. For variety, instead of brown rice, try kamut berries, barley, rye berries, or quinoa.

Eat foods rich in probiotics (see sources on page 45). Consider taking a probiotic supplement that contains several different strains of organisms, and opt for high dosages (at least ten to twenty billion CFUs per day for adults). Check the expiration date. Also include rich dietary sources of prebiotics to keep friendly bacteria well fed (see page 45). Minimize very low-fiber and fiber-free foods that foster the growth of bad bacteria. The worst offenders are refined sugars, white flour products, artificial sweeteners, fried foods, meat, and alcohol.

Fiber is commonly divided into two categories: soluble and insoluble. Solubility is determined by whether the fiber dissolves in water. Although these terms are useful, the health benefits of fiber are thought to be related more to viscosity (whether fiber becomes gel-like or gummy when mixed with water) and fermentability (whether the fiber can be fermented by gut bacteria, producing short-chain fatty acids and gas by-products). Although many soluble fibers are both viscous and fermentable, and insoluble fibers are often nonviscous and nonfermentable, this is not always the case. However, for the sake of simplicity, we will refer to fiber as soluble and insoluble. All fiber-rich foods contain both soluble and insoluble fibers. Table 5.5 (opposite page) provides a list of common types of fiber and sources.[66,8]

Insoluble, nonviscous, less fermentable fiber is more strongly associated with a reduced risk of developing type 2 diabetes. Soluble, viscous, fermentable fiber improves postprandial (after meal) blood glucose because it slows the absorption of sugars into the bloodstream.[69] For people who have type 2 diabetes, foods rich in soluble fiber, such as legumes, oats, barley, flaxseeds, and many fruits and vegetables (asparagus, apricots, Brussels sprouts, citrus fruits, parsnips, passion fruit, roots, and tubers, to mention just a few), are especially helpful.

You may have noticed claims about fiber on food labels of processed and refined foods. Some of these products have isolated, nondigestible carbohydrates, such as inulin, added to boost the fiber content. While adding fiber to packaged foods boosts fiber and makes them appear healthy, products made with refined flour, sugar, and oil are not good choices—even if they are high in fiber!

The recommended intake for fiber is 14 grams per 1,000 calories, or about 25 grams per day for females and 38 grams per day for males.[8] Most Americans consume about half this amount.[70] To kick diabetes, aim to consume at least 45–60 grams of fiber per day (larger individuals can aim for the upper end of the spectrum). This translates to 15–20 grams per meal.

Table 5.6 (pages 90–93) provides a summary of the total, soluble, and insoluble fiber in common foods. When you look at the table, compare the fiber content of foods in different categories. Legumes stand out as fiber superstars. Compare foods within each category to see which ones provide the most total and soluble fiber. For example, in the vegetables group, artichokes and Brussels sprouts are very high in both total and soluble fiber. In the legumes group, lentils are extremely high in total fiber, but most other legumes provide more soluble fiber.

TABLE 5.5. Types of Plant Fiber, Health Effects, and Common Sources

TYPE OF FIBER	HEALTH EFFECTS	COMMON SOURCES
SOLUBLE, VISCOUS, FERMENTABLE		
Beta-glucans	Lower blood glucose and blood cholesterol. Soften stools.	Oats, barley, mushrooms, and seaweed
Gums and mucilages	Lower blood glucose and blood cholesterol. Soften stools.	Seeds, such as flax, psyllium, and guar seeds (guar gum); some sea vegetables; roots; and tubers
Nondigestible oligosaccharides	Some are prebiotics, feeding friendly bacteria. Soften stools, increase stool bulk, and improve laxation.	Jerusalem artichokes, asparagus, Brussels sprouts, cabbage, whole grains, legumes, jicama, and some other fruits and vegetables
Pectins	Lower blood glucose and blood cholesterol. Soften stools.	Berries and fruits (especially apples, apricots, citrus fruits, and passion fruit) and some vegetables
INSOLUBLE, NONVISCOUS, LESS FERMENTABLE		
Celluloses*	Increase stool bulk and improve laxation. No significant effect on blood glucose or blood cholesterol levels.	Grains, fruits, vegetables, legumes, nuts, and seeds
Hemicelluloses**	Increase stool bulk and improve laxation. Not all are nonviscous; those that are may improve blood glucose or cholesterol levels.	Fruits, whole grains (especially outer husks), legumes, nuts, seeds, and vegetables
Lignins	Increase stool bulk and improve laxation. No significant effect on blood glucose or blood cholesterol levels.	Stringy vegetables and the outer layer of cereal grains
Resistant starches	Beneficial effect on blood glucose, insulin sensitivity, and cholesterol levels. Some increase in stool bulk and laxation.	Corn, legumes, potatoes (especially if they are cooked, then cooled), underripe or green bananas, whole grains

Sources: [66,8,67,68]

*Cellulose accounts for about 25 percent of the fiber in grains and fruits and 33 percent in vegetables and nuts.

**Hemicellulose accounts for about 33 percent of the fiber in plants.

Can you eat too much fiber? Although it's possible to eat too much fiber, it's unlikely if you are consuming whole plant foods and drinking sufficient fluids. Most instances of excessive fiber are generally related to taking fiber supplements, eating too much wheat bran, or not drinking enough. It is surprising to learn that during Paleolithic times, humans consumed an estimated 70–150 grams or more of fiber per day![74] This is more than the highest fiber levels eaten today.

TABLE 5.6. Fiber in Common Foods

KEY			
	GOOD SOURCE	HIGH SOURCE	VERY HIGH SOURCE
Total Fiber	2–3.9 g	4–6.9 g	7+ g
Soluble Fiber	1–1.9 g	2–2.9 g	3+ g
Insoluble Fiber	1.5–2.9 g	3–4.9 g	1.5–2.9 g

FOOD	PORTION SIZE	GRAMS TOTAL FIBER	GRAMS SOLUBLE FIBER	GRAMS INSOLUBLE FIBER
FRUITS				
Apple, raw	1 medium	3.7	1	2.7
Apricots, raw	1 cup (250 ml)	3.7	2	1.7
Avocado, raw, California	1 medium	9.2	3.4	5.8
Banana, raw	1 medium	2.8	0.7	2.1
Blackberries, raw	1 cup (250 ml)	7.6	1.4	6.2
Blueberries, raw	1 cup (250 ml)	3.9	0.4	3.5
Cantaloupe, raw	1 cup (250 ml)	1.3	0.3	1
Cherries, raw	1 cup (250 ml)	3.3	1	2.3
Figs, dried	3	4.6	2.2	2.4
Grapefruit	1 medium	2.8	2.3	0.5
Grapes, raw	1 cup (250 ml)	1.6	0.2	0.4
Mango, raw	1 medium	3.7	1.5	2.2
Nectarine, raw	1 medium	2.2	0.8	1.4
Orange	1 medium	3.1	1.8	1.3
Passion Fruit	1 medium	1.9	1.4	0.5
Peach, raw	1 medium	2	0.8	1.2
Pear, raw	1 medium	4	2.2	1.8
Peppers, red, sweet, raw	1 cup (250 ml)	3	1.1	1.9
Pineapple	1 cup (250 ml)	1.9	0.2	1.7
Plums	1 medium	2.5	1.3	1.2
Raspberries	1 cup (250 ml)	8.4	0.9	7.5
Strawberries	1 cup (250 ml)	3.3	0.9	2.4
Watermelon	1 cup (250 ml)	1.4	0.6	0.8

FOOD	PORTION SIZE	GRAMS TOTAL FIBER	GRAMS SOLUBLE FIBER	GRAMS INSOLUBLE FIBER
VEGETABLES				
Artichokes	1 medium	6.5	4.7	1.8
Asparagus, cooked	1 cup (250 ml)	5.6	3.4	2.2
Beets, cooked	1 cup (250 ml)	3.4	1.4	2
Broccoli, cooked	1 cup (250 ml)	4.6	2.3	2.3
Brussels sprouts, cooked	1 cup (250 ml)	6.4	3.9	2.5
Cabbage, cooked	1 cup (250 ml)	3.4	1.5	1.9
Carrots, raw	1 medium	2.3	1.1	1.2
Cauliflower, cooked	1 cup (250 ml)	3.4	0.9	2.5
Celery, raw	1 cup (250 ml)	2	0.7	1.3
Corn	1 cup (250 ml)	3.9	0.5	3.4
Cucumber	1 cup (250 ml)	0.8	0.2	0.6
Green beans, cooked	1 cup (250 ml)	4	1	3
Kale, cooked	1 cup (250 ml)	2.6	1.4	1.2
Kohlrabi, raw	1 cup (250 ml)	4.9	3.4	1.5
Lettuce, romaine	1 cup (250 ml)	0.9	0.3	0.6
Mushrooms, cooked	1 cup (250 ml)	3.4	0.3	3.1
Peas, frozen	1 cup (250 ml)	8.8	2.6	6.2
Potato, boiled with skin	1 cup (250 ml)	3	1.2	1.8
Spinach, cooked	1 cup (250 ml)	5.4	1.1	4.3
Squash, winter, cooked	1 cup (250 ml)	6.7	3.8	2.9
Sweet potato, cooked	1 cup (250 ml)	7.6	2.8	4.8
Tomato, raw	1 cup (250 ml)	2	0.2	1.8
Turnip, cooked	1 cup (250 ml)	3.1	1.1	2
Zucchini, cooked	1 cup (250 ml)	2.5	1.1	1.4
LEGUMES				
Black beans, cooked	1 cup (250 ml)	12.2	4.8	7.4
Black-eyed peas, cooked	1 cup (250 ml)	9.4	1	8.4
Chickpeas, cooked	1 cup (250 ml)	8.6	2.6	6

FOOD	PORTION SIZE	GRAMS TOTAL FIBER	GRAMS SOLUBLE FIBER	GRAMS INSOLUBLE FIBER
Edamame, cooked	1 cup (250 ml)	7.6	3.4	4.2
Kidney beans, cooked	1 cup (250 ml)	11.4	5.7	5.7
Lentils, cooked	1 cup (250 ml)	15.6	1.2	14.4
Lima beans, cooked	1 cup (250 ml)	13.2	2.7	7.2
Navy beans, cooked	1 cup (250 ml)	11.7	4.4	7.3
Pinto beans, cooked	1 cup (250 ml)	14.7	3.8	10.9
Split peas, cooked	1 cup (250 ml)	6.2	2.2	4
NUTS AND SEEDS				
Almonds	¼ cup (60 ml)	4	0.4	3.6
Brazil nuts	¼ cup (60 ml)	1.9	0.5	1.4
Cashews	¼ cup (60 ml)	1.2	0.1	1.1
Coconut, dried	¼ cup (60 ml)	3.3	0.3	3
Flaxseeds	¼ cup (60 ml)	6.4	3.5	2.9
Hazelnuts	¼ cup (60 ml)	2	0.8	1.2
Macadamia nuts	¼ cup (60 ml)	3.1	2.4	0.7
Peanuts	¼ cup (60 ml)	3.3	0.7	2.6
Pecans	¼ cup (60 ml)	2	0.3	1.7
Pistachios	¼ cup (60 ml)	3.5	0.9	2.6
Sunflower seeds	¼ cup (60 ml)	1.5	0.6	0.9
Walnuts	¼ cup (60 ml)	1.5	0.5	1
WHOLE GRAINS				
Barley, cooked	1 cup (250 ml)	8.5	1.8	6.7
Brown rice, cooked	1 cup (250 ml)	3.5	0.2	3.3
Bulgur, cooked	1 cup (250 ml)	7.9	1.3	6.6
Millet, cooked	1 cup (250 ml)	6.5	1.2	5.3
Oatmeal, cooked	1 cup (250 ml)	4	1.9	2.1
Popcorn, popped	3 cups (750 ml)	2	0.1	1.9
Quinoa, cooked	1 cup (250 ml)	5.2	0.7	4.5
Wheat berries, cooked	1 cup (250 ml)	7.6	0.9	6.7
Wild rice, cooked	1 cup (250 ml)	2.9	0.3	2.6

FOOD	PORTION SIZE	GRAMS TOTAL FIBER	GRAMS SOLUBLE FIBER	GRAMS INSOLUBLE FIBER
PACKAGED FOODS				
Bread, white	1 slice	0.6	0.3	0.3
Bread, whole wheat	1 slice	2	0.4	1.6
Cornflakes	1 cup (250 ml)	0.8	0.1	0.7
Crispy rice cereal	1 cup (250 ml)	0.7	0.2	0.5
Donut, cake	1 medium	0.6	0.2	0.4
Fruity presweetened cereal	1 cup (250 ml)	0.6	0.1	0.5
Granola bar	1	1	0.2	0.8
Puffed rice	1 cup (250 ml)	0.3	0.1	0.2
Puffed wheat	1 cup (250 ml)	1.1	0.5	0.6
Shredded wheat, spoon-sized	1 cup (250 ml)	6.2	0.9	5.3
Spaghetti, white noodles, cooked	1 cup (250 ml)	1.8	1.1	0.7
Spaghetti, whole-wheat noodles, cooked	1 cup (250 ml)	3.9	0.8	3.1
Sugars	Any	0	0	0
Vegetable oil	Any	0	0	0
White rice, cooked	1 cup (250 ml)	0.6	0.1	0.5
ANIMAL PRODUCTS				
Meat, poultry, fish, eggs	Any	0	0	0
Dairy products	Any	0	0	0

Sources: [71,72,73]

For some individuals, however, a sudden increase in fiber intake may cause abdominal discomfort, cramping, bloating, gas, and diarrhea. It is even possible to become constipated when consuming a lot of fiber without enough fluids. In the most severe cases, it's possible to develop an intestinal blockage. This can happen if the fiber becomes a hard, dry mass in the intestine, blocking the passage of food. The best way to prevent the adverse effects of a high-fiber diet is to increase your intake gradually (over several weeks) and boost your fluid intake along with it.

Another concern is that very high fiber intakes can reduce the absorption of minerals. While research has shown a reduction in the absorption of some minerals, the impact tends to be fairly small. Also, it's not clear if fiber itself is the culprit or if phytates and oxalates, which can bind to minerals, bear more of the responsibility.[75] Although this is a valid concern, these minerals can be liberated, at least partly, during fermentation in the large intestine. Short-chain fatty acids (also products of fermentation) help to facilitate their absorption from the large intestine.[66] In addition, when compared to refined foods, high-fiber whole foods generally provide enough extra minerals to compensate for any losses incurred. Regardless, it is advised to limit concentrated fiber, such as wheat bran, and to minimize the use of fiber supplements when eating a plant-based diet. The best balance of healthful fiber and nutrients comes naturally with a varied whole-foods, plant-based diet.

REDUCE THE GLYCEMIC LOAD (GL) OF YOUR DIET

The glycemic index (GI) is a measure of how carbohydrates impact blood sugar levels. Carbohydrates with a high GI are more quickly digested, absorbed, and metabolized, causing a rapid and dramatic rise in blood glucose. Foods with a high GI usually trigger an exaggerated insulin response, adversely affecting long-term blood glucose control, increasing triglycerides, and reducing protective HDL cholesterol. Carbohydrates with a low GI are more slowly digested, absorbed, and metabolized, causing a lower and more gradual rise in blood glucose. Foods with a low GI may positively affect insulin response, triglycerides, and HDL cholesterol levels (see figure 5.2, opposite page).[76,77,78,79] Replacing high GI foods with low GI foods improves blood sugar control, reduces a hsCRP (a measure of inflammation), and significantly reduces the risk of developing type 2 diabetes.[3]

To determine the glycemic index of a food, several people eat a sample of the food providing 50 grams of carbohydrate. For each study participant, changes in blood glucose are monitored over time (usually two hours). The values from all of the participants are averaged to obtain the glycemic index of the food. The GI uses a scale of 0 to 100, with higher values given to foods that cause the most rapid rise in blood sugar. Pure glucose serves as a reference point and is given a GI of 100. White bread has a glycemic index of 75 relative to glucose, which means that the blood sugar response to the carbohydrate in white bread is 75 percent of the blood sugar response to the pure glucose. By comparison, barley has a glycemic index of 28 relative to glucose.[78]

The glycemic index tells us how a serving of food containing 50 grams of carbohydrates affects our blood sugar. However, we rarely consume exactly 50 grams of carbohydrate from any food. Therefore a more practical tool called the glycemic load (GL) was created so the glycemic impact of a food could be estimated based on the car-

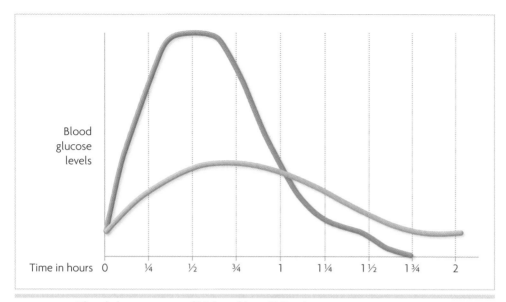

FIGURE 5.2 Blood glucose curve of high and low GI foods.

Note: The amount of carbohydrate in two test foods containing 50 grams of carbohydrates.

bohydrate in a typical serving size (based on the USDA food database). GL is calculated by multiplying the glycemic index by the grams of carbohydrate provided in a portion of the food and dividing the total by 100. The formula for calculating GL is as follows:

Glycemic Load (GL) = GI x CHO content per portion of food ÷ 100

So, for example, the GL of brown rice with a GI of 66 and 52 grams of carbohydrate per a 1-cup (250-ml) serving would be: 66 x 52 ÷ 100 = 34.

The critical point about GL is that serving size matters. For example, if you ate ½ cup (125 ml) of the brown rice (GI = 66; 26 g carbohydrate), the GL would be 17 (66 x 26 ÷ 100 = 17). If you ate 2 cups (500 ml) of brown rice (GI = 66; 104 g carbohydrate), the GL would be 68 (66 x 104 ÷ 100)! Both the GI and GL are rated as being low, medium, or high, according to their impact on blood glucose. A GI of 55 or less is low, 56–69 is medium, and 70 or more is high. A GL of 10 or less is low, 11–19 is medium, and 20 or more is high.

Foods that have a high glycemic index do not always have a high glycemic load. For example, watermelon has a glycemic index of 72; however, a 4-ounce (120-g) serving of watermelon provides only 6 grams of carbohydrate. You would need to eat over eight servings (2 lbs/960 g) of watermelon to get the 50 grams of carbohydrates needed to determine its glycemic index. A 4-ounce (120-g) serving of watermelon has a glycemic load of 4 (72 x 6 ÷ 100), which is low. Table 5.7 (pages 99–100) provides the glycemic index and glycemic load of several common foods.

The impact of decreasing the GL of the diet is measurable and proportionate. One study reported that the risk of developing diabetes is increased by 45 percent for every 100-gram increment of GL. (To get the total GL for the day, add up the GL of each food consumed).[80] To put this into perspective, 100 grams of GL is equal to 100 grams of carbohydrate from food with a GI of 100, 200 grams of carbohydrate from food with a GI of 50, and 300 grams of carbohydrate from food with a GI of 33. The lesson here is that the glycemic impact from a small serving of food with a high GI can be remarkably similar to a much more generous serving of a food with a low GI.

The GI of various foods is not as predictable as one might expect. For example, sucrose (white table sugar) has a glycemic index of 68—lower than that of white bread, which has a glycemic index of 75, or whole wheat bread, which has a glycemic index of 74.[78] How can it be that bread, a complex carbohydrate, has a glycemic index that is higher than table sugar, a simple carbohydrate? The reason is that table sugar is half fructose and half glucose, while bread is all glucose. Glucose goes directly into the bloodstream and has the greatest impact on blood sugar. Fructose is metabolized quite differently, and its impact on blood sugar is about one-fifth that of glucose. So while bread may be more slowly digested and absorbed than sucrose, the glucose in bread causes a greater rise in blood glucose than the combination of glucose and fructose present in table sugar. There are several key factors influencing the glycemic index of foods:[78,77,79,81,82,83,84]

TYPE OF SUGAR PRESENT. Glucose has a much greater impact on blood glucose than do fructose or galactose (a sugar in milk). When comparing the glycemic index of various types of natural sweeteners, the differences are determined by the relative amount of fructose contained in the sugars. Sugars with a lower GI contain more fructose. This does not make them more healthful, as was shown in the discussion of fructose on page 76. Although sugar alcohols aren't technically sugars, their GI ranges from zero for erythritol to 36 for maltitol; other sugar alcohols have a GI of 5–12.

TYPE OF STARCH PRESENT. The two principal starches in foods—amylopectin and amylose—are digested at very different rates. Amylopectin is a highly branched chain of glucose molecules that are rapidly absorbed into the bloodstream. Amylose, a more compact, straight chain of glucose molecules is broken down relatively slowly. Foods that are higher in amylose have lower GIs. If you look at very detailed GI charts, you will notice that the GI of different types of rice varies wildly, with those low in amylose and high in amylopectin having a much higher GI.

AMOUNT AND TYPE OF FIBER PRESENT. Fiber resists the work of digestive enzymes, so it slows the digestion and absorption of sugars from foods, reducing GI. Foods rich in soluble, viscous fiber reduce the glycemic index to a greater extent than foods rich in insoluble, nonviscous fiber. Beans and barley are good examples of foods rich in viscous fiber. Wheat bran is a good example of a food rich in nonviscous fiber. Refined foods that have had most or all of their fiber removed have a higher GI, as they are more rapidly absorbed.

PHYSICAL BARRIER AROUND THE FOOD. Beans and whole grains are surrounded by a fibrous coating that serves as a physical barrier to protect the seed. This barrier makes it more difficult for enzymes to break the food down, reducing the GI.

RIPENESS OF THE FOOD. As foods ripen, starches turn into sugars that are more rapidly digested, increasing their GI. For example, a banana that is slightly green or underripe has a GI of about 30, while an overripe banana has a GI of about 50.

EXPOSURE TO HEAT. Raw foods have a lower GI than the same foods cooked. Cooking increases GI because it breaks down the plant's cell walls, increasing the rate at which its starches and sugars are absorbed. Lightly steaming vegetables to the tender-crisp stage will result in a lower GI than very well-cooked vegetables.

PARTICLE SIZE. Whenever particle size is reduced, the surface area of the food is increased, and it is more rapidly digested and absorbed. Thus, intact whole grains (such as wheat berries and barley) have a much lower GI than ground grains (flours), and whole fruits have a lower GI than fruit sauces or juices.

DENSITY OF THE FOOD. Dense foods containing little air have a lower GI than foods that are light and fluffy. Even though white flour is the main ingredient in white bread and white pasta, the bread has a much higher GI than the pasta because it is light and fluffy and quickly broken down. Puffed cereal grains also have a much higher GI than cooked grains.

CRYSTALLINITY OF THE FOOD. When a starch is raw, it is crystalline; its molecules are organized in a sequence that repeats. When it is cooked, this order is lost; it becomes more easily broken down and digested, and the GI increases. However, when the food cools, it recrystallizes, reducing its GI. For example, red potatoes cubed and boiled in their skin have a GI of 89. When the potatoes are stored overnight in the refrigerator and eaten cold the next day, the GI drops to 56.

ACIDITY. The addition of vinegar, lemon, or lime, ideally near the beginning of your meal (perhaps on a salad), can reduce the glycemic impact of the meal. Even 2–3 teaspoons (10–15 ml) is often enough for an effect. Fermentation also produces acid, reducing the GI. Yogurt has a lower GI than fluid milk, and sourdough bread has a lower GI than conventional bread.

Another important consideration is that people tend to eat foods in combination. For example, baked potatoes have a very high GI and GL, so some health authorities suggest they be avoided. Potatoes, like rice or other starchy staples, are high-carbohydrate foods that when eaten alone are rapidly absorbed into the bloodstream. However, if a baked potato is eaten with a black bean–peanut sauce and broccoli, or a lentil loaf and kale salad, the absorption of the sugars in the potato will be much more gradual. Potatoes (with skin) are high in fiber, cholesterol-free, very low in fat and sodium, and good sources of potassium, manganese, vitamin C, and vitamin B_6. The point is that these whole plant foods with concentrated carbohydrates can be included in a healthy diet when they're consumed as part of a high-fiber, whole-foods, plant-based diet and portion sizes are controlled.

GI and GL are two tools among many that can help you compare and select foods for preventing and treating diabetes. However, foods with a low GI or GL don't automatically acquire a health halo. While the GI and GL can help you choose foods that improve blood glucose control, these tools tell you nothing about the fiber, phytochemicals, antioxidants, pre- or probiotics, essential fatty acids, vitamins, and minerals provided. Nor do they provide information about the harmful contaminants or the products of oxidation that may be present.

Foods that contain little, if any, carbohydrate, such as fried bacon, have a very low GI and a negligible GL. This doesn't make it a healthy choice for people with diabetes. Although protein and fat have minimal impact on blood glucose levels in the short term, they have the potential to significantly increase insulin resistance and produce adverse effects on blood glucose control in the long term.[85,86] Likewise, the GI of potato chips is lower than baked potatoes, while candy bars, cupcakes, and ice cream also frequently fall within the low glycemic index range. In contrast, plenty of nutritious, higher carbohydrate whole foods, such as some fruits, starchy vegetables, and whole grains, have relatively high glycemic indexes (particularly watermelon) or glycemic loads (brown rice), but that does not make them off-limits.

Also, remember that the GI of sugar is determined by the amount of fructose in the mix. As the amount of fructose in a sugar source rises, its glycemic index falls. With most foods, a lower glycemic index is desirable, but when it comes to sugar, a lower GI (as we see with the listing of agave syrup in table 5.2, page 79) means more fructose. So, with sugars, low GI is not a particularly favorable attribute.

While GI and GL have limitations, they are very useful when appropriately used. Among the best ways to use these tools is to compare similar foods or foods from the same category. Compare different intact grains, such as barley (GI = 28) and millet (GI = 71) or different types of nondairy milks, such soy milk (GI = 21) and rice milk (GI = 86).

Foods with a low GL have a relatively small impact on blood glucose, so these should be featured strongly in your diet. Fill your plate with legumes, nonstarchy vegetables, and fruits, along with smaller portions of nuts and seeds. Include moderate servings of high-carbohydrate foods, such as starchy vegetables and whole grains.

TABLE 5.7. GI and GL of Common Foods

KEY TO TABLE 5.7	
Glycemic Index (GI)	Glycemic Load (GL)
Low (white) = 55 or less	Low (white) = 10 or less
Medium (light gray) = 56–69	Medium (light gray) = 11–19
High (dark gray) = 70 or more	High (dark gray) = 20 or more

FOOD	GI	SERVING SIZE	GL	FOOD	GI	SERVING SIZE	GL
GRAINS				Rice, white	43–109	5 oz (150 g)	15–46
Barley, cooked	28	5 oz (150 g)	12	Rice cakes, puffed	82	25 g/.9 oz	17
Bread, sourdough rye	48	1 oz (30 g)	6	Spaghetti, white	49	6 oz (180 g)	24
Bread, white	75	1 oz (30 g)	11	Spaghetti, whole wheat	42	6 oz (180 g)	17
Bread, whole wheat	74	1 oz (30 g)	9	**LEGUMES**			
Bread, 80% intact kernels	41	1 oz (30 g)	5	Beans, black, cooked	20	5 oz (150 g)	5
Buckwheat groats	45	5 oz (150 g)	13	Beans, butter beans, cooked	32	5 oz (150 g)	7
Cereal, bran flakes	63	1 oz (30 g)	12	Beans, kidney, cooked	22	5 oz (150 g)	6
Cereal, cornflakes	81	1 oz (30 g)	20	Beans, navy, cooked	31	5 oz (150 g)	9
Cereal, crispy rice	88	1 oz (30 g)	23	Beans, pinto	33	5 oz (150 g)	8
Cereal, shredded wheat	67	1 oz (30 g)	13	Chickpeas, canned	38	5 oz (150 g)	9
Crackers, rice	91	25 g/.9 oz	23	Hummus	6	1 oz (30 g)	0
Crackers, rye with sesame	57	25 g/.9 oz	9	Lentils	29	5 oz (150 g)	5
Millet, boiled	71	5 oz (150 g)	26	Soybeans, cooked	14	5 oz (150 g)	1
Oatmeal (instant)	79	8 oz (240 g)	21	Split peas, yellow, cooked	25	5 oz (150 g)	3
Oatmeal (traditional)	55	8 oz (240 g)	13	**VEGETABLES***			
Quinoa, cooked	53	5 oz (150 g)	13	Carrots, boiled	39	5 oz (150 g)	2
Rice, brown	50–87	5 oz (150 g)	16–33	Corn	52	2.7 oz (80 g)	9

FOOD	GI	SERVING SIZE	GL
Parsnips	52	2.7 oz (80 g)	4
Peas, frozen, boiled	51	2.7 oz (80 g)	4
Potato, baked	86	5 oz (150 g)	22
Potato, boiled	82	5 oz (150 g)	21
Squash, butternut	51	2.7 oz (80 g)	3
Sweet potatoes	70	5 oz (150 g)	22
Taro	53	5 oz (150 g)	4
FRUITS			
Apple, Golden Delicious	39	4 oz (120 g)	6
Apricots, raw	31	4 oz (120 g)	7
Banana, raw	47	4 oz (120 g)	11
Blueberries	53	4 oz (120 g)	5
Cherries, dark	63	4 oz (120 g)	9
Dates	42	2 oz (60 g)	18
Grapes, black	59	4 oz (120 g)	11
Mango	51	4 oz (120 g)	8
Nectarines	43	4 oz (120 g)	4
Oranges	40	4 oz (120 g)	4
Papaya	56	4 oz (120 g)	5
Pineapple	66	4 oz (120 g)	6
Raisins (sultanas)	57	2 oz (60 g)	25
Strawberries	40	4 oz (120 g)	1
Watermelon	72	4 oz (120 g)	4
NUTS			
Cashews	25	1.7 oz (50 g)	3
Nuts, mixed	24	1.7 oz (50 g)	4
Peanuts	7	1.7 oz (50 g)	0

FOOD	GI	SERVING SIZE	GL
DAIRY AND ALTERNATIVES			
Cow's milk, full fat	31	1 cup (250 ml)	4
Rice milk	86	1 cup (250 ml)	23
Soy milk, regular	21	1 cup (250 ml)	2
Ice cream, French vanilla	38	1.7 oz (50 g)	3
Yogurt, natural	19	1.7 oz (50 g)	3
SUGARS			
Agave	13	.35 oz (10 g)	1
Fructose	19	.35 oz (10 g)	2
Glucose	103	.35 oz (10 g)	10
Honey	61	.35 oz (10 g)	12
Maple syrup	54	.35 oz (10 g)	10
SNACK FOODS			
Chocolate, dark	23	1.7 oz (50 g)	6
Chocolate, milk	43	1.7 oz (50 g)	12
Chocolate, Mars bar	68	2 oz (60 g)	27
Energy bar, Cliff	57	2.2 oz (65 g)	22
Jelly beans	80	1 oz (30 g)	22
Popcorn, plain	65	.7 oz (20 g)	7
Potato chips	56	1.7 oz (50 g)	12
Pretzels	84	1 oz (30 g)	20

Source:[77,78]

Chapter 6

Managing Protein and Fat

Like most people, Diane always thought that protein was the one macronutrient that could do no wrong. She believed that protein from animal sources—meat, poultry, fish, and eggs—was best for people with diabetes because they were carbohydrate-free. She had learned years ago that not only is the protein in plant foods minimal, but it's also inferior. So boiled eggs and yogurt became her breakfast staples, chicken and fish topped her salads, and beef and pork were the usual stars of the dinner show. While she worried about eating too much fat when she was first diagnosed, her internet searches taught her that fat, even saturated fat, had been vindicated as a cause of heart disease, diabetes, and other chronic diseases. The evidence was everywhere—on the covers of magazines, in newspapers, and on almost every website she visited. It was a relief because fat made food taste better. So when everything she thought she knew about protein and fat was turned on its head in her plant-based diabetes program, she was blown away. She wondered how the media could have strayed so far from science.

THE POWER OF PROTEIN FROM PLANTS

Many popular diabetes diets are low in carbohydrates and high in meat. Meat is emphasized because it is essentially carbohydrate-free. But is being carbohydrate-free all it takes to make food diabetes-friendly? The answer is an unequivocal *no*. When you look at the evidence, meat doesn't measure up to expectations. Many studies have examined the link between meat intake and diabetes risk, and they consistently report higher rates of diabetes with higher meat intakes (see pages 53–54). The strongest link is for processed meats and red meat.

Other studies have examined how different protein sources influence diabetes risk. Many of these studies have divided protein into animal versus plant protein. In 2016, a US study of over 200,000 participants reported that those eating the highest amounts of animal protein had a 13 percent increased risk of type 2 diabetes compared with those eating the least.[1] Those eating the most plant protein had a 9 percent risk reduction relative to those eating the least. Replacing just 5 percent of calories from animal protein with plant protein resulted in a 23 percent reduced risk of type 2 diabetes.

In the same year, an Australian study reported a 29 percent increased risk of type 2 diabetes with the highest versus lowest intakes of animal protein and a 40 percent risk reduction in women eating the most versus the least plant protein.[2] The researchers also reported on a meta-analysis of eleven studies with over 500,000 participants. Those consuming highest versus lowest intakes of meat had a 19 percent increased risk, while those eating the highest versus lowest intakes of plant protein had a 5 percent risk reduction.

A 2017 Finnish study examined the effect of protein sources in men who were followed for almost twenty years.[3] Replacing 1 percent of energy from animal protein with energy from plant protein was associated with an 18 percent decreased risk of type 2 diabetes. A 2014 Canadian study examined the risk associated with high-protein intakes. (Recall that keto weight-loss diets suggest 20 percent of calories from protein, and paleo diets suggest 30 percent of calories from protein—both relying mainly on animal protein.)[4] In participants ages fifty to sixty-five, those with intakes exceeding 20 percent had an increased risk of developing type 2 diabetes that was four times higher, while those over sixty-five had a risk that was ten times higher. However, in both cases the associated risk was eliminated or greatly reduced when the source of the protein was plants.

Why the discrepancy between animal and plant protein sources? Protein-rich plant foods are excellent sources of fiber, phytochemicals, antioxidants, and other protective compounds, whereas meats have little to none of these healthful components. In addition, animal protein sources, especially red and processed meats, are high in substances associated with inflammation and oxidative stress, such as saturated fat, heme iron, Neu5Gc, carnitine (which forms TMAO), and chemical contaminants (see table 6.1, opposite page).

What this means in practical terms is that replacing even a small amount of meat with legumes will help to reduce diabetes risk, regardless of the fact that meat is carbohydrate-free and legumes are relatively rich in carbohydrates. How is this best accomplished? Instead of bacon and eggs for breakfast, try scrambled tofu or add some cooked or sprouted lentils to your breakfast bowl. Rather than chicken noodle soup at lunch, opt for a split pea or bean soup. At dinner, swap out meat for beans or tofu in family favorites, such as stews, chili, pasta dishes, or wraps. Experiment with

TABLE 6.1. Plant Protein versus Animal Protein

FOOD COMPONENT	PLANT PROTEIN SOURCES (LEGUMES, SEEDS, NUTS)	ANIMAL PROTEIN SOURCES (MEAT, PROCESSED MEATS)
PROTECTIVE		
Fiber	high	none
Phytochemicals	high	none
Antioxidants	high	minimal
Plant sterols	high	none
Pre- or Probiotics	high	minimal
POTENTIALLY HARMFUL		
Cholesterol	none	moderate
Solid fats (saturated fat)	low	high
Heme iron	none	high
Industrial pollutants	low	moderate/high
Neu5Gc	none	highest in red meat
Endotoxins	low	varies; highest in ground or processed products
Glycotoxins (advanced glycation end products)	low to moderate depending on cooking conditions	highest in processed meat; high in well-cooked meat

legume-, nut-, and seed-based veggie loaves and patties, or try some of the delicious ready-made options that are widely available in the marketplace. Try more bean-based foods with multicultural flavors.

FAT FACTS AND FAIRY TALES

The science is crystal clear: there is a broad spectrum of fat intake that can support and promote excellent health. This is beautifully illustrated by the Blue Zones (see page 111), where the longest-living, healthiest populations reside. In Okinawa, fat intake is only 6–11 percent of calories; in Ikaria, Greece, it is about 50 percent. Intake in other Blue Zones range from 20–30 percent of calories from fat. The most salient lesson these populations teach is that the sources of macronutrients (fat, carbohydrate, and protein) matter more than the relative percentages of those macronutrients.

There is good evidence supporting the use of very low-fat plant-based diets as a therapeutic treatment for diabetes. For example, in studies by the Physicians Committee for Responsible Medicine, good results were achieved using plant-based diets that provided only about 10 percent of calories from fat.[5,6] On the other hand, higher-fat plant-based diets have also been shown to be effective. For example, a Finnish study reported favorable findings using diets that provided approximately 25 percent of calories from fat.[7] An American study that did not specify percentages of calories from macronutrients achieved remarkable success using a plant-based diet that included moderate amounts of higher-fat plant foods, such as nuts, seeds, and avocados.[8]

There may be advantages to including some higher-fat plant foods within the framework of a whole-foods diet. In establishing appropriate guidelines for people who are fighting cardiometabolic diseases, such as diabetes and heart disease, many factors need to be considered. Sufficient fat is necessary for the body to properly accomplish these functions:

- provide structure and function for cell membranes and the brain
- make hormones and bile acids
- maximize absorption of critical fat-soluble nutrients and phytochemicals
- maintain skin and hair
- regulate gene expression
- ensure a sufficient supply of essential fatty acids

There is a fine balance between keeping fats low enough to reduce lipotoxicity and exposure to potentially harmful fats while keeping them high enough to not compromise optimal body functioning. One of the advantages of including some higher-fat plant foods, such as nuts, seeds, and avocados, is that these foods have a very low glycemic index, so they'll help to lower the glycemic load of the total diet. On the other hand, higher-fat foods are more calorically dense. When you eat less fat, you can eat more food. For example, you get 120 calories from 1 tablespoon (15 ml) of oil or 14 cups (3.5 L) of greens; you get 400 calories from ½ cup (125 ml) of nuts or four bananas.

Most major health and diabetes organizations suggest a range for recommended fat intake from a low of 15–20 percent of calories to a high of 30–35 percent of calories from fat.[9,10] In practical terms, if you are overweight or obese, you would be well advised to stay at the lower end of the range. This will allow you to enjoy a larger volume of food. Although very low-fat diets (10 percent fat) may be appropriate for some individuals, most will need slightly higher intakes to maximize protective dietary components and provide sufficient raw materials for body maintenance. Still others may be well advised to aim for 20–25 percent of calories from fat, especially if they are carbohydrate sensitive.

TABLE 6.2. Fat Limits at Differing Levels of Total Fat Intake

TOTAL PERCENT OF CALORIES FROM FAT	1,600 CALORIE DIET MAXIMUM FAT (G)	1,800 CALORIE DIET MAXIMUM FAT (G)	2,000 CALORIE DIET MAXIMUM FAT (G)
10	18	20	22
15	27	30	33
20	36	40	44
25	44	50	55
30	54	60	66

The bottom line is that there is some flexibility in the percentage of calories that comes from fat, and what is optimal can vary from one individual to the next. However, there is much less flexibility in terms of the quality of fat. When fat comes from whole plant foods, it is naturally packaged with fiber, phytochemicals, antioxidants, plant sterols, and other protective components. Thus, the impact fat from whole foods has on health tends to be favorable, even when intakes are at the high end of the recommended range. Conversely, when fats are derived from highly processed foods, fast foods, convenience foods, and refined fats and oils, negative health consequences can occur even when fat intakes are relatively low. Table 6.2 (above) provides the upper limit of fat grams at varying levels of fat intake (as a percentage of calories). Maximum fat grams are provided for three levels of caloric intake: 1,600 calories, 1,800 calories and 2,000 calories.

If your diet consists exclusively of legumes, grains, vegetables, and fruits, your calories from fat will hover around 10 percent. This is a diet with no added fat and very limited, if any, higher-fat plant foods. In some cases, 1 tablespoon of ground flaxseeds is included to ensure a source of omega-3 fatty acids. One serving of a higher-fat plant food provides about 14 grams of fat—the amount in 1 tablespoon (15 ml) of oil. Adding one serving of higher-fat plant food will bring your fat intake to about 15 percent of calories. One and one-half servings will get you to about 20 percent, two servings to about 25 percent, and two and one-half to three servings to 30 percent. One serving, or approximately 14 grams of fat, can be found in the following foods:

- ¼ cup (60 ml) nuts or seeds
- 2 tablespoons (30 ml) nut or seed butter
- ½ medium avocado
- 1 ounce (30 g) shredded coconut
- 20 large olives
- 1 cup (250 ml) medium-firm tofu

For most people who are trying to lose weight, adding one to two servings (but not more than that) is a reasonable target, depending on energy requirements and weight-loss goals. It's best to avoid or minimize the use of oil and other concentrated fats. That's because these foods provide about 120 calories per tablespoon (15 ml), yet they have a very low nutrient density (few nutrients per calorie). When fighting diabetes, especially if you are overweight, you want every calorie that crosses your lips to be bursting with protective components. Table 6.3 (below) provides a nutritional comparison between sunflower seeds and sunflower seed oil. You will see at a quick glance why eating whole foods makes good sense!

There are two additional considerations that must be factored in to ensure the highest-quality fat for health and healing:

1. Harmful fats must be minimized. These include saturated fats, trans-fatty acids, and damaged fats (such as rancid or oxidized fats).

2. Sufficient essential fatty acids must be present.

TABLE 6.3. Nutrients in Sunflower Oil versus Sunflower Seeds

NUTRIENTS	NUTRIENT CONTENT OF SUNFLOWER OIL 1 Tbsp/15 ml	NUTRIENT CONTENT OF SHELLED SUNFLOWER SEEDS 2.5 Tbsp/0.7 oz (37 ml/21 g)
Calories	120	120
Fat (g)	13.6	10
Protein (g)	0	4
Fiber (g)	0	2.3
Thiamin (mg)	0	0.2
Riboflavin (mg)	0	0.05
Niacin (mg)	0	1.7
Folate (mcg)	0	49
Vitamin E (mg)	5.6	5.4
Calcium (mg)	0	14
Iron (mg)	0	0.8
Magnesium (mg)	0	27
Potassium (mg)	0	176
Zinc (mg)	0	1.1

Oils are refined foods. When they are extracted from whole foods, the fiber and protein get left behind, as do almost all of the vitamins and minerals (with the exception of vitamins E and K) and many of the phytochemicals. While oils are not poison, getting fat from whole foods naturally increases the nutrient density of the diet while reducing the caloric density. Unsaturated vegetable oils are more healthful than solid fats high in saturated fats or trans-fatty acids.

Like sugars, if oils are used, they should be incorporated only as a flavoring and in the smallest amounts possible. Oils actually have more nutritional value than sugar because they can be significant sources of vitamin E (and in some cases vitamin K), and if they are well chosen (as with flaxseed or hemp seed oil), they can also be rich sources of omega-3 fatty acids. In addition, oils enhance the absorption of many protective fat-soluble nutrients, antioxidants, and phytochemicals. By contrast, most refined sugars have no nutritional attributes to speak of. Many people eating very low-fat diets use sugar as the primary condiment, which may not be the best choice, especially for people with diabetes. A sugar-based, fat-free dressing is not as nutritious as a dressing that includes higher-fat whole foods, such as hemp seeds, avocado, walnuts, or tahini. The bottom line is this: to reduce disease risk or to treat current disease, avoid the use of concentrated fats and oils and instead rely on whole foods for your fat.

Putting a Lid on Harmful Fats

There are some types of fat that are associated with protection against disease and others that tend to increase risk. All whole foods contain saturated, monounsaturated, and polyunsaturated fats in varying amounts. Some foods also contain trans-fatty acids that are artificially created by the partial hydrogenation of oils or are naturally present in meat and dairy products. Of all fats, trans-fatty acids and saturated fat are the most strongly associated with cardiometabolic disease risk (see pages 48–49).

There is no level of intake of trans-fatty acids that is safe. Because the evidence against trans-fatty acids is so strong, the US Food and Drug Administration banned manufactured trans-fatty acids from the food supply in 2018. Although this dramatically reduces trans-fatty acids in foods, small amounts are still present in meat, poultry, and dairy products and in some processed foods. People who eat a 100 percent plant-based diet and who don't consume any processed foods with trans-fatty acids effectively eliminate trans-fatty acids from their diets.

How have manufacturers responded to the ban on trans fats? In most cases they have simply substituted other hard fats that have a long shelf life, such as coconut oil, palm oil, lard, or fully hydrogenated oils (while partial hydrogenation produces trans fats, full hydrogenation produces saturated fats). The American College of Cardiology and the American Heart Association recommend limiting saturated fat to not more than 5–6 percent of total calories for people at risk for heart disease, which includes anyone with diabetes.[11] This means 9–11 grams per day for a 1,600-calorie diet, 10–12 grams for an 1,800-calorie diet, and 11–13 grams for a 2,000-calorie diet.

Table 6.4 (opposite page) lists amounts of saturated fat in common animal and plant foods. As you can see, saturated fat adds up quickly if you are consuming animal products, especially those that are high in fat. Just one fast-food entrée or 1.5 ounces (45 grams) of cheese will put you over the top. Fortunately, most plant foods are low in saturated fat, even those that are high-fat foods, such as nuts and seeds. The exceptions are coconut, coconut milk, and tropical oils, which, as you will see, can also put you over the limit for saturated fat quite quickly.

The other type of fat that should be avoided is damaged fat—rancid fats and fats that are oxidized or otherwise damaged by heat. Clinical studies have demonstrated a link between oxidized fats, insulin resistance, fatty liver, and type 2 diabetes.[13,14] The following tips will help you to minimize your exposure to these harmful compounds.

- Avoid fried foods.
- Minimize or avoid oils in cooking.
- If you use oils, do not allow them to smoke. Keep cooking temperatures as low as possible.
- Do not burn high-fat foods or allow them to blacken.
- Store high-fat foods (including shelled nuts and seeds) in the refrigerator or freezer.
- Minimize processed foods, as many are subjected to very high heat.
- Use moist cooking methods; stew, steam, or sauté in water or broth.

Balancing Essential Fatty Acids

Essential fatty acids are essential because the body can't make them; they must come from your food. There are two essential fatty acids—omega-6 (linoleic, or LA) and omega-3 (alpha-linolenic, or ALA)—and both are polyunsaturated fats. Linoleic acid (omega-6) is pervasive in the food supply. It is the predominant fat in corn, grapeseed, sunflower, safflower, and soybean oils. It's also plentiful in seeds, such as poppy, pumpkin, sesame, and sunflower; in pine nuts and walnuts (other nuts contain mainly

TABLE 6.4. Saturated Fat in Common Foods

FOOD	PORTION SIZE	SATURATED FAT (G)
ANIMAL PRODUCTS		
Meat lover's pizza	3 slices	16
T-bone steak	8 oz (240 g)	15
Fast-food cheeseburger	1	14
Ice cream, premium	½ cup (125 ml)	11
Italian sausage	3.5 oz (100 g)	10
Pork chop, braised	1 chop (7 oz/210 g)	9
Butter	1 Tbsp (15 ml)	7
Cheddar cheese	1 oz (30 g)	6
Wiener, beef	1 (45 g)	6
Whole milk	1 cup (250 ml)	5
Salmon	3.5 oz (100 g)	4
Chicken thigh	4.4 oz (133 g)	3
PLANT FOODS		
Coconut oil	1 Tbsp (15 ml)	11
Coconut milk, canned	¼ cup (60 ml)	11
Coconut meat, raw	1 oz (30 g)	9
Palm oil	1 Tbsp (15 ml)	7
Dark chocolate	1 oz (30 g)	7
Olive oil	1 Tbsp (15 ml)	2
Avocado	½ medium	2
Nuts and seeds	1 oz (30 g)	1–2
Olives, large	10	1
Tofu	3 oz (90 g)	0.5
Soy milk	1 cup (250 ml)	0.5
Almond or cashew milk	1 cup (250 ml)	0

Source: [12]

monounsaturated fat); and in smaller amounts in grains. Alpha-linolenic acid (omega-3) is less well distributed in nature, although it's plentiful in flaxseeds, chia seeds, hemp seeds, and walnuts. Smaller amounts are found in green leafy vegetables. All plant foods contain a balance of saturated, monounsaturated, and polyunsaturated fats (both omega-6 and omega-3).

Generally, you don't have to worry much about getting enough omega-6 fatty acids, even with low-fat diets. However, getting enough omega-3, or ALA, can be more of a challenge. You need 2–4 grams of ALA a day on a plant-based diet. One day's supply of ALA can be obtained from 1.5 tablespoons (22 ml) of ground flaxseeds or chia seeds, 1 ounce (30 g) of walnuts, or 2–3 tablespoons (30–45 ml) of hemp seeds. Surprisingly, you can also get a day's requirement from about 25 cups (6.25 L) of leafy greens. On average, about half of the fat in greens is omega-3, but greens are so low in fat that you would need to eat a lot of them to get enough. See table 6.5 (at left) for the essential fatty acid content of selected foods.

People with diabetes have a diminished ability to convert the plant omega-3 fatty acids into the more biologically active long-chain omega-3s, EPA and DHA.[15] For this reason, fish (which contains EPA and DHA) is often touted as a superfood for people with diabetes. While fish is more healthful than meat, it's one of the most concentrated sources of environmental contaminants. A safer source of EPA and DHA is microalgae—tiny plants in the sea that manufacture EPA and DHA. In fact, microalgae are the source of the EPA and DHA in fish! Microalgae are commonly cultured for their omega-3 content, and the EPA and DHA are extracted and sold in supplement form. If you take 300–500 milligrams daily, or even just two or three times a week, you would get about the same amount of EPA and DHA as you would if you ate fish—without the concerns about contaminants.

TABLE 6.5. The EFA Content of Selected Omega-3-Rich Plant Foods

FOOD	SERVING SIZE	OMEGA-6 (grams per serving)	OMEGA-3 (grams per serving)
Chia seeds	2 Tbsp/30 ml (20 g)	1.2	3.6
Flaxseeds, ground	2 Tbsp/30 ml (14 g)	0.8	3.2
Walnuts, English	¼ cup/60 ml (30 g)	10.8	2.6
Hemp seeds	2 Tbsp/30 ml (20 g)	5.5	2.0
Tofu, firm	½ cup/125 ml (126 g)	5.5	0.7
Kale, raw	1 c/250 ml (50-60 g)	0.06	0.08

Source: [12]

Chapter 7

Other Dietary Heavyweights

Diane spotted the magazine through the corner of her eye while picking up a bottle of water at the airport. It was an entire issue dedicated to the Blue Zones. She was instantly intrigued, as the Blue Zones were referred to in her plant-based diabetes program. The Blue Zones are places where there are more centenarians than anywhere else on the planet. She made the purchase and spent the entire three-hour flight poring over the magazine's contents.

Diane was fascinated by the stories of elders from Okinawa, Japan; Sardinia, Italy; Ikaria, Greece; Loma Linda, California; and the Nicoya Peninsula of Costa Rica. These individuals don't just live to be one hundred years old but are also remarkably vital and sharp at advanced ages; they garden, walk up mountains, and play chess. Diane could not help thinking about the contrast between these people and those she knew of a similar vintage.

But what really impressed her was the simplicity of the lifestyle factors that are thought to be responsible for their health and longevity. People of the Blue Zones put family first, are strongly socially engaged, and have a deep sense of purpose. They are moderately physically active throughout the day and tend not to smoke. Where food is concerned, every Blue Zone population consumes a largely unprocessed, plant-based diet featuring legumes as a staple. It all made so much sense. She was essentially practicing the lessons taught for decades by the people of the Blue Zones. Plant-based diets are loaded with protective dietary components, such as phytochemicals and antioxidants. They are low in dietary components that are associated with increased risk of disease, including environmental contaminants and harmful chemicals formed from high-temperature cooking, such as deep-frying.

Diane wished she could share her newly acquired knowledge with the entire world. She began by launching a plant-based support group in her community, along with a lively website. She shared her excitement, her newfound knowledge, and her delicious culinary adventures. Diane decided that if she could not live in one of the five known Blue Zones, she would do her best to create a little Blue Zone in her small corner of the world.

PROTECTION FROM PLANTS: PHYTOCHEMICALS AND ANTIOXIDANTS

To enhance their own survival, all plants produce compounds called phytochemicals (from the Latin word *phyto*, meaning "plant"). Some phytochemicals are responsible for a plant's color, flavor, texture, and fragrance, and they play a critical role in attracting pollinators and seed dispersers. Other phytochemicals act as an internal defense system that protects plants from pests, pathogens, and potentially hostile environments. Because of the particular requirements individual plants have, there may be as many as one hundred thousand different kinds of phytochemicals. Often, thousands of copies of each different phytochemical can be found in a single plant.[1]

Fortunately, when you eat plants, the phytochemicals they contain continue to work their magic in your body. Whether serving as antioxidants (see page 43), mimicking hormones, reducing inflammation, blocking tumor formation, eradicating carcinogens, stimulating enzymes, or destroying bacteria, phytochemicals have hundreds of mechanisms that help to prevent the onset of diseases and fight existing diseases. Although some phytochemicals are antioxidants, not all antioxidants are phytochemicals. Some vitamins, such as vitamins C and E, and the mineral selenium also act as antioxidants.

Many factors can affect the quantity of phytochemicals in food as well as their bioavailability. For example, agricultural factors, such as soil, water, climate, and the use of chemicals, influence phytochemical content. Organically grown produce must develop a more robust defense against assailants than plants protected by chemical pesticides, so its phytochemical content is correspondingly higher.[2,3,4] Conversely, storage methods after harvest can diminish phytochemical concentrations.

Food-refining methods can dramatically reduce phytochemical content, especially when the most phytochemical-rich parts of plants are removed (such as the germ and bran from wheat grains) or when the processing involves exposure to harsh chemicals, heat, or pressure. Food preparation methods, such as cooking, sprouting, fermenting, blending, juicing, and processing, can also significantly affect phytochemical content and bioavailability, in either direction.

Most phytochemicals are more efficiently absorbed from raw foods. For example, the absorption of isothiocyanates can be significantly higher from raw cruciferous vegetables than cooked cruciferous vegetables.[5,6,7,8] In general, cooking foods tends to decrease phytochemical content; the greater the intensity and duration of heat exposure, the more significant the phytochemical losses. Not surprisingly, water-soluble phytochemicals are more readily lost when food is boiled. On the other hand, cooking softens or ruptures plant cell walls, making it easier for the body to extract and absorb certain types of phytochemicals, particularly carotenoids.[9,10] For example, more lycopene is bioavailable from cooked tomatoes than from raw tomatoes, and more beta-carotene is bioavailable from cooked carrots than from raw carrots.[11,12,13,14]

Adding even a small amount of fat from high-fat whole foods, such as avocado, improves carotenoid absorption from foods, whether the foods are raw or cooked.[15,16,17,18,19]

The bioavailability of phytochemicals from raw foods can be maximized by reducing the particle size and increasing the surface area of the food by chopping, puréeing, processing, milling, mashing, grating, or chewing well.[20,17,21] Juicing is even more effective because the process removes the plant's cell walls, which contain fiber and other components known to reduce the bioavailability of nutrients and phytochemicals. For this reason, some carotenoids, such as alpha-carotene, beta-carotene, and lutein, appear to be more bioavailable from vegetable juice than from raw or cooked vegetables.[22,23]

Sprouting and fermenting significantly enhance a plant food's phytochemical content.[24,25,26,27] Scientific studies have shown that for a variety of food plants, germinating yields remarkable increases in phytochemicals.[27,28,29,30,26,7,31] This rise in phytochemical content is predictable because the life of a new plant depends on the support and protection from these compounds. One notable example is broccoli sprouts, which were found to contain ten to one hundred times more glucoraphanin (a glucosinolate and the precursor of sulforaphane) than mature broccoli.[26,7] Sulforaphane is a potent natural inducer of the body's detoxifying phase II enzymes, which process and eliminate carcinogens. Sulforaphane has also been shown to be an impressive antimicrobial agent; it's highly effective against *Helicobacter pylori* (*H. pylori*), an infectious bacteria associated with gastritis, peptic ulcers, and stomach cancer.[32,33] Recent evidence has also shown that broccoli sprouts may improve insulin resistance in patients with type 2 diabetes.[34] Finally, sulforaphane appears to reduce oxidative stress and tissue damage associated with a variety of disease states.[35]

Maximizing Phytochemicals and Antioxidants in the Diet

While vegetables and fruits are commonly regarded as the primary suppliers of phytochemicals and antioxidants, these compounds are also plentiful in all whole plant foods. The most effective way to maximize phytochemical and antioxidant intake is to fill your plate with a wide variety of colorful plant foods that cover the entire spectrum of the rainbow. For example, red or black rice, quinoa, or beans will typically have more phytochemicals than brown or white rice.

In addition to eating more organic, raw plant foods and breaking them down during food preparation, regularly include sprouted and fermented foods in your diet to boost phytochemical intake. When you do cook, keep cooking times short and temperatures low.

Drinking vegetable juices can be a practical way to boost antioxidant and phytochemical intake. Enjoy the juice on an empty stomach prior to eating breakfast. Stick to juices that are freshly pressed, and to keep calories down, don't include fruits and use only small amounts of carrots or beets. A great combination is dark leafy greens, celery, cucumber, ginger, turmeric root, and lemon or lime.

As a general rule, rely on foods, *not* supplements, for phytochemicals. When phytochemicals are isolated and concentrated, their effects can be vastly different than when they are consumed in whole foods. In some cases, supplements can be harmful. One possible explanation for this is that phytochemicals in foods have synergistic effects that do not occur when the phytochemical is consumed in isolation.

Among the most celebrated phytochemical and antioxidant superstars are dark-green leafy vegetables, cruciferous vegetables, sprouts, purple and blue fruits, herbs and spices, deeply colored legumes, nuts and seeds, garlic, cocoa beans, citrus fruits, tea, and tomatoes. Remember, the absorption of fat-soluble nutrients is enhanced when a source of fats is consumed, although only small amounts are needed. Higher-fat foods, such as nuts and seeds, are the richest sources of the important antioxidant vitamin E. Table 7.1 (below) highlights the phytochemical and antioxidant superstars for fighting diabetes, along with their sources and mechanisms of action. Incorporate a variety of these foods into your daily diet!

TABLE 7.1. Phytochemical and Antioxidant Superstars for Fighting Diabetes

PHYTOCHEMICAL/ ANTIOXIDANT	FOOD SOURCES	MECHANISM OF ACTION
Allicin	Garlic Onions Leeks	May improve blood glucose. May improve cardiovascular risk factors.
Anthocyanins	Berries (açai, raspberries, blueberries, black currants, blackberries) Cherries Eggplant Red and purple cabbage Black plums Purple sweet potatoes Pecans	Antioxidant. Anti-inflammatory. Reduce insulin resistance.

PHYTOCHEMICAL/ ANTIOXIDANT	FOOD SOURCES		MECHANISM OF ACTION
Bioflavonoids (e.g., hesperidin and naringin)	Citrus fruits Peppermint	Peppers Broccoli	Anti-inflammatory. May prevent the progression of hyperglycemia.
Capsaicin	Hot chiles Sweet peppers		Increases energy expenditure. Enhances insulin response. Reduces inflammation and lipid oxidation. Promotes weight loss.
Carotenoids	Orange, yellow, and red vegetables Dark-green vegetables		Antioxidant. Enhance insulin sensitivity. Some carotenoids are associated with reduced diabetes risk.
Catechins	Tea (green, matcha, black, white, and fruit) Fresh fruit (apples, apricots, cherries, peaches, berries) Cocoa Broad beans, fava beans Some nuts		Reduce insulin resistance. Increase glucose uptake. May improve diabetic wound healing.
Curcumin	Turmeric		Anti-inflammatory. Anti-obesity.
Gingerol	Ginger		May suppress formation of advanced glycation end products. Improves blood glucose levels and glucose tolerance.
Isoflavones	Soybeans		May improve beta cell function and insulin sensitivity.
Proantho-cyanidins	Almonds, hazelnuts, peanuts, pecans, pistachios (much higher in raw than roasted)		Anti-inflammatory. Antioxidant. May improve glucose uptake.
Quercetin	Apples Onions, scallions	Broccoli Tea	Anti-inflammatory. Antioxidant. May improve blood glucose levels and insulin production. May lower triglycerides and cholesterol.
Resveratrol	Grapes, grape juice Some berries	Peanuts, pistachios Red wine	Reduces fasting blood glucose. Reduces insulin resistance.
Sulforaphane	Broccoli sprouts Broccoli		Improves fasting glucose in people with poorly controlled type 2 diabetes.

Source: 36,37,38,39,40,41,42,43,44,45,46,47,48

CHEMICAL CONTAMINANTS: HIDDEN HARMS IN FOOD

hemical contaminants, both those that get into food through the environment and products of high-temperature cooking, can wreak havoc in your body. They can promote oxidative stress, fuel inflammation, promote fat accumulation (by disrupting hormones), and damage vital organs, DNA, and the central nervous system. All of these effects increase the risk of type 2 diabetes and its complications.[49] Reducing exposure to these compounds is an important step toward correctly abnormalities of metabolism. (See pages 49–50 in chapter 3.)

Environmental contaminants can be effectively minimized by making three significant dietary changes:

1. **Dramatically reduce or eliminate animal products.** Heavy metals and persistent organic pollutants (POPs) are concentrated in animal foods as they move up the food chain. One notable exception is arsenic, which is concentrated in chicken, rice products (organic or conventional; whole or refined), and hijiki seaweed. Although it is not necessary to eliminate rice, reducing your intake and varying your grains makes good sense. Hijiki seaweed is particularly high in arsenic and is best avoided or greatly minimized.[50,51,52,53]

2. **Buy organic.** Pesticides are most concentrated in conventional produce. While organic produce is not entirely free of pesticides, levels are significantly lower than they are in conventional produce.[54,55,56] An excellent resource put out every year by the Environmental Working Group ranks produce based on pesticide data from the US Department of Agriculture (USDA). The twelve products with the greatest level of contamination are known as the "Dirty Dozen," and the fifteen least contaminated foods are crowned the "Clean 15." If you can't afford to buy everything organic, select organic for products that fall within the "Dirty Dozen" and conventional for those that fall within the "Clean 15." Generally, foods that are eaten with the skin (such as apples, peaches, pears, and berries) pose a greater risk than those eaten with the peel removed (such as pineapple, bananas, kiwi, and melons). Washing does not completely remove pesticides, though washing for at least thirty seconds does reduce pesticide content somewhat. A well-diluted solution of salt or baking soda appears to be even more effective than plain water.[57] Produce from local farmers' markets may have lower levels than conventional supermarket produce, even when it's not organic. If you can, grow some of your own food. If you don't have a yard, consider using containers on a porch or deck.

3. **Minimize the use of foods packaged in plastic or in cans lined with BPA.** When purchasing food, opt for glass or paper instead of plastic. Use glass for storage and reheating as well. Look for cans with BPA-free liners. Avoid imported

canned foods (due to potential lead seams) and foods stored in lead-glazed or leaded glassware.

PATHOGENIC PRODUCTS OF HIGH-TEMPERATURE COOKING

Products of high-temperature cooking include heterocyclic amines, polycyclic aromatic hydrocarbons, advanced glycation end products, and acrylamide (see pages 50–51). These compounds increase oxidative stress and inflammation and can increase the risk of diabetes and its complications.[58,59] There are ways of minimizing exposure to each of these chemicals:

- **Use mostly fresh, whole plant foods.** These foods will have the lowest levels of the chemicals formed from high-temperature cooking.
- **Avoid meat, especially processed meats.** Heterocyclic amines can only be formed in meat, poultry, and fish; plants lack the compounds necessary for its formation.[60,61] Meat is often fried or grilled, also producing polycyclic aromatic hydrocarbons and aldehydes.[62,63] Processed meats and fried meat are also the most concentrated sources of advanced glycation end products.[64,65]
- **Minimize ultraprocessed foods.** Some foods, such as chips and other salty snacks or puffed cereals, are processed at very high temperatures and for significant periods of time. Even foods that are slightly processed, such as whole-grain crackers, cereals, and tea and coffee, can be significant sources of acrylamide, advanced glycation end products, or polycyclic aromatic hydrocarbons.[64,66,67]
- **Eat more raw foods.** When your diet is high in raw foods, you automatically put a lid on the products of oxidation formed from cooking.
- **Avoid fried foods.** Frying is a potent producer of all products of oxidation.[68] If you do use oil in cooking, do not allow the oil to smoke.
- **Be cautious with air-frying.** Using an air-fryer is a fun way to create crispy foods without the oil. However, high temperatures are employed, so products of oxidation, such as acrylamide and advanced glycation end products, will form.[69] If you make air-fried food, reserve it as an occasional treat.
- **Use wet cooking methods.** Primarily steam, stew, boil, or sauté in a little water.
- **Be savvy with dry heat.** Use lower temperatures, limit the cooking time, and don't blacken or overcook foods.
- **Store foods properly.** To retain freshness and minimize products of oxidation, keep perishables in the refrigerator and dry foods in cool, dark places. Use foods before the "sell by" or "use by" date. Nuts and seeds are protected by hard shells in nature. When the shells are removed, their oils are susceptible to oxidation from light, heat, and oxygen, especially nuts and seeds that are rich in omega-3

fatty acids.[70] Nuts and seeds are protected when stored in the freezer or refrigerator. Using mason jars for storage allows for easy access. Frozen nuts do not require thawing before use.

SLASHING SALT

Restricting sodium can reduce blood pressure and lower the risk of cardiovascular disease in people with type 2 diabetes (see page 52). One teaspoon (5 ml) of salt has about 2,300 milligrams of sodium, which is considered a safe upper limit for healthy adults. However, for people with diabetes, it is recommended that sodium be slashed to 1,500 milligrams, or about two-thirds of a teaspoon (3 ml) per day.[71] A study looking at sodium intakes of Americans with type 2 diabetes reported average intakes of over 3,200 milligrams, with just over 20 percent of participants consuming less than 2,300 milligrams, and only 2.4 percent meeting the recommended limit of 1,500 milligrams per day.[71]

Salt added to foods prepared outside the home accounts for an estimated 70 percent of sodium in the American diet.[72] This salt comes predominantly from processed foods and restaurant meals. Sodium that occurs naturally in foods accounts for close to 15 percent, followed by salt added in home food preparation and use at the table (at about 5 percent each).

The amount of salt in processed foods and restaurant meals may surprise you (see table 7.2, below). Ounce for ounce, cornflakes have more salt than potato chips. Two slices of pepperoni pizza contain over 1,500 milligrams of sodium, and a fast-food cheeseburger and fries have over 1,100 milligrams. A medium-sized dill pickle packs over 800 milligrams of sodium. The suggestions provided in Sodium Smarts (page 120) will help you to keep your sodium intake within the recommended limit of 1,500 milligrams.

TABLE 7.2. Sodium Content of Common Foods

(Compare to the recommended day's maximum sodium intake of 1,500 milligrams.)

FOOD	SERVING SIZE	SODIUM CONTENT (MG)
Salt	1 tsp (5 ml)	2,300
Ramen noodles, with flavor packet	1 package (86 g)	1,611
Pepperoni pizza	2 slices	1,520
Cheeseburger and fries	1 burger/1 medium fries	1,127
Fast-food biscuit with egg/bacon	1	1,266

FOOD	SERVING SIZE	SODIUM CONTENT (MG)
Fried chicken, fast food	3.5 oz (100 g)	1,042
Canned beans	1 cup (250 ml)	750–950
Soup	1 cup (250 ml)	600–900
Ham	3 oz (90 g)	880
Macaroni and cheese, boxed	1 cup (250 ml)	869
Pickles, dill	1 medium	833
Miso	1 Tbsp (15 ml)	634
Tomato sauce	½ cup (125 ml)	450
Cottage cheese	½ cup (125 ml)	410
Veggie burger pattie	1	398
Pretzels	1 oz (30 g)	352
Canned corn, drained	1 cup (250 ml)	336
Soy sauce or tamari	1 tsp (5 ml)	300–350
Canned beans, low sodium	1 cup (250 ml)	250–350
Olives	10 large	320
Sauerkraut	¼ cup (60 ml)	320
Canned tuna	3 oz (90 g)	301
Italian dressing, reduced fat	2 Tbsp (30 ml)	268
Canned tomatoes	½ cup (125 ml)	225
Cornflakes	1 oz (30 g)	204
Cheese, Cheddar	1 oz (30 g)	185
Ketchup	1 Tbsp (15 ml)	178
Bread, whole wheat	1 slice	150
Potato chips	1 oz (30 g)	148
Soda crackers	5	140
Peanuts, dry-roasted, salted	1 oz (30 g)	116

Source: [73]

Sodium Smarts

- Use unprocessed, whole plant foods as the foundation of your diet—whether you purchase them or grow them in your garden.
- Prepare foods at home from scratch.
- Eat out less often. If you have a restaurant meal, ask the chef to go lightly on the salt.
- If you use processed foods, read the label, and choose products that are low in sodium. Look for products labeled "low-salt" or "reduced-sodium."
- Look for salt-free herb blends for cooking, and select seasonings that don't list sodium in the ingredients.
- Use smaller amounts of sodium than recipes call for.
- Use fresh or frozen vegetables and beans instead of canned whenever possible.
- If you use jarred or canned foods, rinse the food well to remove some of the sodium.
- Limit your use of pickled and fermented vegetable products—they're soaked in salt!
- Go lightly on added salt while cooking and at the table.
- When cooking, add salt near the end—you can use less because the taste will be more pronounced.
- Squeeze lemon or lime juice on foods instead of salt.
- Avoid eating salty snacks. If you really want a crunchy snack, make your own popcorn and flavor it with nutritional yeast and herbs.
- Reduce your portion sizes; eating less food means you'll consume less salt.

NUTRITION KNOW-HOW

Many people with diabetes need more of certain vitamins and minerals to enhance insulin sensitivity and promote healing. Vitamins that deserve special attention for people with diabetes are vitamins B_{12} and D and the antioxidant vitamins, which include vitamin A (as carotenoids) and vitamins C and E. Minerals that are most often in short supply are chromium, magnesium, and potassium. Eating plant-based foods will help you get many of these nutrients, but to be sure you get enough, here are simple steps you can take:

Vitamin B_{12}

Having insufficient vitamin B_{12} can negatively affect fasting blood glucose, oxidative stress, and inflammation in individuals with diabetes.[74] A lack of vitamin B_{12} can present as peripheral neuropathy or dementia, so it is important for people with diabetes to check their vitamin B_{12} status.[75] People who are taking metformin are at increased risk because metformin reduces vitamin B_{12} absorption.[76] In addition, if you are over fifty years of age, animal products are not considered reliable sources of vitamin B_{12}.[77] This is because as you age, your ability to cleave the B_{12} off the protein it is bound to in animal foods is diminished. Whole plant foods are *not* reliable sources of vitamin B_{12}. The most reliable sources of vitamin B_{12} are supplements or foods fortified with vitamin B_{12}.

To ensure you're getting adequate amounts, have your physician monitor your status and adjust your supplements accordingly. Most people will be able to maintain adequate vitamin B_{12} levels by taking a supplement of 1,000 mcg daily or two to three times a week. The foods most commonly fortified with vitamin B_{12} are nondairy milks, meat analogs, cereals, and nutritional yeast. For detailed B_{12} guidelines, see page 128.

Vitamin D

A growing number of Americans get less vitamin D than they need—over 40 percent of adults overall, over 80 percent of black adults, and almost 70 percent of Hispanic adults.[78] There's mounting evidence that the lack of vitamin D can increase the risk for developing diabetes and its progression.[79,80] While it's possible to produce enough vitamin D with adequate exposure to warm sunshine, people who live more than 30 degrees north or south of the equator will need another source during the cooler months of the year. Also, cloud cover, sunscreen, dark skin, clothing, aging, and excess body fat all negatively influence vitamin D production.

Vitamin D fortification of foods is not generally sufficient to meet recommended intakes. Many people will need a supplement to optimize their vitamin D status, and the amount required will depend on that status. The RDA is 15 micrograms (600 IU) for everyone one to seventy years of age and 20 micrograms (800 IU) for people over seventy. However, higher amounts in the range of 25–100 micrograms (1,000–4,000 IU) may be necessary to achieve recommended blood levels.[81,82,83]

Antioxidant Vitamins

Impaired antioxidant status is a common feature of type 2 diabetes and has been shown to play a role in the development of insulin resistance.[84,85] Adults with a history of prediabetes, diabetes, and obesity have increased vitamin C requirements.[86] Vitamin C is found almost exclusively in vegetables and fruits, so shifting to a plant-based diet boosts intake and status. The richest food sources include sweet peppers, citrus fruits, kiwis, tomatoes, papayas, broccoli, Brussels sprouts, strawberries, passion fruit, guavas, mangoes, and cauliflower. High serum carotenoid concentrations are associated with a reduced risk of insulin resistance and diabetes. Carotenoids are found in orange, yellow, red, and green vegetables and fruits, with the richest sources being sweet potatoes, carrots, squash, pumpkins, dark leafy greens, and peppers. Vitamin E is most concentrated in higher-fat plant foods, so people who eat very low-fat diets can fall short. The most plentiful sources are sunflower seeds, almonds, peanuts, pine nuts, Brazil nuts, wheat germ, and avocados. Smaller amounts are present in a variety of vegetables and fruits, such as dark greens, broccoli, kiwis, red peppers, and butternut squash.[87]

Chromium

Chromium enhances the action of insulin and plays an important role in the metabolism of carbohydrates, fat, and protein. Although recommended dietary allowances have not been established for chromium, adequate intakes (AIs) have been set at 35 micrograms a day for men up to age fifty and 30 micrograms thereafter, and 25 micrograms for women up to age fifty and 20 micrograms thereafter. Broccoli is a chromium superstar with about 22 micrograms per cup (250 ml). Other rich plant sources of this nutrient include Brazil nuts, green beans, lentils, oats, pears, potatoes, prunes, strawberries, tofu, tomatoes, and whole grains (especially barley and oats).

Research regarding the benefits of chromium supplementation in people with diabetes is conflicting and inconclusive, so it is not routinely recommended. Many medications interact with chromium, so be sure to check with your physician before supplementing. There is no controversy, however, about ensuring adequate dietary chromium intakes, so go ahead and binge on broccoli![88,89,90]

Magnesium

Magnesium helps to control blood sugar by regulating insulin secretion from the pancreas. Reduced dietary intakes serve as a risk factor for impaired glucose tolerance and type 2 diabetes.[91] People with diabetes are more likely to be low in magnesium because high blood glucose causes magnesium to be excreted in the urine.[92] The recommended dietary allowance (RDA) for magnesium is 420 milligrams per day for men age thirty-one or older and 320 milligrams per day for women age thirty-one or older.[93] The best magnesium sources are cooked spinach, green soybeans, lima beans, pumpkin seeds, teff, and tofu. Other good sources include almonds, black turtle beans, black-eyed peas, breadfruit, dark chocolate, dried apricots, hazelnuts, peanuts, plantains, tomato sauce, and winter squash.

Potassium

Normal body function depends on the tight regulation of potassium, both inside and outside of cells. Potassium is an important electrolyte, but it also has many other critical roles in the body, including stimulating insulin production. While there is no RDA for potassium, the AI is set at 2,600 milligrams for adults.[94]

Potassium is a nutrient that many people fall short on, but people who eat plant-based diets have higher intakes than other dietary groups.[95] If you're on blood pressure medication, your potassium levels may fall, so you may be asked to increase your intake of potassium-rich foods. However, if you have kidney disease due to your diabetes, your potassium levels can escalate to dangerous levels, so you may be asked to reduce your intake of potassium-rich foods. Generally, though, most people should maximize potassium intake, as high intakes are associated with reduced risk of hypertension, stroke, and kidney stones.[96] The richest food sources of potassium are fruits and vegetables. Bananas are often touted as the best source, but many foods outrank them, including acorn squash, bamboo shoots, black turtle beans, black-eyed peas, Chinese cabbage, green soybeans, kiwis, lima beans, potatoes, sweet potatoes, taro, and tomato sauce.

WATER WORKS

People with diabetes are at a higher risk for dehydration because high blood sugar levels deplete fluids. In an effort to get rid of excess glucose, the kidneys pass it out in the urine, which requires fluids. The higher your blood sugar, the more you need to drink to aid the body in ridding itself of the excess glucose and to ensure adequate hydration. Other factors that can increase your risk of dehydration are excessive sweating, illness with vomiting or diarrhea, and alcohol consumption. Common symptoms of dehydration include extreme thirst, headache, dry mouth and eyes, dizziness, fatigue, and dark-colored urine. In severe cases, blood pressure can dip, heart rate can speed up, and confusion can set in. Dehydration can cause your skin to become dry and itchy and crack, increasing the risk of infection. In all, for people with diabetes, dehydration can be dangerous.

Water is the ideal hydrator, as it won't raise your blood sugar, and it has zero calories. A good target is six to eight glasses a day for women and eight to ten glasses a day for men. The best way to reach these numbers is to begin your day with a large glass of water (add lemon if you like). Then, be sure to drink water between meals—aim for about 2 cups (500 ml) between each meal. Keep a water bottle handy.

If plain water doesn't do it for you, try adding a few slices of citrus fruit or cucumber, a sprig of fresh mint or lemon balm, or a few frozen berries to either still or carbonated water. Other healthful options are teas (especially green teas, but also herbal, black, or white tea); vegetable juices made with celery, cucumber, leafy greens, ginger, and lemon or lime; and unsweetened nut or soy milk. If you're a coffee drinker, monitor your blood sugar levels after you drink coffee; if you have a particularly negative reaction, switch to decaf or tea. If you do drink coffee, stick to black. Absolutely avoid all beverages with added sugars.

Studies of Western populations commonly report that moderate alcohol consumption reduces diabetes and cardiovascular risk, while heavy drinking increases risk.[97,98] However, studies of Asian populations report an increased diabetes risk with alcohol intake.[99,100] There are many reasons to minimize your intake if you do indulge. Excessive alcohol can raise blood pressure and triglycerides, damage the liver, weaken the heart muscle, and contribute to pancreatitis.[101] Alcohol increases the risk for cancer, particularly cancers of the upper digestive tract, liver, colon, rectum, and breast.[102] According to the World Cancer Research Fund International and the American Institute for Cancer Research, there is no safe level of intake.

If you take insulin or certain types of diabetes medications, alcohol can cause hypoglycemia, and this is particularly problematic if you drink on an empty stomach. The body views alcohol as a poison, and the liver gets right to work trying to eliminate it. Of course, when your liver is busy with that work, it may be less able to perform other tasks, such as releasing glucose into the bloodstream. Some evidence suggests that alcohol may stimulate the release of insulin, which can compound the problem.

Typical alcohol guidelines are no more than one drink a day for women and two for men. The difference is because men tend to be able to process alcohol more efficiently than women. However, less is better, and none is likely best. If you do indulge, keep intake as low as possible and avoid making alcohol part of your daily routine. Also, be very selective about the type of alcohol you drink. Lower-calorie and lower-carbohydrate choices are preferable. Dry wine, light beer, or distilled spirits are preferred over sweet wines, regular beers, liqueurs, and fancy mixed drinks. One 12-ounce (375-ml) bottle of stout or ale can clock in at nearly 200 calories!

Chapter 8

The Diet Blueprint

At first Diane was nervous about making the monumental diet changes recommended by her plant-based support program, especially while she was living among family and friends who ate so differently. Would her husband like the foods she prepared? What would she order at restaurants? How would she participate in family celebrations?

She started out slowly, replacing eggs with oats, cow's milk with cashew milk, and beef with beans. She soon discovered that many of her favorite recipes could be reinvented with whole-foods, plant-based ingredients. What really took her by surprise was how much her food preferences changed. What once tasted divine now tasted sickeningly sweet. Cravings for cookies gave way to greens.

Diane's progress in three months was staggering. She lost eighteen pounds (8 kg), her fasting blood sugar dropped to 104 mg/dl (5.8 mmol/l), and her doctor took her off all her diabetes medications. Within a year, Diane had shed forty-three pounds (20 kg); her fasting sugar was 87 mg/dl (4.8 mmol/l), and her BMI was 22. Although she might not be pegged as svelte by passersby, she felt svelte for the first time in her life, and for Diane, that was good enough.

The basic formula was simple: healthy, delicious, plant-based food and daily physical activity. Sure, there were other fine details, but Diane's success rested largely upon these two critical changes. The dietary protocol that follows provides the blueprint that led Diane to reclaim her health. It will do the same for you.

THE KICK DIABETES DIET PROTOCOL

When you suffer from diabetes, your body might be compared to a house on fire. Food can serve as gasoline or water. Processed foods and fatty animal products fuel the drivers of diabetes like gasoline fanning the flames. Whole plant foods suppress the drivers of diabetes like water dousing the flames. When your goal is reversal, you need to pull out all the stops. That is exactly what the following dietary protocol does.

The next steps toward kicking diabetes involve choosing the best foods within each food group and answering common, pressing questions. It can take three to four weeks to rewire your taste buds and for your gut bacteria to adjust to the increased amount of fiber in a whole-foods, plant-based diet. Be prepared for sensory adjustments that take a little time. Once your taste buds become accustomed to the new normal, foods that are fatty, sugary, and salty will lose their luster, and you'll love the amazing flavors, textures, and aromas of fresh, whole foods.

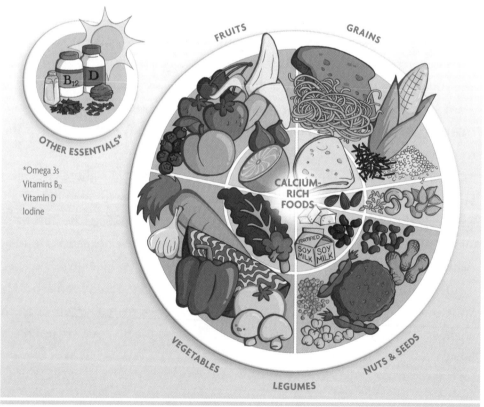

FIGURE 8.1 The Kick Diabetes Plant-Based Plate.

TABLE 8.1. Kick Diabetes Food Groups: Optimal Servings and Serving Sizes

FOOD GROUP	OPTIMAL SERVINGS PER DAY	FOOD EXAMPLES AND SERVING SIZES	CALCIUM-RICH FOODS 5–8 SERVINGS PER DAY
Nonstarchy Vegetables	5 or more 7+ even better!	Raw or cooked vegetables, ½ cup (125 ml); raw leafy vegetables, 1 cup (250 ml); vegetable juice, ½ cup (125 ml)	Bok choy, broccoli, collard greens, kale, napa cabbage, okra, 1 cup (250 ml) cooked, or 2 cups (500 ml) raw
Fruits	3 or more	Whole fruit, medium-sized; fruit, raw or cooked, ½ cup (125 ml); dried fruit, ¼ cup (60 ml)	Oranges, 2; dried figs, ½ cup (125 ml)
Legumes	3 or more	Cooked beans, peas, or lentils, bean pasta, or tofu or tempeh, ½ cup (125 ml); raw peas or sprouted lentils, mung beans, or peas, 1 cup (250 ml); vegetarian meat substitute, 1 oz (30 g); fortified soy milk, 1 cup (250 ml)	Black or white beans, 1 cup (250 ml); calcium-set tofu, ½ cup (125 ml); fortified soy milk or soy yogurt, ½ cup (125 ml)
Whole Grains and Starchy Vegetables	2 or more	Cooked whole grains or starchy vegetables, ½ cup (125 ml); 1 oz (30 g) very dense whole-grain bread (see page 142)	—
Nuts and Seeds	2–3	2 Tbsp (30 ml) nuts or seeds; 1 Tbsp (15 ml) nut or seed butter	Almonds or chia or sesame seeds, ¼ cup (60 ml); almond butter or tahini, 2 Tbsp (30 ml)
Herbs and Spices	3 or more	¼–½ tsp (1–2 ml) ground spice; 1 tsp (5 ml) dried herbs; 1 Tbsp (15 ml) fresh herbs	—

Design Your Own Kick Diabetes Plant-Based Plate

Food guides are meant to help you design a diet that ensures all your nutrient needs are met on a daily basis. The Kick Diabetes Plant-Based Plate is intended specifically for adults with type 2 diabetes. It's rich in protective nutrients, minimizes harmful components, and meets the recommended nutrient intakes. What follows is an overview of the foods in each group and two menus that are adjusted for different activity levels.

When you follow this guide, you don't need to meet the minimum recommended servings from every food group every day. Instead, reach those average intakes over time. You can arrange meals or snacks in various ways and still meet recommended intakes for all nutrients, so there's plenty of flexibility. Calcium-rich foods are highlighted in the central circle of the plate because calcium-rich foods are found within every group. The third column in table 8.1, above, lists the foods that qualify as good calcium sources, providing 100–150 milligrams of calcium per serving. Special guidelines are given for calcium and four other nutrients—vitamin B_{12}, vitamin D, iodine, and omega-3 fatty acids—in a section on page 128 called Essential Extras.

You'll see that certain foods that may have shown up regularly in your meals are missing from the Kick Diabetes Plant-Based Plate. This guide is built around whole plant foods while excluding the two categories most strongly linked to increased diabetes risk: highly processed foods and animal products.

ESSENTIAL EXTRAS

Vitamin B$_{12}$

People age sixty-five or older or adults of any age on metformin:

- Daily: Take a supplement providing 100–1,000 micrograms vitamin B$_{12}$. (Monitor your status; your physician will adjust your requirements accordingly.)

Adults under age sixty-five, choose *one* of the following:

- Daily: Take a supplement providing 25–100 micrograms vitamin B$_{12}$.
- Two or three times a week: Take a supplement providing 1,000 micrograms vitamin B$_{12}$.
- Daily: Consume at least three servings of foods fortified with vitamin B$_{12}$ that provide at least 2 micrograms vitamin B$_{12}$ per serving. The Daily Value (DV) for vitamin B$_{12}$ used on food labels is 6 micrograms, so if a food provides 33 percent of the DV, it provides 2 micrograms.

Omega-3 Fatty Acids

Include at least *one* of the following daily; each serving provides about 2.5 grams of omega-3s:

- 1½ tablespoons (22 ml) ground flaxseeds
- 1½ tablespoons (22 ml) chia seeds
- 3 tablespoons (45 ml) hemp seeds or walnuts

Along with the smaller amounts of omega-3s from other plant foods, this will meet the needs of both women and men. People with diabetes may also be well advised to take a supplement of 200–300 milligrams microalgae-based EPA/DHA at least two or three times a week.

Iodine

You can get your day's recommended intake of 150 micrograms of iodine from a multivitamin-mineral supplement or from about ⅓ teaspoon (2 ml) iodized salt. Salty seasonings, such as Bragg Liquid Aminos, soy sauce, tamari, and Celtic, Himalayan, or sea salt are not sources of iodine. Sea vegetables are rich in iodine. For example, kelp powder is loaded with about 150 mcg in 1/16 teaspoon (0.3 ml). Other types of seaweed provide less. The upper limit is 1,100 mcg, so don't overdo it!

Vitamin D

Get daily vitamin D from sunlight, fortified foods, a supplement, or a combination of all three.

- **Sunlight.** Expose the face and forearms to *warm* sunlight (from 10:00 a.m. to 2:00 p.m.) without sunscreen for at least fifteen minutes for light-skinned people, twenty minutes for dark-skinned people, or thirty minutes for people over the age of seventy.
- **Fortified foods or supplements.** The minimum recommended intake for vitamin D is 15 micrograms (600 IUs) up to age seventy and 20 micrograms (800 IUs) over age seventy. For people with diabetes, especially if they're overweight, a vitamin D supplement of 25–50 micrograms (1,000–2,000 IUs) per day is advised.

Calcium

The calcium-rich foods are those foods in other food groups that are particularly high in this mineral. These are shown in the inner circle of the Kick Diabetes Plant-Based Plate. In table 8.1 (page 127), Kick Diabetes Food Groups, they appear in the column at the right. Become familiar with high-calcium plant foods and incorporate them into your meals regularly. Recommended intakes for calcium are as follows:

- 1,000 milligrams per day for women age nineteen to fifty and men age nineteen to seventy
- 1,200 milligrams per day for women over fifty and men over seventy

To meet recommendations, aim for five to eight servings of high-calcium plant foods daily. (The balance will come in smaller amounts from other plant foods.) Each serving of the following foods provides approximately 150 milligrams of calcium:

- 2 cups (500 ml) raw bok choy, broccoli, collard greens, kale, or napa cabbage
- 1 cup (250 ml) cooked bok choy, broccoli, collard greens, kale, mustard greens, napa cabbage, okra, or black or white beans
- ½ cup (125 ml) calcium-set tofu, dried figs, fortified nondairy milk, cooked soybeans, or soy nuts
- ¼ cup (60 ml) almonds or chia or sesame seeds

- 2 tablespoons (30 ml) almond butter or tahini
- 2 oranges

If you fall short of the recommended number of servings of calcium-rich foods, you can top up your intake with a calcium supplement.

GETTING THE MOST FROM EACH FOOD GROUP

Kicking diabetes is possible, but it takes a solid commitment to lifestyle changes. It doesn't, however, require perfection. It's a process. The target servings shown on the Kick Diabetes Plant-Based Plate (page 126) are your ultimate goal, but you can get there one step at a time. For each food group, there are three suggested possible steps to your goal. If you need to take smaller steps, that's all right. Do what works for you. If you slip up, don't worry; that's normal. Just get back on track right away. Extend your walk an extra fifteen minutes; cut back on calories a little at your next meal. Trust the process, and trust yourself.

NONSTARCHY VEGETABLES

KICK DIABETES TARGET 7 or more servings per day (include a rainbow of colors)

LEVEL 1: 5 servings per day (1–2 leafy greens; 3–4 other vegetables)

LEVEL 2: 6 servings per day (2 leafy greens; 1 yellow or orange vegetable; 3 other vegetables)

LEVEL 3: 7 or more servings per day (3 or more leafy greens; 1 or more each of yellow or orange, red, purple or blue, and white or beige vegetables)

Best Choices

- Dark leafy greens are the most nutrient dense of all foods, with broccoli, bok choy, collard greens, kale, mustard greens, and okra being good calcium sources. Some others are high in oxalates that reduce calcium absorption; beet greens, spinach, and Swiss chard are healthy options but not good sources of calcium.
- All other nonstarchy vegetables are great choices—eat them to your heart's content.
- Organic vegetables are preferred; minimize your exposure to potentially harmful chemicals.
- Eat a rainbow of colors to maximize the quantity and variety of protective compounds.
- The fresher, the better. Nothing beats homegrown vegetables, so if you can, frequent farmers' markets and produce stands or start gardening.

Tips for Success

- *Grow more, buy more, eat more.* As the junk food is banished, load up on the healthiest foods of all—vegetables. Some can be washed and precut for instant use. Store in a glass or BPA-free container.

- *Make it easy.* Buy some of your produce already prepared, such as grated carrots, triple-washed greens, or frozen greens.

- *Make a huge bowl of salad to last a few days.* Have a giant salad for one meal a day. Include a variety of greens, a rainbow of vegetables, a protein source, and something filling, such as a cooked or sprouted grain or steamed starchy vegetable.

- *Sneak in veggies.* Dice veggies into soups and scrambles, chop veggies into stews and casseroles, grate veggies into loaves and patties, and blend veggies into sauces, dips, and dressings.

- *Get creative.* Add veggies to savory oatmeal, replace rice with cauliflower rice, or use collard leaves to make a wrap.

- *Have ½ cup (125 ml) of steamed dark leafy greens seasoned with lemon juice or balsamic vinegar three times a day.* This is powerful medicine!

- *Drink your veggies.* One way of getting a powerful antioxidant boost is to start your day with a green juice about one hour before breakfast. (See Green Giant Juice, page 190.)

- *Add veggies to smoothies.* If you have a smoothie meal, be sure to add loads of greens and frozen peas. Throw in a small carrot, a small beet, or a few slices of red, orange, or yellow peppers.

Common Questions

Are frozen, canned, and jarred vegetables good choices?

Fresh is generally best for maximum nutrition. However, vegetables are usually frozen soon after they've been picked, so their nutrients are well preserved, and they are super-convenient. Canned vegetables lose some of their water-soluble nutrients during processing, are often high in added sodium, and may have added sugar, so they are less-desirable choices. If used, select low- or no-sodium options canned in glass jars or BPA-free cans.

What are the best ways to cook vegetables?

Steaming results in the greatest nutrient retention (see table 8.2, page 132). If you're steaming several different types of vegetables for one meal, begin with the ones that take the longest time to cook, and add others accordingly. (While you can steam all vegetables, roasting or sautéing may be preferable for onions, garlic, mushrooms, and peppers for

TABLE 8.2. Guide to Steaming Vegetables

VEGETABLE	SIZE	TIME (IN MINUTES)
Asparagus	Whole spears or 2-inch (5-cm) pieces	7–10 for spears, 5–6 for pieces
Bean sprouts	As is.	1–2
Beans, green or yellow (wax)	Whole beans or 2-inch (5-cm) pieces	6–10 for whole beans, 5–7 for pieces
Beets	½-inch (1-cm) cubes, grated	12–15 for cubes, 5 for grated
Bell peppers	Strips or pieces	2–3
Broccoli, broccolini	Florets	5–7
Brussels sprouts	Halved	7–10
Cabbage	Small wedges	7–10
Carrots	Thin slices, grated	6–9 for slices, 3 for grated
Cauliflower	Florets	5–7
Celery	½-inch (1-cm) slices	5–7
Daikon radishes	Peeled and sliced	5
Greens (except spinach and kale)	Washed and chopped	2–4
Kale and collards	Trimmed and shredded or broken into pieces	5–7
Kohlrabi	½-inch (1-cm) cubes	5–8
Parsnips	Slices	10–12
Peas, sugar snap	Washed	4–5
Radishes	Halved	5–7
Spinach	Washed and trimmed	2–3
Squash	¾-inch (2-cm) cubes	7–10
Sweet potatoes	¾-inch (2-cm) cubes	7–10
Zucchini	Slices	3–5

maximum retention of flavor.) Microwaving and blanching also minimize nutrient losses. Boiling causes greater losses of vitamins and minerals through heat and discarded water. Baking or roasting can destroy vitamins (but not minerals) and create harmful by-products (see page 50), especially if foods are overcooked or blackened. The least-desirable methods are those that use very high temperatures and concentrated oils, such as deep-frying. Although a quick sauté can preserve nutrients, it can add a lot of fat and calories if oils are liberally used. For sautéing, replace oil with vegetable broth, water, or wine.

How can I make tough greens more enjoyable in salads?

The easiest way is to slice the greens matchstick thin and distribute them through the salad with more tender greens. Another option is massaging the sliced kale with a little lemon juice and letting it sit for twenty minutes before adding it to the salad. You could also dice and lightly steam the kale before using it. This works especially well in a salad rich in grains or legumes.

FRUITS

KICK DIABETES TARGET   3 or more servings per day

   LEVEL 1:   2 servings per day (any fresh fruit)

   LEVEL 2:   3 servings per day (any fresh fruit)

   LEVEL 3:   3 or more servings per day (1 of berries, 1 of citrus, 1 or more of other fruit)

Best Choices

- Berries provide a lot of fiber and phytochemicals and have a low glycemic index, so they're an exceptional choice.
- Citrus fruits are high in protective phytochemicals and have less impact on blood sugar than some other fruits.
- All other fresh fruits are healthy options, although bananas and dates contain more carbohydrates and calories than most other fruits, so they have a higher glycemic load.
- Fresh fruits are best, but frozen fruits are also good choices. Canned or jarred fruits are acceptable if they're packed in water, although there are greater nutrient losses with canned fruits, and the sugars in them are more rapidly absorbed into the bloodstream. Avoid fruits that are canned in syrup or contain added sugar.
- Opt for organic whenever possible.

Tips for Success

- *Have fruit with your morning meal.* Have at least two servings (a total of 1 cup/250 ml) of fruit with breakfast.
- *Use fruit as your go-to dessert.* Fresh fruit (sliced or whole), fruit salad, fruit-based ice cream, and baked fruit make delectable treats.
- *Add fruit to salads.* Enjoy some berries or sliced mango, apples, pears, oranges, or grapefruit on your salad.

- *Pick fruit if hunger strikes.* If you are famished, make fruit your go-to snack. To make the fruit even more filling, add a little natural nut butter or tahini, and top it with a sprinkle of cinnamon (see page 145).
- *Use fruit as your sweetener of choice in treats.* Both fresh and dried fruits are the most healthful substitutes for sugar in recipes.
- *Stew fruit in season and then freeze it for amazing breakfasts and dessert toppings.* Fruit can be stewed with just enough water to prevent sticking and cooked over a very low temperature. Wonderful choices are Italian prune plums, blueberries, apricots, peaches, and nectarines.
- *Keep some precut fruit in the refrigerator for easy use.* This works only for choices that do not brown, such as melons, pineapples, mangoes, papayas, and strawberries.

Common Questions

How much fruit is too much?

It depends on what else you're eating. If you're trying to lose weight and are eating all the recommended servings of other food groups, three or four servings of fruit is a reasonable target. If you're eating fewer calories than you need, there's no set limit on whole fresh fruits.

Is the fructose in fruit a problem?

The short answer is no. The body's ability to handle fructose is seldom overwhelmed by consuming whole fruit. Fruits also are loaded with protective phytochemicals, antioxidants, vitamins, and minerals, as well as the valuable fiber that slows absorption of the sugars. In fact, the more fruit that people consume, the lower their risk of diabetes.

Are dried fruits OK for people with diabetes?

Dried fruits are much higher in calories and have a greater impact on blood sugar than fresh fruits, so although they're healthy, they should be used sparingly. Avoid dried fruits with added sugars. Read the label, as many dried fruits have added sweeteners.

Are fruit juices OK for people with diabetes?

Fruit juices are best avoided because they're quickly absorbed into the bloodstream and lack the fiber of whole fruits. In addition, it's easy to drink a lot of juice in a short time. You can get through 1 cup (250 ml) of orange or apple juice in a minute, but it would take much longer to eat two oranges or apples. Fruit water is a wonderful option. Simply add citrus slices, strawberries, or other fruit or berries to a pitcher of water and let the water steep for eight to twelve hours in the refrigerator for a refreshing, fruity-tasting, sugar-free beverage.

Should I avoid watermelon because it has a high glycemic index?

No, it is not necessary to avoid watermelon even though it has a high glycemic index. Because the carbohydrate content of watermelon is low, it has low glycemic load. However, if you do eat it, eat a small serving—not half the watermelon!

LEGUMES (BEANS, LENTILS, SPLIT PEAS)

KICK DIABETES TARGET   3 or more servings per day

> **LEVEL 1:** 2 servings per day (beans, lentils, peas, soy milk, split peas, tempeh, tofu, veggie meats)
>
> **LEVEL 2:** 3 or more servings per day (at least 1 serving of whole legumes, lentils, or split peas)
>
> **LEVEL 3:** 3 or more servings per day (at least 2 servings of whole legumes, lentils, or split peas)

Best Choices

- Whole beans, chickpeas, split peas, and fresh peas are exceptional choices, brimming with fiber, plant protein, vitamins, minerals, and phytochemicals. Their consumption is strongly associated with diabetes risk reduction. For preparation, see table 11.2 (page 186) and pages 182–185, plus see the outstanding recipes in this book and in the *Kick Diabetes Cookbook*.

- Sprouted mung beans, peas, and lentils are good choices and safe to consume raw. Larger beans need to be cooked after sprouting.

- Traditional soy products are very healthful, with organic options recommended. Tofu and tempeh are protective against disease and have a long history of use in long-living populations. Tempeh, a fermented product, is relatively high in fiber. Tofu is extremely versatile and provides readily available plant protein.

- Hummus is popular and available in many flavors and variations, and it's super-easy to prepare at home. Commercial varieties can be high in sodium, so always read the labels.

- Bean pasta is a rapidly rising star, with types based on a variety of legumes. The advantages over traditional pasta are extensive, especially for people with diabetes. Bean pasta provides about half the carbohydrate, double the fiber, and triple the protein of regular pasta.

- Select organic whenever you can.

Tips for Success

- *Have beans for breakfast.* Many people around the world enjoy beans or lentils with their morning meals. If this strikes you as unusual, think of beans on toast, breakfast burritos, or scrambled tofu. Add lentils to your breakfast grains (you can cook them together) or beans to savory steel-cut oats.

- *Add legumes to salads.* Add chickpeas, black beans, grilled tempeh, smoked or baked tofu, or peas to a full-meal salad. Make a bean-based side salad.

- *Add a bean, lentil, or pea soup to your meal.* Bean soups are comfort foods—think split pea soup, lentil soup, or bean and barley soup. Enjoy them along with a salad, or add loads of veggies and greens for a one-bowl main dish.

- *Make legumes the main event.* Get creative when it comes to lunches and dinners. For centuries, numerous cultures have relied on these as dietary staples. Mexican, Indian, South American, Asian, and African cuisines include many delicious legume dishes.

- *Spice it up.* Beans can be bland, so add a burst of flavor with herbs and spices, such as garlic, ginger, curry, and smoked paprika.

- *Eat beans and greens.* When it comes to fighting diabetes, the heavy hitters are beans and greens, so eat them together. Steam greens, throw in some white beans, and top with garlic and lemon juice or balsamic vinegar.

- *Make bean-based spreads, dips, and dressings.* Make hummus or bean-based dips with chickpeas, black beans, or white beans. Use lentils as a base for a spread and white beans or chickpeas in a salad dressing.

Common Questions

How can I get more comfortable eating beans and lentils when they cause gas?

Beans and lentils cause gas because they contain a very healthy type of carbohydrate (oligosaccharides) that isn't broken down and digested in the small intestine. It makes its way into the large intestine and provides a feast for the bacterial inhabitants. Gas is a by-product. The following suggestions will help to keep gas production tolerable:

- *Reduce the oligosaccharides in beans.*
    - Use the hot-soak method for cooking dried beans (see page 185). This involves bringing beans to a boil and then letting them soak for twenty-four hours. Discard the soaking water and use fresh water to cook. The hot-soak method reduces oligosaccharides more than the traditional soaking method, which doesn't involve pre-boiling.

- Buy only as many dried beans as you can use within a few months and throw out beans that are older than one year.
- Sprout legumes before cooking them. Sprouting converts oligosaccharides into more-digestible sugars.
- Some canned beans have less oligosaccharides because they are very well cooked, so they may be a good option for some people (though they are more costly). Rinse them well before using.

- *Start with small portions*, then gradually increase your intake. In this way, healthy gut flora will flourish and become accustomed to the dietary shift, and unhealthy flora will get crowded out.
- *Cook beans thoroughly.* When beans are undercooked, they're more difficult to digest and cause more gas.
- *Select small legumes*, as they are easier to digest. The least problematic are skinless, split legumes, such as mung dal (split mung beans), red lentils, and split peas. In general, these will produce less gas than large beans, such as lima or kidney beans.
- *Pick options with fewer oligosaccharides.* Choose tofu and bean products that are fermented, such as tempeh.
- *Use seasonings that counteract the production of intestinal gas.* Black pepper, cinnamon, cloves, garlic, ginger, turmeric, and the Japanese seaweed kombu are all prized for their ability to diminish gas production.
- *Improve your gut flora.* Take probiotics in supplement form or use them in the preparation of fermented foods, such as vegan cheeses, yogurts, and other dishes.
- *Avoid overeating.* Eat smaller meals; stop eating when you are 80 percent full.
- *Consider a digestive enzyme supplement.* Find one that is targeted toward bean digestion.

Are canned beans OK for people with diabetes?

Canned beans are definitely OK, but they can be high in sodium and some have added sugar, so read labels. Canned baked beans typically have added sugar; it's wise to make baked beans at home so you can control the ingredients. Your best options are no- or low-sodium products in BPA-free cans. You can reduce the sodium by about 40 percent by rinsing canned beans well before using them. A good alternative to canned beans is cooking your own beans in large batches and freezing them in 1½- or 2-cup (375- or 500-ml) portions in freezer bags or jars. If you have an Instant Pot or similar pressure cooker, cooking beans is a breeze.

Are beans safe for people who have a history of gout?

Yes, in most cases. Gout is often referred to as the "disease of kings" because it is associated with an overindulgence in rich foods. It is triggered by chronic elevation of uric acid in the blood. While most foods contain purines, high intakes boost uric acid levels. For this reason, purines are restricted in people with gout. The most concentrated purine sources are organ meats and small fish. These foods contain 200–400 milligrams of purines per serving of 3.5 ounces (100 g). Other meat products (fish, beef, pork, and chicken) are moderately high in purines, averaging 100–200 milligrams per serving of 3.5 ounces (100 g). Beans are moderate in purines, with 50–100 milligrams per serving of ½ cup (125 ml) of cooked beans. For example, lentils contain 74 milligrams of purines per serving; small white beans, 68 milligrams per serving; and red beans, 55 milligrams per serving. Also, the absorption of purines from plant foods is lower. So if you have active gout, you will want to moderate your bean intake somewhat, but it is not necessary to eliminate beans.

Aren't the lectins in beans dangerous for people?

They can be. For example, the type of lectins in raw, sprouted, or undercooked kidney beans can cause a violent reaction akin to food poisoning. Other lectins, however, have been shown to reduce cancer risk. The bottom line is that the dangerous lectins in some legumes are easily destroyed by sufficient cooking. Thirty minutes of cooking gets rid of most lectins, and pressure cooking pretty much wipes them out.

Are veggie meats an acceptable option?

Yes, but if you use them, do so only occasionally. Veggie meats are concentrated sources of plant protein, and they are very low in carbohydrates, so they have a very low glycemic index. However, they are relatively processed products and often are high in sodium and fat. Read the label. In some products the protein used has been extracted with toxic chemicals, such as hexane. To eliminate this concern, select organic products. Some veggie meats are based on whole foods (such as burgers made with black beans and quinoa); these are great options. You also can assemble your own homemade versions.

WHOLE GRAINS AND STARCHY VEGETABLES

KICK DIABETES TARGET 2–4 servings per day (more or less depending on energy needs and weight-loss goals).

LEVEL 1: Eliminate white rice and processed foods made with refined flour. Include moderate amounts of whole grains and starchy vegetables.

LEVEL 2: If you include starchy vegetables and grains, select at least 1 serving of colorful starchy vegetables (corn, sweet potato, winter squash) and 1 serving of intact whole grains. If you consume any additional whole grains, stick mainly to those listed with or above rolled whole grains in the whole-grain hierarchy (see figure 8.2, page 140).

LEVEL 3: If you include starchy vegetables and grains, select 1 or more servings of colorful starchy vegetables and 1 or more servings of intact whole grains. If you consume additional whole grains, eat mainly intact grains.

In some cases, it is appropriate to eliminate this group entirely for a short time. During intensive weight-loss efforts, eliminating grains and starchy vegetables drops glycemic load dramatically, so it can be quite an effective strategy. However, these foods are healthy options; they contribute significantly to fiber and micronutrient intakes, as well as to satiety. Portion control is important for this food group. Stick mainly to starchy vegetables and whole grains that have a lower glycemic index and load. Products with a high glycemic index produce a rise in blood sugar similar to or higher than that of refined products. For example, millet has a glycemic index of 71, which is considerably higher than white pasta with a glycemic index of about 49. Starchy vegetables, such as breadfruit, corn, plantains, potatoes, pumpkins, sweet potatoes, taro, and winter squash, are high in carbohydrates. While nonstarchy vegetables provide about 5 grams of carbohydrate per serving, starchy vegetables provide triple that amount, similar to that of whole grains. Yellow and orange starchy vegetables provide two nutrients not available from whole grains: vitamin A (as carotenoids) and vitamin C.

Best Choices

- Colorful starchy vegetables (orange, yellow, or purple) and colorful grains (red or black quinoa and rice) have the greatest antioxidant and phytochemical content.
- Starchy vegetables with their skin on have more fiber, nutrients, and phytochemicals than peeled vegetables.
- Intact grains, as they are picked off the plant, are higher in nutrients, fiber, phytochemicals, and other protective components than more processed grains, such as flour (see the whole-grain hierarchy, figure 8.2, page 140). They also have the lowest glycemic index of all grains.
- Grains with lower arsenic content are preferable to rice as dietary staples.
- Organic grains are safest; this is especially true for wheat or oats. Conventional wheat and oats are commonly sprayed with a pesticide that contains glyphosate, which is a probable human carcinogen.

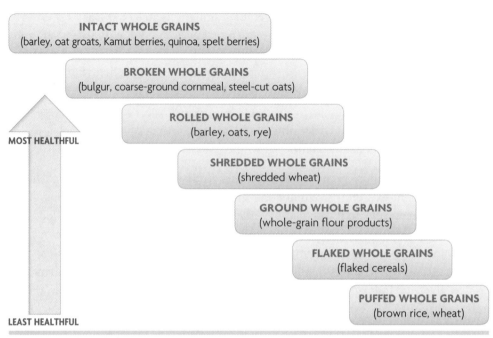

FIGURE 8.2 The Whole-Grain Hierarchy.

Tips for Success

- *Include a starchy vegetable or intact whole grain at each meal.* This will make meals more satisfying and will help to avoid the temptation to eat between meals. Keep portions moderate.

- *Get familiar with intact grains.* You can cook up a batch and use it as a breakfast cereal, as a topping for salads, or as a hearty addition to soups and stews. You'll find information on cooking intact grains on page 186.

- *Replace higher glycemic index grains with those that are low.* For example, instead of brown rice, serve barley. If using bread, opt for extremely heavy breads or sprouted-grain breads rather than lighter whole-grain breads.

- *Add whole grains or starchy vegetables to soups and salads.* For lunch, sprinkle intact whole grains or steamed squash cubes on your salad. Add corn or barley to soup.

- *Stuff baked potatoes or yams with beans and vegetables.* Stuffed sweet potatoes or yams offer a nutritional advantage, but regular baked potatoes are fine too, especially when they're topped or filled with high-fiber beans. And be sure to eat the skin! Serve steamed dark leafy greens or a salad on the side.

- *Enjoy a vegetable curry or stir-fry over a healthy whole grain, such as black rice, red quinoa, or another intact whole grain.*

- *Minimize whole-grain flour products (such as whole-grain bread and crackers).* Many products labeled "whole grain" contain added fat, sugar, salt, flavors, colors, and preservatives; read labels carefully.

- *Include a variety of grains, as each one has its own strengths.* Among the true grains, Kamut, oats, spelt, and wheat are the richest in protein. The pseudograins, quinoa and buckwheat, are great choices too. Each starchy vegetable has its unique advantages. Sweet potatoes are the highest in carotenoids and trace minerals; winter squash provides more folate.

Common Questions

Are whole grains healthy foods?

Absolutely! Whole grains provide about half the world's protein and fiber. They're rich in B vitamins (especially thiamin and niacin) and vitamin E. They're good sources of copper, iron, manganese, magnesium, phosphorus, selenium, and zinc, plus a variety of phytochemicals and antioxidants.

Are grains essential for a healthy diet?

No. There are no nutrients in grains that can't be derived from other foods. One approach is to eat your daily quota of vegetables, fruits, legumes, nuts, and seeds, and then vary your grain intake based on your energy (caloric) needs. If your energy needs are very low, your allowance for grains will be low. If you're moderately or very active, you can afford to eat more grains.

Should everyone avoid gluten?

No. While the 1 percent of the population with celiac disease must be vigilant about avoiding gluten, and another estimated 6–10 percent may suffer from non-celiac gluten sensitivity, most people can tolerate gluten. Vary the grains you eat, and include several gluten-free grains, such as amaranth, buckwheat, millet, quinoa, and teff in your rotation. Opt for organic grains when possible.

Are starches for thickening sauces off-limits because they're refined?

No. While these are highly refined, generally only a small amount is required per serving. If you use 2 tablespoons (30 ml) of arrowroot starch, cornstarch, or potato starch to thicken a sauce, it typically amounts to about ¾ teaspoon (4 ml) per person.

Are foods derived from grains (oat bran, wheat bran, wheat germ) healthy choices?

Although oat bran, wheat bran, and wheat germ aren't technically whole grains, they do have nutritional benefits. Oat bran can provide viscous fiber, which helps to control blood sugar. Wheat bran can be useful for people who suffer from constipation; however, caution is warranted because it can reduce mineral absorption. Wheat germ can add vitamin E to granola or muesli. Nevertheless, eating the whole grain is the best option.

Is it OK to include bread?

Yes, but very selectively. Because bread is often yeasted to make it light and fluffy, the carbohydrate in bread is rapidly absorbed and has a big impact on blood sugar. Bread can also be high in sodium and low in fiber. Sprouted breads (made from sprouted grains rather than flour, and dehydrated or baked at a low temperature) are reasonable choices. Breads made from sprouted-grain flours are also preferable to conventional whole-grain breads. Those that contain sprouted legumes have the lowest GI of all breads.

Usually, the denser the bread, the more slowly the nutrients are absorbed and the more healthful it is. Very heavy breads (those that you can practically stand on!) are best, such as German pumpernickel. Light, fluffy, whole wheat bread might have a GI of 74, while heavy German pumpernickel has a GI of about 48. The bottom line is that most of the grains you eat should be intact whole grains. If you include bread, pick wisely and have it infrequently, not daily.

NUTS AND SEEDS

KICK DIABETES TARGET   2–3 servings per day

LEVEL 1:   1–2 servings per day, including ½ or 1 serving of an omega-3-rich choice (chia seeds, ground flaxseeds, hemp seeds, or walnuts)

LEVEL 2:   2–3 servings per day, including 1 serving of an omega-3-rich choice

LEVEL 3:   2–3 servings per day, including 1 serving of an omega-3-rich choice plus 1 serving of a vitamin E-rich choice (almonds, hazelnuts, sunflower seeds)

Note: In this guide we include peanuts and peanut butter in the nuts and seeds group. Although peanuts are botanically legumes, they're used like nuts for culinary and nutritional purposes.

Best Choices

■ Omega-3-rich options include walnuts and chia, flax, or hemp seeds. The absorption of omega-3 fatty acids is improved by grinding chia seeds and flaxseeds.

- Seeds are higher in protein and fiber and more concentrated in essential fatty acids (both omega-6 and omega-3 fatty acids) than nuts (except for walnuts). The seeds highest in protein are hemp and pumpkin seeds.
- Go for variety, as the nutrition contribution of nuts and seeds is quite diverse. Almonds and sunflower seeds are the vitamin E superstars. Almonds and chia, poppy, and sesame seeds are rich in calcium. Most seeds, pine nuts, and cashews are rich in iron and zinc. Brazil nuts are selenium superstars, and chia and pumpkin seeds are richest in magnesium. Walnuts and pecans appear to be champions in terms of antioxidant content. Peanuts are particularly high in protein.
- Choose nuts and seeds that are raw, soaked, or lightly roasted. Soaking (and dehydrating, if you like) increases the content and availability of nutrients, phytochemicals, and antioxidants. Roasting can cause the formation of products of oxidation, so keep temperatures below 250 degrees F (120 degrees C) if possible. Do not allow nuts and seeds to get dark brown.
- Select organic, especially for peanuts.

Tips for Success

- *Add omega-3-rich seeds or walnuts to a breakfast bowl (see Whole-Food Breakfast Bowl, page 196).* You'll need about 1 tablespoon (15 ml) of ground flaxseeds, 1½ tablespoons (22 ml) of chia seeds, or 3 tablespoons (45 ml) of hemp seeds or walnuts to fulfill your omega-3 requirement. Make a mix of seeds, and store the mixture in a mason jar in the refrigerator so you can enjoy the combined benefits of many different seeds. (See Omega-3-Rich Seed Mix, page 197.)
- *Add 1–2 tablespoons (15–30 ml) nuts or seeds to salads.* Almonds, pumpkin seeds, and sunflower seeds are excellent choices.
- *Use seeds, nuts, or their butters as your salad-dressing base.* These are the perfect nutrient-rich replacements for oils in dressings (see the dressing recipes on pages 217–221).
- *Use nuts or seeds in main dishes.* Add walnuts or sunflower seeds to patties or loaves, add pine nuts or hazelnuts to pilafs, or throw a few peanuts or cashews into a stir-fry.
- *Enjoy a few unshelled nuts for a snack or dessert.* Crack open two or three walnuts or five or six other nuts and serve them with sliced fresh fruit for a simple but satisfying snack or dessert.
- *Use nuts or seeds to top fruit salad, fruit-based ice cream, or baked fruit.* Sprinkle nuts or seeds on fruit desserts for added flavor and nutrient absorption and to slow the absorption of fruit sugar.

Common Questions

Aren't nuts and seeds high in fat and calories?

Yes, 75–85 percent of the calories in nuts and 55–75 percent of the calories in seeds are from fat. They provide 500–800 calories per cup (250 ml)! So although they're valuable foods, they should be eaten in small amounts, not by the bowlful.

Are nuts and seeds OK for people with diabetes?

Absolutely! In fact they're more than OK—they're important. Among all the plant-based foods, nuts have the least impact on blood sugar. In addition, they deliver essential nutrients, fiber, phytochemicals, and antioxidants.

Is coconut a healthy choice?

Yes, it's acceptable, but only in small amounts, primarily as a flavor booster. Unlike true nuts, which feature monounsaturated fats, and seeds, which have mostly polyunsaturated fats, coconut contains mostly saturated fat. To enhance the flavor of foods without adding much fat, sprinkle 1 tablespoon (15 ml) of unsweetened shredded dried coconut over a breakfast bowl (see page 196) or fruit dessert. If a recipe calls for coconut milk (which has about 450 calories per 1 cup/250 ml), replace it with thick unsweetened soy or cashew milk, or add 1 teaspoon (5 ml) of coconut extract per 1 cup (250 ml) of nondairy milk.

HERBS AND SPICES

KICK DIABETES TARGET   3 or more servings per day

Herbs and spices are of tremendous value in a diabetes-reversal diet because of the wealth of protective phytochemicals and antioxidants they contain.

> **LEVEL 1:** 1 or more servings per day
>
> **LEVEL 2:** 2 or more servings per day
>
> **LEVEL 3:** 3 or more servings per day

Best Choices

- Cinnamon seems to show the most promise for slowing blood glucose absorption or stabilizing blood sugar, although cayenne, cloves, curry powder, fenugreek, garlic, ginger, marjoram, rosemary, and sage may also be of value.
- Turmeric is the anti-inflammation superstar. Basil, black pepper, cardamom, cinnamon, cloves, garlic, ginger, fennel, nutmeg, and rosemary all have inflammation-quenching abilities.

- For the greatest antioxidant action, cloves lead the pack. Allspice, basil, bay leaves, chiles, cinnamon, curry powder, ginger, lemon balm, marjoram, mint, dry mustard, oregano, paprika, saffron, sage, thyme, and turmeric are in the running too.

Tips for Success

- *Spice up breakfast.* Allspice, cinnamon, cloves, ginger, and nutmeg combine well with sweet breakfasts. Basil, cayenne, garlic, oregano, rosemary, thyme, and turmeric are great additions to savory breakfasts.
- *Infuse hot teas with herbs or spices.* Use cinnamon, cloves, fennel, ginger, lemon balm, mint, or turmeric.
- *Add fresh herbs to salads.* Basil, chives, cilantro, dill, mint, parsley, oregano, and thyme are wonderful herbs for salads.
- *Add herbs and spices to salad dressings.* Basil, cayenne, garlic, ginger, mustard, and turmeric all add a welcome jolt of flavor. Prepared mustard also acts as an emulsifier.
- *Season soups, stews, and other dishes with plenty of herbs and spices.*

Common Questions

Does it matter if herbs are fresh or dried?

Both are excellent choices. For a salad or as a garnish, fresh is best. If you're cooking herbs for fifteen minutes or longer, either fresh or dried will do. Whole dried spices will keep for three to four years, ground spices for two to three years, dried herbs for one to three years, and seasoning blends for one to two years. Store dried herbs and spices in a cool, dry spot, away from heat.

Are some types of cinnamon potentially toxic?

Yes. The cinnamon that's commonly used throughout North America is called cassia cinnamon and contains a compound called coumarin, which is toxic to the liver, especially in large amounts. Some countries have suggested upper intake limits of no more than ⅓–1 teaspoon (2–5 ml) daily for a 176-pound (80-kg) person. Either limit your intake of cassia cinnamon or use Ceylon cinnamon instead. Although less widely available (it can be purchased online) and more expensive, Ceylon cinnamon contains very little coumarin. The taste is milder but pleasant. Although most studies on cinnamon and blood sugar reduction were done using cassia cinnamon, there is evidence that Ceylon cinnamon provides similar advantages.

TABLE 8.3. Top Ten Diabetes Friends and Foes

DIABETES FOOD FRIENDS	DIABETES FOOD FOES
Beans, peas, and lentils	Alcohol
Berries	Beverages with added sugar
Fresh fruit	Full-fat dairy products
Green leafy vegetables	Deep-fried foods
Herbs and spices	Grilled meat or poultry
Intact whole grains (such as barley and oats)	Red and processed meats
Nuts (such as walnuts and almonds)	Ultraprocessed foods
Other vegetables	Solid fats
Seeds (such as flax, chia, and hemp)	Sugar, syrups, and sweets
Water	White flour, white rice products

Now that you know what to eat, let's look at some of the other aspects of lifestyle that can augment a well-planned diet. You'll see how exercise, rest, and stress reduction combine to provide a winning combination for kicking diabetes.

Chapter 9

The Lifestyle Blueprint

Diane had never been a fitness enthusiast. Although rescuing a dog was something that she had always wanted to do, she knew that having a dog meant walking a dog, and that would motivate her to get outside. She liked her Pilates class, but she managed to wiggle her way out of it more often than she cared to admit. Diane's sleep was not what she knew it should be. She watched too much TV, and she wondered if her daily glass of wine morphed into two or three glasses too often on weekends. When she committed herself to a plant-based diet, she also committed herself to upping her game in other areas of her lifestyle. She started by walking after every meal—even on her weekday lunch hours at work. Sometimes they were short walks, but they were still walks, and they got progressively brisker as the excess weight fell away. Diane didn't like the idea of taking spin and cardio classes, as she felt self-conscious and a little embarrassed by her fitness level. But when she arrived, she discovered that she was not alone. After just a few weeks, her stamina increased, along with her confidence level. As her fitness improved, the quality of her sleep followed, and she had less desire to watch TV or to indulge in wine. Somehow, she was remaking herself, and she was feeling pretty comfortable in her new skin.

I have a vivid memory of my dad when he was in his late forties, smiling at me as he slowly sauntered by with a big bag of chips in one hand, a bottle of cola in the other, and two cigarettes hanging out of his mouth. No matter how hard I tried to convince him to make healthier choices—whether I used fear or guilt— he dismissed me. This day was no different. When I challenged him, his response was predictable. "I would rather live fifty years having the freedom to do what I love than live seventy-five years having to avoid the things I most enjoy." He added, "After all, I could be hit by a truck tomorrow." I responded in frustration, "That may be true, but it doesn't mean you should walk out in front of one."

As fate would have it, just shy of his fiftieth year, my dad had a stroke. His blood pressure, cholesterol, and blood sugar were so high that he was told he would die within three months if he continued to smoke, and that if he did stop smoking, he might have three years. I think that was the moment he recognized that life was more precious than cigarettes, cola, and potato chips. Although my dad never made the radical changes I had hoped for, he made enough of them to dance with his sweetheart at their fiftieth wedding anniversary and see his grandchildren graduate. However, while moderate changes can delay the onset of complications, as he gratefully experienced, it takes more significant changes, like those made by Carlos (see page 25), to reverse diabetes.

TAKING ON THE LIFESTYLE CHALLENGE

Now you have a game plan for improving your dietary habits and overcoming the food challenges that might come your way. The next step is to implement a new lifestyle routine and understand the challenges that might sabotage that routine. In this chapter, you'll set achievable goals and get flexible guidelines for adopting a healthy lifestyle that will help you conquer diabetes for good.

GETTING STARTED

Before you begin on the road to recovery, prepare for the journey. Determine, as my dad did, why it is you want to get healthy and then be specific about the health targets you want to reach. Following each of these steps will greatly enhance your odds of success.

1. **DETERMINE YOUR DESTINATION.** Before heading out on your journey, determine your final destination or your ultimate goal, so you'll have a path or general direction. Write it down. It could look something like this.

   Ultimate Goal: To achieve excellent lifelong health, including freedom from diabetes. Think about the reasons you want to achieve these goals. Although health goals are often about adding years to your life, they're even more about adding life to your years. Write down the reasons for your ultimate goal. These are your primary motivations; they provide the fuel you need to make the journey. You may have dozens of these. List them all and keep them beside your bed or somewhere handy so you can look at them regularly. Here are some examples:

- I want to live to see my grandchildren graduate.

- I want to start riding a bicycle again.

- I want to travel to Europe and be able to walk through streets, museums, art galleries, and churches all day long.

- I want to go to my fortieth high school reunion and feel proud of the way I look.

- I want to feel cheerful and energetic.

- I want to be less of a burden on my partner and my family.

- I want to write an article to be published in a magazine.

- I want to dance at my daughter's wedding.

- I'd like to find a partner with whom to enjoy my future years.

2. **SET MAJOR GOALS.** Your major goals break your ultimate goal into more-manageable pieces. They will move you further along your journey and are a critical piece of your road map to health. Think carefully about what needs to be accomplished in order to arrive at your final destination. Write down your major goals. They could look something like this:

MAJOR GOALS:

- Overcome insulin resistance.

- Get off medications.

- Achieve a healthy body weight.

- Achieve a normal blood pressure.

- Get physically fit.

3. **DEVELOP A PLAN OF ACTION.** Once your goals are set, you're ready to write out a plan of action. Goals are general intentions—they provide direction, but your plan of action is made up of all the little routines that you repeat on a regular basis and that get you to your final destination. They're objectives that must be achieved in order to reach your goals.

RECOGNIZING THE BARRIERS TO SUCCESS

Even with your new goals in hand, it's important to understand the obstacles you must overcome in order to reach those goals. As a species, we're programmed to respond to threats in a way that preserves life and health. So why, you may wonder, are obesity, diabetes, and heart disease spiraling out of control? The barriers to health are sometimes so powerful that they can override your body's innate instinct to survive.

Fortunately, if you recognize the barriers, you can hold firm and steer clear. The first order of business is to learn to spot the barriers.

Your social environment is one of the trickiest to maneuver. Your relationships have a profound influence on your health behaviors, affecting what you eat, your physical activity, your sleep, and many other lifestyle choices. Research has shown that the more friends and family members you have who are obese, the greater your odds are of becoming obese yourself, unless you take conscious steps to make more healthful choices. One study reported that having a single friend who became obese in a given interval would increase your risk of becoming obese by 57 percent.[1] Social environments can serve as stressors, affecting your mental and emotional health, as well as your ability to make decisions that support and promote health.

Even your physical environment can incite overeating and underactivity. In other words, your physical environment can be obesogenic (produce obesity) and diabetogenic (produce diabetes). The design of your neighborhood, including transportation systems, access to healthy foods, food advertising, and proximity to fast-food restaurants, corner stores, and liquor stores can all factor in, as well as can the distance to walking and cycling infrastructures, recreation areas, and fitness facilities. Easy access to processed foods, which are high in fat, sugar, and salt, presents a monumental hurdle for many individuals. Humans are hardwired to be attracted to these substances because they can be protective in times of famine. However, when you're drowning in foods that have been manufactured to enhance taste appeal, this hardwiring can work against you.

While these challenges may seem overwhelming at times, your awareness of them is also incredibly empowering. The bottom line is simple: When it comes to lifestyle changes, the more you change, the more you heal. Other factors that significantly affect health are also things you can control: physical fitness, stress management, social engagement, and rest and relaxation (see figure 9.1, below).

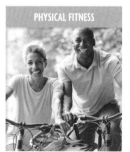 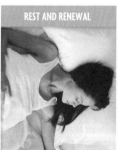 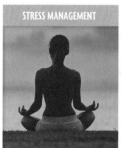 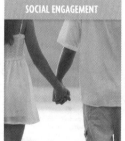 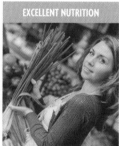

PHYSICAL FITNESS · REST AND RENEWAL · STRESS MANAGEMENT · SOCIAL ENGAGEMENT · EXCELLENT NUTRITION

FIGURE 9.1. Factors affecting health that you can control.

PHYSICAL FITNESS

I f you're trying to restore insulin sensitivity and defeat diabetes, regular exercise is not an option; it's an imperative. Exercise lowers blood glucose by increasing your muscles' need for glucose and stimulating a mechanism that allows your cells to use glucose without using insulin. As a bonus, physical activity after a meal prevents excess sugar from being stored as fat. Even light activity, such as walking at a slow pace, can lower blood glucose as effectively as oral medications. Exercise helps you achieve and maintain a healthy body weight and reduces the risk of the major complications of diabetes, including heart disease.[2]

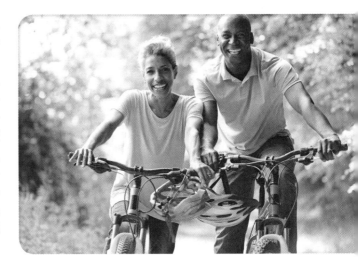

The official position statement of the American Diabetes Association (ADA) on physical activity recommends daily physical activity, including a minimum of 150 minutes of exercise per week. A mix of both aerobic and resistance training are suggested, and not allowing more than two days between exercise sessions is advised. Additionally, the ADA recommends that prolonged sitting be interrupted with bouts of light activity every thirty minutes for blood glucose benefits.[2]

KICK DIABETES RECOMMENDATION Make exercise as much a part of your daily life as eating, sleeping, and breathing.

LEVEL 1: Walk or be otherwise physically active for 10–15 minutes (or longer) after every meal.

LEVEL 2: Add 30 minutes of exercise at least five days per week, in addition to after-meal walks.

LEVEL 3: Increase exercise to 45–60 minutes at least five days per week, in addition to after-meal walks.

Any amount of exercise is better than none, but to kick diabetes, commit to *at least* 10–15 minutes (longer duration is even more effective) of movement after meals. This can be a walk around the block or a few minutes on an exercise bike. It can even be sweeping the floor or working around the yard. Just move your body rather than sitting. Once after-meal movement becomes a consistent part of your daily routine, add in other exercise. Begin with 10–15 minutes, slowly working your way up to 30 minutes and eventually to 45–60 minutes. If you're a senior, the rules of the game stay the same, unless it isn't possible for you. In this case, be as active as your body allows. Exercise doesn't have to happen all at once to reap the benefits. You can break your routine down and do three 10- or 20-minute sessions if that works better for you. Get creative—pool or chair exercises can be helpful if joint pain is an issue.

The best kind of exercise is movement you'll do consistently and willingly. If you enjoy it, you're much more likely to stick with it. While all forms of exercise afford health benefits, there are three main types of exercise that work together to help restore and maintain health.

Aerobic (Cardio) Activity

Aerobic activity is any movement that relies on your large muscle groups to get your heart and lungs working harder than they do when you're sedentary. This type of exercise improves blood sugar control, insulin sensitivity, endothelial function, blood lipids, blood pressure, endurance, circulation, and heart health. Examples of aerobic exercise are jogging, brisk walking, cycling, swimming, skating, climbing stairs, cross-country skiing, and jumping rope. It's best to include some form of aerobic activity every day.

Resistance (Strength) Training

Diabetes is associated with low muscle strength and accelerated decline in muscle strength and function.[2] Resistance training builds, strengthens, firms, and tones your muscles and improves bone density, balance, and coordination. Because muscle is so important for burning fat and glucose, strength exercises improve blood sugar control and decrease insulin resistance. Examples include push-ups, lunges, and pull-ups and the use of resistance bands, dumbbells, or weight machines. Include resistance training at least twice and preferably three times a week.

Flexibility Exercises

Many people with diabetes have limited joint mobility. This may be a product of higher levels of advanced glycation end products, also known as AGEs (see page 51). These accrue with aging, but they also accumulate rapidly in the presence of high blood glucose levels.[2] Flexibility exercises are activities that improve range of motion and lengthen muscles. In addition, they help to keep you limber, reducing stiffness, aches, and pains. Good examples of exercises that promote flexibility are yoga, pilates, tai chi, and stretching routines. Although flexibility exercises do not appear to improve glycemic control or diabetes outcomes as much as cardio and strength exercises, they definitely improve the ability to do all forms of movement. Aim for a 15–20 minute (or longer) session of deep stretching twice a week and 10 minutes on all other days.

Creating an Exercise Schedule

Ideally, you'll want to include all three types of exercise in your weekly routine. If you're concerned about injury or have physical limitations, a personal trainer or exercise physiologist can set up a program that suits your lifestyle and abilities. Table 9.1, below, provides a sample exercise schedule for levels 1, 2, and 3.

Every physical movement that helps increase your energy expenditure contributes to your overall fitness. Thus, everyday activities can count toward your movement tally for the day: gardening, walking at work or while shopping, hanging laundry, cleaning house, making your bed, and watering your plants—even tapping your foot while seated! In one study, obese individuals sat for 2.5 hours more each day than their lean counterparts. Even though obese individuals have resting metabolic rates that are similar to non-obese individuals, they are more sedentary and expend less energy in daily activities. If obese individuals adopted similar activity patterns and movements as leaner individuals, they would expend an additional 300 calories per day.[3] The take-home message is to do whatever you can to add more movement to your day. Throw on some dance tunes to motivate you to embrace your housework with vigor. Use stairs instead of elevators, walk to your postal box, cut and grate vegetables by hand, or do a seated light-dumbbell workout while watching TV.

Fortunately, age need not be a barrier to fitness. Even people who are one hundred years old can improve their fitness level with training. Start off slowly and gradually build intensity and endurance.

TABLE 9.1. Sample Exercise Schedule

	LEVEL 1	LEVEL 2	LEVEL 3
Type of Activity	**Aerobic** three times a day (after each meal); 10–15 minutes per session	**Aerobic** three times a day (after each meal); 10–15 minutes per session	**Aerobic** three times a day (after each meal); 10–15 minutes per session
		Plus 20 minutes higher-intensity aerobics three times a week	**Plus** 30 minutes higher-intensity aerobics three or more times a week
		Strength 20 minutes strength training two times a week	**Strength** 30 minutes strength training three times a week
		Flexibility 10–20 minutes per day	**Flexibility** 15–30 minutes per day

No matter how much you recognize the need for exercise, getting going can be tough. You may feel too sore, weak, or tired. You may be in a slump or feel embarrassed about your appearance. A good book or a favorite show may seem infinitely more attractive. When it comes to exercise, make your decisions based on your long-term goals rather than your current state of mind. These ten simple strategies will help you to find your fitness mojo and will be your keys to an active lifestyle:

1. *Schedule your workouts.* This may well be the deciding factor in your fitness success. Life is busy, so if you don't make exercise a priority and schedule it into your day, it may not happen. Schedule walks, fitness classes, cycling, and other activities every day of the week. Establish a routine so you don't even have to think about it—you just know what activity you're doing on any given day. You might enjoy adding in a pre- and or post-workout routine. This could be having an energy-boosting tea while reading your favorite magazine before the workout and getting in a hot tub afterward.

2. *Find a buddy.* One of the most tried and true tactics for staying accountable to your exercise commitments is to work out with a friend. You may not find someone to do everything with, but you may find someone to be your walking partner, another person to be your biking buddy, and yet another to be your yoga pal. If you lack friends and family who want to join you in your quest for a more active lifestyle, make friends through walking clubs, fitness classes, or other organized recreational activities. Working out with others provides huge motivation.

3. *Establish a five-minute rule.* When you're feeling especially unmotivated, tell yourself that you only have to exercise for five minutes. Set a timer, and once it goes off, you have permission to stop your workout. More often than not, the biggest barrier to completing a workout is getting started. Once you get going, you'll feel fired up and ready to continue.

4. *Be an early bird.* Energy tends to diminish as the day goes on. If you're able to exercise first thing in the morning, you can get your day off to a great start. An early start also means you'll be done sooner and can get on with your day.

5. *Play outside.* Sometimes the thought of a class indoors can seem ho-hum, especially when the sun is shining outside. Scope out the parks in your area, and get out for a bike ride, walk, or jog. Start cross-country skiing, take up pickleball, or join a hiking club. Consider outdoor tai chi or fitness boot camps.

6. *Put your money where your mouth is.* When you pay a monthly fee for a gym or an exercise program, the best way to get your money's worth is to use it often. Simply reminding yourself of your financial sacrifice may provide motivation for getting there. If you're doing free stuff, consider paying yourself a dollar or two every time you do a workout. At the end of the month, treat yourself to a massage or a special outing with a friend.

7. *Double your pleasure.* If you're using an exercise machine, such as a treadmill, elliptical machine, or exercise bike, take in a favorite podcast, audiobook, or comedy show while you're working out.

8. *Mix it up.* Instead of sticking to one activity day in and day out, have a different routine for each day. This will help keep things fresh and interesting. Perhaps Monday is yoga day, Tuesday is fitness boot camp, Wednesday is your walking group, Thursday is spin class, Friday is pickleball, and weekends are your days to get outside and swim, bike, hike, or ski.

9. *Use visual aids.* Put a favorite photo of yourself at your fittest, or of someone who inspires you to get fit, on your refrigerator, mirror, smartphone, or computer.

10. *Get a gadget.* Having a fitness tracker, watch, pedometer, or other gadget can push you a little harder than you might otherwise do on your own. Even buying a new yoga mat, free weights, or running shoes can make exercise more exciting.

Precautions

People with diabetes are at higher risk for some health problems with physical activity. These risks are easily averted with the proper precautions.

1. Get the green light from your physician or health-care provider before you begin a new exercise regimen, especially if the activities are significantly more vigorous than brisk walking.

2. Take your blood sugar reading before and after your exercise session. This is particularly important if you're on insulin or some types of oral diabetes medications. Exercise helps your body use glucose more effectively, and if you're taking these medications, your blood glucose could dip too low, causing a hypoglycemic reaction. Once you begin a daily exercise program, work closely with your health-care provider to adjust your medications so hypoglycemic reactions are avoided. While hypoglycemia is not common in people with diabetes who aren't on medications or insulin, a condition called reactive hypoglycemia is an early symptom of insulin resistance in prediabetes. Sometimes after a meal, especially one that is high in refined carbohydrates, the pancreas releases so much insulin that blood glucose dips too low. This could be exacerbated by physical activity that further lowers blood sugar.

3. Gradually increase the intensity of your exercise program so your body adjusts over time. If you feel breathless, dizzy, nauseous, or otherwise unwell or uncomfortable, stop your activity until that discomfort has passed and resume it at a less vigorous level. If problems persist with exercise, contact your health-care provider.

4. Ensure appropriate footwear for each activity. People with diabetes are at a much higher risk of complications due to blisters and other foot injuries. Be sure to do a daily foot check.

REST AND RENEWAL

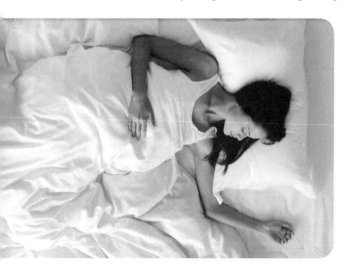

Lack of sleep or poor-quality sleep affects your health, mood, and general well-being. It can also lead to weight gain, reduced physical and mental performance, and increased risk of chronic diseases and premature death.[4] People who sleep for fewer than five to six hours a night or who have poor-quality sleep are at a higher risk of obesity and diabetes, and people with diabetes have an increased risk for sleep disorders, such as sleep apnea and restless legs syndrome.[5] One meta-analysis reported that a lack of sleep (fewer than five hours per day) increased diabetes risk by 48 percent, while poor-quality sleep increased risk by 40 percent.[6] For people who have diabetes, suboptimal sleep has been shown to increase insulin resistance and adversely affect blood glucose control and HbA1c.[7,8] Both high and low blood sugar can disrupt sleep, as can other ailments that disproportionately affect people with diabetes, such as chronic pain, depression, heartburn, and peripheral neuropathy. If kicking diabetes is your goal, sufficient, high-quality sleep is a critical part of the plan.

According to the National Sleep Foundation, adults eighteen to sixty years of age need seven or more hours of sleep. People who are sixty-one to sixty-four years of age require seven to nine hours, and those over sixty-five need seven to eight hours.[9]

KICK DIABETES RECOMMENDATION Make getting sufficient sleep a health priority.

LEVEL 1: Establish an environment that supports a good night's sleep. Practice a relaxing bedtime routine and avoid distractions and stimulants.

LEVEL 2: Follow a sleep schedule. Go to bed at the same time each night, and rise at the same time each morning. Stick to within one hour of this routine on weekends.

LEVEL 3: Get seven to nine hours of high-quality sleep each night if you're an adult under sixty-five years of age. Get seven to eight hours if you're age sixty-five or older.

Like every other aspect of a healthy lifestyle, quality sleep requires conscious preparation. Playing a computer game or watching television while sipping an espresso coffee before you head to bed will not work in your favor. Relax before bedtime. For at least thirty to sixty minutes before bedtime, turn off all technology—no computer screens or televisions. The light from these devices delays the release of the sleep-inducing hormone melatonin. Avoid intense exercise and demanding errands in the late evening. Say no to stimulating beverages, such as coffee, colas, energy drinks, and alcohol. Eat your last meal no later than two hours before bed.

To ensure quality sleep, establish a bedtime routine. Personal care, including a warm bath followed by reading a favorite book, is a great start. Set up a supportive sleep environment. Noise and light both interfere with quality sleep. Even a little light shining into your room reduces rest. Wearing an eye mask is helpful when it's impossible to eliminate light. Keep your room clean and uncluttered and invest in a comfortable pillow and mattress. Be consistent with your sleep hours and aim for as much sleep before midnight as possible; these hours tend to be the most restorative.

If you have difficulty falling asleep or staying asleep or suffer from a sleep disorder, seek the assistance of a sleep specialist. A sleep study in a special laboratory may be advised so that the doctor can determine the cause of your sleep problems. Whether the issue is your sleep environment, your bedtime routine, or a more troublesome issue, such as sleep apnea, the good news is that all of these can be improved upon or fixed. Sleep apnea can often be overcome by achieving a healthy body weight. It can also be managed with the use of a sleep apnea device; these have become much more comfortable and easier to use than earlier models. Rest and renewal can be achieved with preparation and wise choices.

SEVEN STEPS TO SOUND SLEEP

1. Establish a regular time for going to bed and waking.
2. Adopt a regular pre-sleep routine.
3. Create a comfortable sleep environment.
4. Allow for some time between consuming meals, caffeinated beverages, and/or alcohol and going to bed.
5. Steer clear of sleep disruptors, such as computer or TV screens, for at least thirty to sixty minutes before bedtime.
6. Turn off your cell phone and other noisemakers.
7. Read a book the old-fashioned way.

STRESS MANAGEMENT

Stress is the body's way of managing changes that require a response. The body reacts according to the form of stress and your state of health. Generally, we're well equipped to handle stress, as it's a normal, healthy part of daily life. Stress can be a motivator, pushing us to do our best. However, excessive stress can take a physical, mental, and emotional toll, and that toll rises sharply for people with diabetes. In addition to the standard laundry list of daily stressors, people with diabetes face the added pressure of managing and monitoring blood sugar, medications, meal planning, and often multiple complications associated with the disease.

When faced with challenges, your body sets in motion a series of responses geared toward survival. The brain sends out a distress signal, the nervous system is activated, and hormones that help kick your body into high gear are released. Adrenaline, the fight-or-flight hormone, is responsible for immediate reactions that affect your breathing, muscle tension, and sweat response. Norepinephrine is another immediate responder, increasing focus and awareness.

Cortisol, also known as the stress hormone, takes minutes rather than seconds to take effect. It is responsible for helping to maintain blood pressure and fluid balance. While cortisol is vital in times of danger, persistent stress can produce chronically elevated cortisol levels, suppressing the immune system, reducing libido, and triggering acne. It is particularly problematic for people with diabetes because in times of stress you need ready access to fuel for your muscles, so cortisol triggers the release of stored glucose and blood sugar levels rise.

Elevated cortisol also elicits food cravings, so it is harder to control your intake of problematic foods. It promotes the accumulation of visceral belly fat, which, in turn, exacerbates insulin resistance. Chronically elevated cortisol is linked to depression, blood vessel constriction, and elevated blood pressure. Depression is associated with progressive insulin resistance and type 2 diabetes. High blood pressure aggravates many of the complications of diabetes, such as eye and kidney diseases. All in all, excess cortisol accelerates the progression and complications associated with diabetes.[10,11,12]

KICK DIABETES RECOMMENDATION   Reduce and manage daily stressors.

LEVEL 1: Identify the sources of excess stress in your life. Some will come from external sources, and some will stem from your own negative attitudes or stress-inducing thoughts.

LEVEL 2: Identify your current coping mechanisms and determine which are of benefit and which need to be replaced with ones that are more constructive. Consider ways that stressful situations might be avoided.

LEVEL 3: Alter, avoid, adapt, or accept your stressors. Put in place at least one new daily stress-management practice.

There are two main types of stress—acute and chronic. Acute stress is caused by a single event in your life and is short-lived, so it doesn't affect you for a long enough time to do extensive damage. Such stresses are generally an unavoidable but manageable part of life. Chronic stress results from repeated exposure to situations that cause the relentless release of stress hormones. This type of stress does the most damage because our stress-response systems were designed for occasional, rather than constant, activation. When our stress responses are chronically stimulated, all body systems are on constant overdrive.

Chronic stress often stems from issues of daily life—chaos in the home, an unhealthy relationship, or a miserable work environment. Your first order of business is to identify the sources of harmful stress. It can be helpful to keep a journal to record times of stress, what you believe caused the stress, and the response it elicited. It is easy to blame external sources, but often stress arises from our own stress-inducing negative thoughts and attitudes. In order to manage stress effectively, you need to take responsibility for your own role in fueling it.

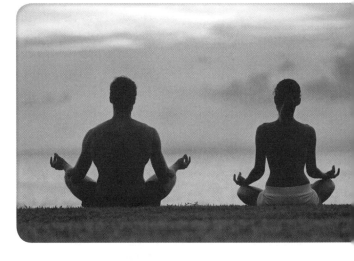

Think about how you currently manage stress and determine whether each response serves you well. Some people deal with stress by relying on addictive substances, such as alcohol, drugs, and cigarettes. These may seem to help in the moment, but the reward is short-lived and the health cost is high. A similar phenomenon occurs with emotional eating. When you deal with stress by eating foods laced with sugar, fat, and salt, your blood sugar control deteriorates, insulin sensitivity declines, and GI distress (gas, bloating, and constipation) intensifies. Whether you have an addiction to a substance or to a food, the worse you feel, the more apt you are to return to your vice, and a downward spiral ensues. Other common stress responses that do not serve you well are oversleeping or not getting enough sleep, overworking, isolating yourself from others, getting angry at others, or treating others unkindly. The best way to deal with stress is by reducing or removing its sources, learning to handle stressors in a healthy manner, doing things that take you away from the stress (even for a short period), and using techniques that build your resiliency and confidence.

No matter what the cause, effective stress-reduction strategies are a must. Get familiar with the four A's—avoid, alter, accept, and adapt—and put them into action.[13]

1. **AVOID.** Lighten your load by thinking ahead and taking ownership of your surroundings. For example, if you're bothered by long lines at your local supermarket, pick a less busy time to shop. If you're put out by the price of lunches at local restaurants, bring your own. Keep your distance from people who trigger your stress. Avoid engaging in conversations about topics that stress you out.

Don't be afraid to say no—you don't have to please everyone all the time. Prioritize your to-do list—stick to things you really want or need to do.

2. **ALTER.** Even if you can't avoid a stressor, you *can* make changes to alter the stressor. Put yourself in the driver's seat, and be assertive rather than aggressive. If the stress is induced by an individual, respectfully express your concerns to that individual. Recognize that compromise may be necessary. Work on time management to alter common daily stressors, and set limits on your time.

3. **ACCEPT.** There are occasions when you need to accept a situation as it is and learn to manage the stress it brings. You can't change the loss of a loved one, the results of the last election, or how certain people behave, but that doesn't mean your feelings aren't valid. You can accept that these things are out of your control and work on managing the stress and pain that they bring. Talk with someone you trust—a family member, friend, colleague, or professional counselor. If the situation involves anger toward someone, forgive and forget so you can move on. Think positively and talk to yourself compassionately. Don't beat yourself up about bad decisions; rather, focus on the lessons they taught you and how they have helped you make wiser decisions today.

4. **ADAPT.** Negative thoughts can add serious stress to your life. Adapting by changing your standards, attitudes, or expectations can bring tremendous relief. If you are a perfectionist, recognize that no one is ever perfect and that striving for perfection is setting yourself up for disappointment. Establish reasonable standards for yourself and for those around you. If you're in a frustrating situation, such as a traffic jam, train yourself to make the most of your time. For example, turn up the music and enjoy the alone time, listen to an engrossing audiobook, or take time to pray or meditate.

When everything seems to be going against you, think about people who are less fortunate—those who aren't sure where their next meal is coming from or whether their family will be able to escape a vicious regime. Think about the wonderful aspects of your life—where you live, your family or friends, your animal companions, or your work.

Stop yourself when you start to think negative thoughts. Adopt a positive mantra. Practice self-care. Daily exercise increases brain chemicals that generate calmness and pleasure. Exposure to warm sunshine produces vitamin D, which elevates a feel-good hormone called serotonin. Creative activities, such as playing a musical instrument, knitting, drawing, or bird-watching, can help you feel calm and collected. Mindfulness or a spiritual practice can help you put things into perspective. Whatever techniques you choose, stick to a routine. This reassures your brain that life is predictable, leading to more confidence and composure.

For some individuals, stress can be so overwhelming it can't be managed alone. In such cases a qualified therapist or counselor can help you learn to cope with stress safely and confidently and slowly build resiliency.

SOCIAL ENGAGEMENT

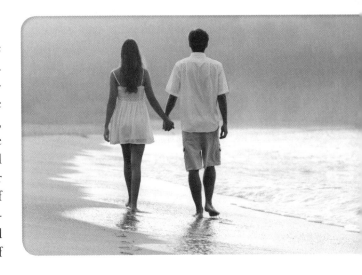

Social connectedness is a prominent feature among the world's healthiest elderly citizens. A meta-analysis of 148 studies involving over three thousand participants reported a 50 percent increase in the likelihood of survival in individuals with the strongest, healthiest social relationships. The most impressive results were for people who had a wide variety of social connections, and the most negative findings were for those who were living alone.[14] A 2018 study out of Denmark reported a 60–70 percent increase in mortality in people who were socially isolated.[15] A twofold increase in mortality was associated with a lack of involvement with clubs or organizations.

Staying socially engaged appears to be on par with other major determinants of health, such as diet, obesity, physical activity, and alcohol abuse. Establishing and maintaining meaningful relationships provides a sense of purpose and fulfillment and reduces the risk of heart disease, dementia, depression, and sleep disorders.

KICK DIABETES RECOMMENDATION   Establish and maintain strong social ties.

LEVEL 1: Purposefully reach out to family, friends, neighbors, colleagues, and others every day. Begin by consciously doing one thing a day to improve your connection with others and build from there.

LEVEL 2: Spend quality time with a cherished friend or friends at least once a week. Have at least one person in your life with whom you communicate daily or very regularly.

LEVEL 3: Increase your social involvement through organizations, volunteer groups, clubs, meetups, and hobbies. Commit to joining at least one new group and becoming an active member.

How often do you feel isolated or lonely? Who do you most love being around? How much effort do you make to nurture these relationships? How often do you see the people with whom you really want to engage? If your social life is lacking, nurture your network of family, friends, neighbors, and colleagues. This can be as simple as a warm smile and a few caring words, a thoughtful deed, or a random act of kindness. Be encouraging and express gratitude. Random acts of kindness may be even more gratifying for the person giving than those receiving. Consider ways that you can add joy to the lives of those around you. Share food that you have grown, gathered, or prepared. Offer to lend a hand to a neighbor or colleague. Let others know how much you appreciate, admire, or value them. Tell them how they inspire you, bring you joy, or make you feel loved or cared for.

Plan a get-together with friends or family at least once a week. Life is so busy; if you don't schedule time for the people who matter to you, days can slip by without any connection. Do something active if possible—a walk in the park, a game of horseshoes, or dancing. If a meal is involved, take the opportunity to share delicious, healthy food or pick a restaurant that serves healthy fare. Establish and maintain a friendship with a family member or a friend that involves a daily visit—even by phone. Select someone with whom you feel safe sharing almost anything and who offers an equal exchange of energy.

Take up a new hobby or rediscover an old one. Join a group that provides social stimulation, such as a book club, or adds exercise to the mix, such as a walking group. If you're a senior, take advantage of your local community's senior center. Become a volunteer. Get involved with literacy programs, animal shelters, soup kitchens, thrift stores, outreach for the homeless, or a foster grandparent program. Offer to help family, friends, or neighbors. Shovel a driveway, water a garden, or invite a lonely neighbor over for tea or coffee. If you enjoy being around young children, offer to babysit once a week—chasing around little ones brings joy and exercise!

When Diane was asked why she wanted to defeat diabetes, she replied, "Because I want to keep my toes, my legs, my eyes, and my kidneys. I want to be able to hike and bike and swim. I don't want to hold anyone else back. I didn't realize I had a choice, but I do now. I choose health."

When she was asked if it was hard to do, she said, "It was the hardest thing I've ever done in my life. I was hooked on foods I didn't know were addictive. It was also, by far, the most rewarding thing I've ever done in my life. Imagine trading in a death sentence—not just any death sentence . . . a slow, painful death sentence—for life, and not just any life . . . the energetic, adventurous, joyful sort of life. I miss nothing; I cherish everything that has brought me to this place."

Menu Planning

When Diane committed to a whole-foods, plant-based diet, she was worried about feeling hungry all the time. She wondered if she would have the willpower to stick with a program that would help her lose the necessary weight. Should she begin with a modified fast or a very low-calorie diet? Would she be able to hold true to such a plan? Would she have enough energy to teach school when she was depriving herself of food? Should she just follow a low-calorie diet and forget about fasting? It was all a little overwhelming.

Ultimately, Diane opted for a one-week modified fast, followed by a 1,600-calorie-per-day diet until her goal weight was reached. Her original goal was 140 pounds (63.5 kg) because she couldn't imagine ever getting below that weight. She reached her goal in five months (a loss of 28 pounds/12.7 kg) and decided to keep doing what she was doing. Within a year, she was down to 125 pounds (56.7 kg), 2 pounds (1 kg) less than she was the day she got married. She felt as though she had successfully scaled a mountain. She pictured herself, arms outstretched, at the top of a mountain with the most breathtaking views. Just thinking about it made her want to be there. So she joined a local hiking club and became a devoted member and an inspiration to the entire group.

DECISIONS, DECISIONS

Your first order of business is to establish a plan of action. This means deciding if you are willing to do a modified fast to jump-start your recovery. It's a highly recommended step, as this type of fast can hasten the reversal of diabetes by helping to reduce inflammation, oxidative stress, lipotoxicity, and glucotoxicity. There are a number of ways to accomplish this task, and your ultimate choice will depend on which feels right for you and your current lifestyle. If you are on any medications for diabetes or other conditions, you will need to work closely with your physician or health-care provider to manage those medications. Many people will either have to reduce or stop medications all together—especially diabetes, blood pressure, and lipid-lowering drugs.

Following a modified fast, your focus needs to shift to developing healthful eating patterns that you will stick with for the rest of your life. This matters even more than calories, but it is still important to produce a caloric deficit if weight loss is needed. The low-calorie, moderate-calorie, and maintenance diets are provided as a guide. They need not be rigidly adhered to, and you will have to play around with them to see what works for you. A tall, large-boned person will need more calories than a small person, so adjust the diet accordingly. If you can, practice time-restricted feeding so that you are not eating after dinner until breakfast and your body has at least twelve to fourteen hours without food in a twenty-four-hour period.

KICK DIABETES MODIFIED FASTING MENUS

If you recall, there are three types of modified fasts: time-restricted feeding, intermittent fasting, and periodic fasting (see pages 61–62). Regardless of which method suits you best, your total caloric intake will be between 600 and 1,000 calories per day, depending on your frame size, height, age, gender, and activity level. If you are small-framed, short, older, and female, you will lean toward the lower end of the range (600–700 calories per day); if you are of average build, middle-aged, and moderately active, aim for the middle of the range (800 calories per day); if you are large-framed, tall, young, and active, aim for the upper end of the range (900–1,000 calories).

Time-restricted feeding can be done at any caloric level and appears helpful whether you are on a modified fast, low-calorie diet, or maintenance program. Generally, with a modified fast, the time restriction on eating would increase. For example, on a 1,600-calorie weight-loss diet, you might fast for twelve to fourteen hours, while on a modified fast you might fast for sixteen to eighteen hours and eat only two meals a day. In this case, you could stop eating at 6:00 p.m., have your first meal of the day at 11:00 a.m., and then have your second meal at 5:00 p.m.

Intermittent fasting is an option that requires a very low-calorie intake for one to three days a week (or on alternate days). For example, you might eat 1,600 calories a day for six days of the week, and on one day of the week you would do a juice fast. This would be a 6:1 intermittent fast.

The third option is periodic fasting or modified fasting during which you might eat 1,600 calories for twenty-five days of the month and 800 calories for five days of the month. You could continue this for three cycles or until your weight goals are achieved, or you could simply do it once or twice and move to a low-calorie weight-loss diet.

There are three menus provided for the modified fasts (see table 10.1, page 16). Recipes are provided for all menus in the recipe section (chapter 12, pages 189–230). The first menu is a juice fast, so most of your calories would come from vegetable juice. This type of modified fast is best used with intermittent fasting no more than one day per week. If you are on anticoagulant medications, juicing is not recommended because of the high levels of vitamin K the juice provides (this can also apply to other foods, such as smoothies and large salads). Juices are low in protein and some other nutrients, so it's best not to be on them for extended periods of time unless you are under close medical supervision. Even when you're doing a juice fast one day a week, having one meal with Chia Pudding (page 191) is suggested to boost protein, fiber, and other nutrients.

The second menu is smoothie-based. For some individuals, doing a smoothie modified fast is appealing for convenience. It's quick and easy to prepare, so it naturally limits your time in the kitchen and your temptation around food. While smoothies can be packed with high-quality ingredients, the fiber in smoothies doesn't have the same impact on regularity as solid food. Also, liquid meals can be less satisfying. For these reasons, smoothie fasts are more appropriate as intermittent fasts just one or two days per week. To boost fiber and nutrition, make smoothie bowls (see page 195).

The third menu is based on solid foods, and this is the preferred modified fast, as fiber, protein, and nutrients are maximized. The solid-food menu provides three light meals and can be cut to two meals if preferred to allow more generous portions.

You will notice that in all menus, you start the day with Turmeric Tea Elixir (page 189). This will provide fluids and an impressive antioxidant boost. The menus are all 800 calories, so for people who need more or less, portion sizes will need to be adjusted accordingly. For 600–700 calories per day, reduce portion size by one-quarter to one-eighth. For 900–1,000 calories per day, increase portions by one-quarter to one-eighth. Food should stay consistent from day to day. Modified fasts are not meant to serve as your daily diet; instead, they help to jump-start the process of reversal and regeneration. It's not possible to meet all nutritional requirements eating only 800 calories per day, so malnutrition will result if such a diet is used for an extended period of time.

TABLE 10.1. Modified Fasting Menus

MEAL	MENU 1 VEGETABLE JUICE FAST	MENU 2 SMOOTHIE FAST	MENU 3 SOLID-FOOD FAST
Breakfast	Turmeric Tea Elixir (page 189) Chia Berry Bowl (page 191), 2 cups/500 ml	Turmeric Tea Elixir (page 189) Green Smoothie (page 194) or Green Smoothie Bowl (page 195), 16 oz/500 ml	Turmeric Tea Elixir (page 189) Green Giant Juice (page 190), 8–12 oz/250–375 ml (optional) Chia Berry Bowl (page 191), 2 cups/500 ml
Midmorning	Green Giant Juice (page 190), 16 oz/500 ml		
Lunch	Green Giant Juice (page 190), 16 oz/500 ml	Green Smoothie (page 194) or Green Smoothie Bowl (page 195), 16 oz/500 ml	Full-Meal Rainbow Salad (page 209) with balsamic vinegar, 6 cups/1.5 L
Midafternoon	Green Giant Juice (page 190), 16 oz/500 ml		
Dinner	Green Giant Juice (page 190), 16 oz/500 ml	Green Smoothie (page 194) or Green Smoothie Bowl (page 195), 16 oz/500 ml	Healing Greens, Beans, and Vegetable Soup (page 204), up to 4 cups/1 L OR Green Smoothie (page 194) or Green Smoothie Bowl (page 195), 16 oz/500 ml
Water	6–8 glasses (1.5–2 quarts/1.5–2 L) a day recommended		
Supplements	High-quality multivitamin-mineral supplement (with at least 25 mcg B_{12} and 150 mcg iodine) 300–1,000 mg EPA/DHA Vitamin B_{12} (if not 25+ mcg in the multivitamin-mineral supplement) 1,000–2,000 IU Vitamin D		

Nutritional Analysis for Modified Fast Menus

Menu 1 (Vegetable Juice Fast)

CALORIES: 802, protein: 42 g, fat: 26 g, carbohydrate: 100 g, dietary fiber: 46 g, calcium: 1625 mg, iron: 16 mg, magnesium: 347 mg, potassium: 4,798 mg, sodium: 113 mg, zinc: 5.8 mg, thiamin: 2.3 mg, riboflavin: 2.8 mg, niacin: 23 mg, folate: 595 mcg, vitamin A: 62 mcg RAE, vitamin C: 99 mg, omega-6 fatty acids: 5.6 g, omega-3 fatty acids: 12.4 g

PERCENTAGE OF CALORIES FROM: protein 21%, fat 29%, carbohydrate 50%

Menu 2 (Smoothie Fast)

CALORIES: 1,000, protein: 59 g, fat: 32 g, carbohydrate: 119 g, dietary fiber: 23 g, calcium: 1,460 mg, iron: 16 mg, magnesium: 602 mg, potassium: 3,591 mg, sodium: 344 mg, zinc: 6 mg, thiamin: 1.6 mg, riboflavin: 1 mg, niacin: 24 mg, folate: 298 mcg, vitamin A: 2,041 mcg RAE, vitamin C: 387 mg, omega-6 fatty acids: 13.4 g, omega-3 fatty acids: 4.8 g

PERCENTAGE OF CALORIES FROM: protein 23%, fat 29%, carbohydrate 48%

Menu 3 (Solid-Food Fast)

CALORIES: 999, protein: 44 g, fat: 23 g, carbohydrate: 154 g, dietary fiber: 59 g, calcium: 1,355 mg, iron: 19 mg, magnesium: 368 mg, potassium: 3,395 mg, sodium: 1,041 mg, zinc: 7.4 mg, thiamin: 1.6 mg, riboflavin: 1.6 mg, niacin: 27 mg, folate: 612 mcg, vitamin A: 3,010 mcg RAE, vitamin C: 421 mg, omega-6 fatty acids: 5.4 g, omega-3 fatty acids: 11.3 g

PERCENTAGE OF CALORIES FROM: protein 18%, fat 20%, carbohydrate 62%

KICK DIABETES WEIGHT-LOSS AND WEIGHT MAINTENANCE MENUS

The following menus are designed to provide powerful results for people with type 2 diabetes. There are seven menus, each of which supply 1,600, 1,800, or 2,000 calories (kcal), depending on the serving sizes consumed. The analyses are done using the 1,600-calorie menu, so nutrient values would be increased accordingly for higher-calorie menus. The menus are all designed to meet or exceed recommended nutrient intakes, as long as reliable sources of vitamin B_{12}, vitamin D, and iodine are provided (see page 128–129).

If you're not losing weight as expected (1–2 lbs /0.5–1 kg a week), you'll need to exercise more, if possible, or slightly reduce your calories. If you cut back to 1,200 or 1,400 calories, you may end up with nutrition shortfalls, so it is preferable to increase exercise to keep the diet nutritionally adequate in the long term. Typically, the 1,600-calorie menus are suitable for weight loss in women. The 1,800-calorie menus are suitable for weight loss in men and weight maintenance in women. The 2,000-calorie menu is suitable for weight maintenance in men. Of course, there are variations in individual need, so adjust accordingly. If you're using a multivitamin-mineral supplement, choose one that includes vitamins B_{12} and D and iodine.

The analyses were done using unsweetened fortified soymilk, which is higher in protein than other nondairy milks. Other unsweetened nondairy milks are lower in calories. In order to provide suggestions for various individuals, each of the seven menus reflects a different eating style (see table 10.2, page 168). You don't have to follow each day in order, and you can use leftovers for the next day. Each day can be used as a template to design similar menus suited to your eating style.

TABLE 10.2. Seven Days of Meals at a Glance

DAY OF THE WEEK	BREAKFAST	LUNCH	DINNER
Monday A+ Alice	Turmeric Tea Elixir (page 189) Whole-Food Breakfast Bowl (page 196) Omega-3-Rich Seed Mix (page 197) unsweetened nondairy milk	Full-Meal Rainbow Salad (page 209) Liquid Gold Dressing (page 221) fresh fruit	Big Green Power Bowl (page 224) Lemon-Tahini Dressing (page 219) fresh fruit
Tuesday Easy Ed	Turmeric Tea Elixir (page 189) Berry Burst Muesli (page 198) ground flaxseeds unsweetened nondairy milk	Healing Greens, Beans, and Vegetable Soup (page 204) Ezekiel Nut Butter and Banana Wrap (page 202)	Black Bean Stuffed Sweet Potato (page 225) Power Greens Salad (page 210) Cheezy Roasted Red Pepper Dressing (page 220) fresh fruit
Wednesday Adventurous Annie	Turmeric Tea Elixir (page 189) Green Smoothie Bowl (page 195)	Power Greens Salad (page 210) Creamy Dill Dressing (page 218) fresh fruit	Gado Gado (page 226) Fruit with Pear Cream (page 192) or unsweetened nondairy yogurt
Thursday Picky Pete	Turmeric Tea Elixir (page 189) Ezekiel Nut Butter and Banana Wrap (page 202) Chia Berry Bowl (page 191)	Old-Fashioned Split Pea Soup (page 206) Cheezy Kale Chips (page 223) raw veggies Creamy Dill Dip (page 218)	Old-Fashioned Bean and Vegetable Stew (page 229) fresh fruit
Friday Spicy Sam	Turmeric Tea Elixir (page 189) Spiced Creamy Barley Bowl (page 199) Very Berry Sauce (page 193) Omega-3-Rich Seed Mix (page 197) unsweetened nondairy milk	Smokin' Lentil Soup (page 205) Cauliflower and Red Quinoa Salad (page 211) fresh fruit	Moroccan Stew (page 227) fresh fruit with Pear Cream (page 192)
Saturday Cozy Rosie	Turmeric Tea Elixir (page 189) Apple Pie Oats (page 200) Omega-3-Rich Seed Mix (page 197) unsweetened nondairy milk	Curry in a Hurry Soup (page 208) Carrot-Raisin Salad (page 213)	Fettuccine Alfredo (page 228) Whole-Food Caesar Salad (page 214) Nut Parmesan (page 216) fresh fruit

DAY OF THE WEEK	BREAKFAST	LUNCH	DINNER
Sunday Foodie Judy	Turmeric Tea Elixir (page 189) Indian Breakfast Lentils (page 201) fresh fruit, chopped Omega-3-Rich Seed Mix (page 197) unsweetened nondairy milk	Queen of Greens Soup (page 207) Chickpea Salad in Endive or Radicchio Cups (page 212) or in a sprouted-grain wrap	Swiss-Style Tofu (page 230) roasted butternut squash steamed broccoli, broccolini, or Brussels sprouts Cheezy Roasted Red Pepper Dressing (page 220) to top veggies

Menu 1 – Monday: A+ Alice

This menu highlights a practically perfect plant-based day. It's jam-packed with fiber, phytochemicals, antioxidants, and plant sterols from a beautiful variety of whole foods. This menu could serve as your everyday template. Add variety by changing up your vegetables, fruits, grains, legumes, nuts, and seeds.

MEAL	FOOD	SERVING SIZE		
		1,600 KCAL	1,800 KCAL	2,000 KCAL
Breakfast	Turmeric Tea Elixir (page 189)	1½ cups (375 ml)	1½ cups (375 ml)	1½ cups (375 ml)
	Whole-Food Breakfast Bowl (page 196)	2 cups (500 ml)	2½ cups (625 ml)	3 cups (750 ml)
	Omega-3-Rich Seed Mix (page 197)	2 Tbsp (30 ml)	2 Tbsp (30 ml)	3 Tbsp (45 ml)
	Unsweetened nondairy milk	1 cup (250 ml)	1¼ cups (310 ml)	1½ cups (375 ml)
Lunch	Full-Meal Rainbow Salad (page 209)	4 cups (1 L)	5 cups (1.25 L)	6 cups (1.5)
	Liquid Gold Dressing (page 221)	3 Tbsp (45 ml)	¼ cup (60 ml)	5 Tbsp (75 ml)
	Fresh fruit	1 medium	1 medium	1 medium
Dinner	Big Green Power Bowl (page 224)	3 cups (750 ml)	3½ cups (875 ml)	4 cups (1 L)
	Lemon-Tahini Dressing (page 219)	3 Tbsp (45 ml)	¼ cup (60 ml)	5 Tbsp (75 ml)
	Fresh fruit	1 medium	1 medium	1 medium

NUTRITIONAL ANALYSIS FOR 1,600 CALORIE MENU: calories: 1,627, protein: 61 g, fat: 39 g, carbohydrate: 258 g, dietary fiber: 70 g, calcium: 1,239 mg, iron: 24 mg, magnesium: 480 mg, potassium: 5,105 mg, sodium: 747 mg, zinc: 8 mg, thiamin: 1.7 mg, riboflavin: 1.6 mg, niacin: 22 mg, folate: 777 mcg, vitamin A: 2,851 mcg RAE, vitamin C: 786 mg, omega-6 fatty acids: 9.5 g, omega-3 fatty acids: 5.7 g

PERCENTAGE OF CALORIES FROM: protein 15%, fat 22%, carbohydrate 63%

Menu 2 – Tuesday: Easy Ed

This menu is an almost-instant day, with minimal food preparation required. It can be used on days you don't have time to cook or as a template for those who don't like to cook.

MEAL	FOOD	SERVING SIZE		
		1,600 KCAL	1,800 KCAL	2,000 KCAL
Breakfast	Turmeric Tea Elixir (page 189)	1½ cups (375 ml)	1½ cups (375 ml)	1½ cups (375 ml)
	Berry Burst Muesli (page 198)	2 cups (500 ml)	2 cups (500 ml)	2½ cups (625 ml)
	Ground flaxseeds	1 Tbsp (15 ml)	1 Tbsp (15 ml)	1½ Tbsp (22 ml)
	Unsweetened nondairy milk	1 cup (250 ml)	1 cup (250 ml)	1¼ cups (310 ml)
Lunch	Healing Greens, Beans, and Vegetable Soup (page 204)	2 cups (500 ml)	2 cups (500 ml)	2 cups (500 ml)
	Ezekiel Nut Butter and Banana Wrap (page 202)	1 wrap; 1 small banana; 2 Tbsp (30 ml) nut butter; 1 Tbsp (15 ml) seed mix	1 wrap; 1 small banana; 2 Tbsp (30 ml) nut butter; 1 Tbsp (15 ml) seed mix	1 wrap; 1 medium banana; 3 Tbsp (45 ml) nut butter; 2 Tbsp (30 ml) seed mix
Dinner	Black Bean Stuffed Sweet Potato (page 225)	1 small potato; ¾ cup (185 ml) beans; ¼ cup (60 ml) corn; ½ cup (125 ml) salsa; ¼ sliced avocado	1 medium potato; 1 cup (250 ml) beans; ⅓ cup (85 ml) corn; ¾ cup (185 ml) salsa; ⅓ sliced avocado	1 large potato; 1 cup (250 ml) beans; ⅓ cup (85 ml) corn; ¾ cup (185 ml) salsa; ⅓ sliced avocado
	Power Greens Salad (page 210)	3 cups (750 ml)	3 cups (750 ml)	3 cups (750 ml)
	Cheezy Roasted Red Pepper Dressing (page 220)	3 Tbsp (45 ml)	3 Tbsp (45 ml)	¼ cup (60 ml)
	Fresh fruit	1 medium	1 medium	1 medium

NUTRITIONAL ANALYSIS FOR 1,600 CALORIE MENU: calories: 1,600, protein: 55 g, fat: 52 g, carbohydrate: 228 g, dietary fiber: 54 g, calcium: 757 mg, iron: 17 mg, magnesium: 320 mg, potassium: 2,654 mg, sodium: 937 mg, zinc: 8 mg, thiamin: 1.1 mg, riboflavin: 1 mg, niacin: 16 mg, folate: 354 mcg, vitamin A: 1,904 mcg RAE, vitamin C: 247 mg, omega-6 fatty acids: 6.9 g, omega-3 fatty acids: 5.9 g

PERCENTAGE OF CALORIES FROM: protein 14%, fat 29%, carbohydrate 57%

Menu 3 – Wednesday: Adventurous Annie

This menu provides some novel options for the more adventurous eater. Lunch is portable, so it's great for people who are heading to work or spending time outdoors. Green smoothie bowls are a delicious way to weave some greens into your day.

MEAL	FOOD	SERVING SIZE		
		1,600 KCAL	**1,800 KCAL**	**2,000 KCAL**
Breakfast	Turmeric Tea Elixir (page 189)	1½ cups (375 ml)	1½ cups (375 ml)	1½ cups (375 ml)
	Green Smoothie Bowl (page 195)	2 cups (500 ml); 1 cup (250 ml) fruit; ¼ cup (60 ml) grains; 2 Tbsp (30 ml) seeds	2½ cups (375 ml); 1 cup (250 ml) fruit; ¼ cup (60 ml) grains; 3 Tbsp (45 ml) seeds	3 cups (750 ml); 1 cup (250 ml) fruit; ¼ cup (60 ml) grains; 3 Tbsp (45 ml) seeds
Lunch	Power Greens Salad (page 210) with beans and butternut squash	4 cups (1 L) salad; ⅔ cup (165 ml) beans; ½ cup (125 ml) butternut squash	4 cups (1 L) salad; ¾ cup (185 ml) beans; ⅔ cup (165 ml) butternut squash	4 cups (1 L) salad; 1 cup (250 ml) beans; ¾ cup (185 ml) butternut squash
	Creamy Dill Dressing (page 218)	¼ cup (60 ml)	¼ cup (60 ml)	¼ cup (60 ml)
	Fresh fruit	1 medium	1 medium	1 medium
Dinner	Gado Gado (page 226)	4 cups (1 L)	5 cups (1.25 L)	6 cups (1.5 L)
	Gado Gado Sauce (page 222)	¼ cup (60 ml)	⅓ cup (85 ml)	½ cup (125 ml)
	Fruit with Pear Cream (page 192) or unsweetened nondairy yogurt	1 cup (250 ml) fruit; 2 Tbsp (30 ml) Pear Cream or ¼ cup (60 ml) unsweetened nondairy yogurt	1 cup (250 ml) fruit; 3 Tbsp (45 ml) Pear Cream or ⅓ cup (85 ml) unsweetened nondairy yogurt	1 cup (250 ml) fruit; ¼ cup (60 ml) Pear Cream or ½ cup (125 ml) unsweetened nondairy yogurt

NUTRITIONAL ANALYSIS FOR 1,600 CALORIE MENU: calories: 1,634, protein: 80 g, fat: 42 g, carbohydrate: 234 g, dietary fiber: 59 g, calcium: 1,545 mg, iron: 28 mg, magnesium: 813 mg, potassium: 6,287 mg, sodium: 1,349 mg, zinc: 11 mg, thiamin: 2.1 mg, riboflavin: 1.8 mg, niacin: 33 mg, folate: 924 mcg, vitamin A: 4,672 mcg RAE, vitamin C: 647 mg, omega-6 fatty acids: 14 g, omega-3 fatty acids: 4 g

PERCENTAGE OF CALORIES FROM: protein 20%, fat 23%, carbohydrate 57%

Menu 4 – Thursday: Picky Pete

This menu is designed for either the picky or more traditional eater who may not be thrilled by salads. While it is important to gradually build up a taste for leafy greens, adding cooked greens to familiar dishes can be a reasonable stepping-stone.

MEAL	FOOD	SERVING SIZE		
		1,600 KCAL	1,800 KCAL	2,000 KCAL
Breakfast	Turmeric Tea Elixir (page 189)	1½ cups (375 ml)	1½ cups (375 ml)	1½ cups (375 ml)
	Ezekiel Nut Butter and Banana Wrap (page 202)	1 wrap; 1 small banana; 2 Tbsp (30 ml) nut butter; 1 Tbsp (15 ml) seed mix	1 wrap; 1 small banana; 2 Tbsp (30 ml) nut butter; 1 Tbsp (15 ml) seed mix	1 wrap; 1 medium banana; 3 Tbsp (45 ml) nut butter; 2 Tbsp (30 ml) seed mix
	Chia Berry Bowl (page 191)	1 cup (250 ml) berries; 2 Tbsp (30 ml) Pear Cream or ¼ cup (60 ml) unsweetened nondairy yogurt	1 cup (250 ml) berries; 3 Tbsp (45 ml) Pear Cream or ⅓ cup (85 ml) unsweetened nondairy yogurt	1 cup (250 ml) berries; ¼ cup (60 ml) Pear Cream or ½ cup (125 ml) unsweetened nondairy yogurt
Lunch	Old-Fashioned Split Pea Soup (page 206)	1½ cups (325 ml)	2 cups (500 ml)	2 cups (500 ml)
	Cheezy Kale Chips (page 223)	1 cup (250 ml)	1 cup (250 ml)	1 cup (250 ml)
	Raw veggies	3 cups (750 ml)	3 cups (750 ml)	3 cups (750 ml)
	Creamy Dill Dip (page 218)	3 Tbsp (45 ml)	¼ cup (60 ml)	¼ cup (60 ml)
Dinner	Old-Fashioned Bean and Vegetable Stew (page 229)	2½ cups (625 ml)	3 cups (750 ml)	3½ cups (875 ml)
	Fresh fruit	1 medium	1 medium	1 medium

NUTRITIONAL ANALYSIS FOR 1,600 CALORIE MENU: calories: 1,629, protein: 65 g, fat: 41 g, carbohydrate: 250 g, dietary fiber: 70 g, calcium: 695 mg, iron: 17 mg, magnesium: 466 mg, potassium: 4,187 mg, sodium: 1,621 mg, zinc: 9 mg, thiamin: 1.6 mg, riboflavin: 1.1 mg, niacin: 22.4 mg, folate: 681 mcg, vitamin A: 2,103 mcg RAE, vitamin C: 486 mg, omega-6 fatty acids: 5 g, omega-3 fatty acids: 3 g

PERCENTAGE OF CALORIES FROM: protein 16%, fat 23%, carbohydrate 61%

Menu 5: Spicy Sam

This menu is simple and flavorful. If you prefer your food on the milder side, decrease the spices in these recipes to suit your taste.

MEAL	FOOD	SERVING SIZE		
		1,600 KCAL	1,800 KCAL	2,000 KCAL
Breakfast	Turmeric Tea Elixir (page 189)	1½ cups (375 ml)	1½ cups (375 ml)	1½ cups (375 ml)
	Spiced Creamy Barley Bowl (page 199)	1 cup (250 ml)	1¼ cups (310 ml)	1½ cups (375 ml)
	Very Berry Sauce (page 193)	½ cup (125 ml)	⅔ cup (165 ml)	¾ cup (185 ml)
	Omega-3-Rich Seed Mix (page 197)	2 Tbsp (30 ml)	2 Tbsp (30 ml)	3 Tbsp (45 ml)
	Fresh fruit	1 cup (250 ml)	1½ cups (375 ml)	2 cups (500 ml)
Lunch	Smokin' Lentil Soup (page 205)	1½ cups (375 ml)	1¾ cups (435 ml)	2 cups (500 ml)
	Cauliflower and Red Quinoa Salad (page 211)	2 cups (500 ml)	2½ cups (625 ml)	3 cups (750 ml)
	Fresh fruit	1 medium	1 medium	1 medium
Dinner	Moroccan Stew (page 227)	2½ cups (625 ml)	3 cups (750 ml)	3½ cups (875 ml)
	Fresh fruit with Pear Cream (page 192)	½ cup (125 ml) fruit; 2 Tbsp (30 ml) Pear Cream	¾ cup (185 ml) fruit; 3 Tbsp (45 ml) Pear Cream	1 cup (250 ml) fruit; 3 Tbsp (45 ml) Pear Cream

NUTRITIONAL ANALYSIS FOR 1,600 CALORIE MENU: calories: 1,590, protein: 64 g, fat: 34 g, carbohydrate: 257 g, dietary fiber: 74 g, calcium: 829 mg, iron: 23 mg, magnesium: 484 mg, potassium: 4,517 mg, sodium: 1,377 mg, zinc: 10 mg, thiamin: 1.7 mg, riboflavin: 1.2 mg, niacin: 21 mg, folate: 776 mcg, vitamin A: 1,664 mcg RAE, vitamin C: 502 mg, omega-6 fatty acids: 7 g, omega-3 fatty acids: 4.5 g

PERCENTAGE OF CALORIES FROM: protein 16%, fat 19%, carbohydrate 65%

Menu 6: Cozy Rosie

This menu is filled with comfort food for the days you crave traditional flavors. These recipes were inspired by less-healthful fare but were reinvented to be 100 percent health-supporting!

MEAL	FOOD	SERVING SIZE		
		1,600 KCAL	**1,800 KCAL**	**2,000 KCAL**
Breakfast	Turmeric Tea Elixir (page 189)	1½ cups (375 ml)	1½ cups (375 ml)	1½ cups (375 ml)
	Apple Pie Oats (page 200)	1 cup (250 ml)	1¼ cups (310 ml)	1½ cups (375 ml)
	Unsweetened nondairy milk	½ cup (125 ml)	¾ cup (185 ml)	1 cup (250 ml)
	Omega-3-Rich Seed Mix (page 197)	1 Tbsp (15 ml)	1½ Tbsp (22 ml)	2 Tbsp (30 ml)
Lunch	Curry in a Hurry Soup (page 208)	2 cups (500 ml)	2 cups (500 ml)	2 cups (500 ml)
	Carrot-Raisin Salad (page 213)	¾ cup (185 ml)	1 cup (250 ml)	1½ cup (375 ml)
Dinner	Fettuccine Alfredo (page 228)	2 cups (500 ml)	2½ cups (625 ml)	3 cups (750 ml)
	Nut Parmesan (page 216)	1 Tbsp (15 ml)	1½ Tbsp (22 ml)	2 Tbsp (30 ml)
	Whole-Food Caesar Salad (page 214)	3 cups (750 ml)	3 cups (750 ml)	3 cups (750 ml)
	Caesar Salad Dressing (page 217)	3 Tbsp (45 ml)	3 Tbsp (45 ml)	3 Tbsp (45 ml)
	Fresh fruit	1 medium	1 medium	1 medium

NUTRITIONAL ANALYSIS FOR 1,600 CALORIE MENU: calories: 1,600, protein: 84 g, fat: 40 g, carbohydrate: 226 g, dietary fiber: 59 g, calcium: 1,023 mg, iron: 27 mg, magnesium: 316 mg, potassium: 5,071 mg, sodium: 1,557 mg, zinc: 7 mg, thiamin: 1.6 mg, riboflavin: 1.2 mg, niacin: 12 mg, folate: 372 mcg, vitamin A: 2,563 mcg RAE, vitamin C: 319 mg, omega-6 fatty acids: 4.2 g, omega-3 fatty acids: 2.1 g

PERCENTAGE OF CALORIES FROM: protein 21%, fat 22%, carbohydrate 57%

Menu 7: Foodie Judy

This flavor-filled menu has a gourmet touch. You will need to allow a little extra time to prepare these meals.

MEAL	FOOD	SERVING SIZE		
		1,600 KCAL	1,800 KCAL	2,000 KCAL
Breakfast	Turmeric Tea Elixir (page 189)	1½ cups (375 ml)	1½ cups (375 ml)	1½ cups (375 ml)
	Indian Breakfast Lentils (page 201)	1 cup (250 ml)	1¼ cups (310 ml)	1½ cups (375 ml)
	Fresh fruit, chopped	1 cup (250 ml)	1 cup (250 ml)	1 cup (250 ml)
	Omega-3-Rich Seed Mix (page 197)	1 Tbsp (15 ml)	1½ Tbsp (22 ml)	2 Tbsp (30 ml)
	Unsweetened nondairy milk	½ cup (125 ml)	¾ cup (185 ml)	1 cup (250 ml)
Lunch	Queen of Greens Soup (page 207)	1½ cups (375 ml)	1¾ cups (435 ml)	2 cups (500 ml)
	Chickpea Salad in Endive or Radicchio Cups (page 212) or in a sprouted-grain wrap	2 cups (500 ml)	2 cups (500 ml)	2 cups (500 ml)
Dinner	Swiss-Style Tofu (page 230)	1 piece	1½ pieces	2 pieces
	Baked butternut squash	¾ cup (185 ml)	1 cup (250 ml)	1 cup (250 ml)
	Steamed broccoli, broccolini, or Brussels sprouts	2 cups (500 ml)	2 cups (500 ml)	2 cups (500 ml)
	Cheezy Roasted Red Pepper Dressing (page 220) to top veggies	2 Tbsp (30 ml)	3 Tbsp (45 ml)	4 Tbsp (60 ml)

NUTRITIONAL ANALYSIS FOR 1,600 CALORIE MENU: calories: 1,607, protein: 81 g, fat: 39 g, carbohydrate: 233 g, dietary fiber: 65 g, calcium: 1,494 mg, iron: 25 mg, magnesium: 456 mg, potassium: 5,112 mg, sodium: 1,722 mg, zinc: 11 mg, thiamin: 2 mg, riboflavin: 1.4 mg, niacin: 26 mg, folate: 714 mcg, vitamin A: 1,333 mcg RAE, vitamin C: 533 mg, omega-6 fatty acids: 12 g, omega-3 fatty acids: 2.5 g

PERCENTAGE OF CALORIES FROM: protein 20%, fat 22%, carbohydrate 58%

MEAL TIMING AND FREQUENCY

Regular mealtimes are important because they help stabilize blood sugars, control appetite, and achieve weight loss. If you put time and thought into planning meals, they tend to be more balanced. With less preparation, there's more of a tendency to eat too much and too quickly.

Ideally, eat your first meal within an hour or two of getting up in the morning. Other meals can be eaten about every four to six hours after that. If you aren't taking diabetes medications or insulin, how often you eat and when you eat are matters of personal preference, as long as you eat healthy foods in reasonable quantities. The important thing is what works for *you*. Some people love a hearty breakfast, while others have limited appetite before noon and a light breakfast works best. Consistency from day to day is what matters.

Regardless of meal timing, learning to recognize and respect hunger is vital to weight management. Avoid overeating or depriving yourself when you're famished. If you think you're hungry, drink a glass of water, then wait fifteen minutes to ensure that you're not mistaking thirst for hunger. If you're really hungry, have a piece of fruit with 2 teaspoons (10 ml) of nut butter or some raw vegetables and hummus. If feelings of hunger are triggered by emotions, explore ways you could respond differently to emotional challenges. For example, if sadness triggers eating, talk to someone or write in your journal. If stress triggers your hunger, go for a long walk, do some deep breathing, or have a bubble bath. If anger triggers your hunger, write a letter to the editor, take it out on a punching bag, or a stomp around the block. If your hunger is linked to environmental stimulants, like the donuts brought into the office, do what you can to transform your environment. Challenge your colleagues to bring in healthier snacks, and lead the charge by bringing in healthy treats, such as kale chips or fresh fruit.

Chapter 11

Whole-Food, Plant-Based Cooking Basics

Diane always considered herself a good cook, and she relished getting into the kitchen and creating a meal. Whether it was simple, everyday food or a gourmet meal for guests, cooking provided stress relief, giving her a chance to unwind. But whole-food, plant-based cooking was unfamiliar territory, and at first she was fumbling. She quickly decided that if plant-based living was to be her new reality, she would do whatever it took to master the art. Her goals went beyond her own health; she wanted to acquire sufficient skill to be able to help others find their way around a plant-based kitchen. Diane signed up for an online whole-food, plant-based cooking course and was smitten with the culinary possibilities it revealed. When she began her journey with a whole-food, plant-based diet, she reconciled herself to a life of culinary deprivation. It felt like punishment for years of overindulgence. But as she progressed with her gastronomic adventure, her biggest surprise was how much she enjoyed the food. She wouldn't trade her new cuisine for her old cuisine for all the tea in China. The experience gave her the courage and confidence she needed to start her plant-based support group.

If you're not used to cooking beans, grains, and vegetables—or doing any cooking from scratch—this preface to the recipes will help get you started on your culinary journey. Even if you're highly skilled in the kitchen, you may be unfamiliar with some of the unique techniques used in whole-food, plant-based cuisine. Be sure to check out the tables for cooking legumes (page 182) and cooking grains (page 186). These handy guides will be your go-to references throughout your plant-based cooking experience.

Before beginning your whole-foods, plant-based culinary adventure, do a kitchen audit and make any necessary adjustments. This will save you time and frustration as you dive into the recipes. This will save you time and frustration.

Gather the essential kitchen equipment. This means having a good chef's knife, a paring knife, a cutting board, mixing bowls, measuring spoons and cups, pots, pans, and baking sheets. Consider investing in a heavy-duty, high-speed blender and a food processor. These will help you prepare dressings, frozen-fruit ice cream, spreads, and sauces in a jiffy. A multipurpose, programmable pressure cooker makes cooking beans a breeze.

Determine the best ways to acquire health-supportive foods in your area. You may find local farmers' markets, organic delivery services, co-ops, bulk stores, buying clubs, international stores, or natural food stores that you can frequent. Consider planting a garden or growing sprouts or herbs at home. For items that are difficult to source locally, seek out great sources online. Stock your pantry well so you are set for food prep. Learn to read labels; compare the total fat, saturated fat, fiber, and sugar content of packaged foods.

Take a plant-based cooking class. Make it a high priority to explore what is available locally or online. A cooking school specializing in plant-based whole foods will familiarize you with ingredients, recipes, and flavor combinations to help you replace favorite comfort foods and broaden your culinary horizons.

Find resources that keep your creative juices flowing. Cookbooks, magazines, websites, and videos can inspire and motivate you to try new things. Embrace the adventure.

Surround yourself with other people who eat plant-based diets. One fundamental requirement for success is gathering a tribe that supports you in your transition. Look for plant-based groups and events in your area. If sources are few and far between, find support online.

GET ORGANIZED FOR COOKING

S ome rudimentary organizational skills can maximize your productivity and efficiency in the kitchen. The following steps can help you attain positive results when using this book and have a more enjoyable experience in the kitchen:

1. Read the recipe before starting.
2. Gather all the needed equipment and ingredients.
3. Set up your counter space. Arrange and organize the ingredients and equipment according to which items you'll use first. If you're short on counter space, consider bringing a small portable table or island on wheels into the kitchen when you need an additional surface on which to organize and prepare ingredients.

EQUIPMENT TO SUPPORT YOUR SUCCESS

Consider kitchen equipment an investment in your health. Working with good equipment of any kind will make you feel capable and will increase your willingness to perform the task at hand. Following is a basic inventory of the tools you will need to prepare all the recipes in this book. Feel free to begin with just a few of these items (you may already have many of them in your kitchen) and add to your collection once you gain experience.

COOKING UTENSILS

- Baking dish, 13 x 9 inches (33 x 23 cm) and 8-inch (20-cm) square
- Baking sheets, 2
- Muffin pan (standard 12-cup pan)
- Loaf pans, 2 medium (6-cup/1.5-L capacity)
- Nonstick frying pan, skillet, saucepan
- Pots with lids, 3 (small, medium, and large)
- Skillets, 2 (small and large)
- Steamer basket
- Stockpot with lid (12 quart/36 L)

ELECTRIC APPLIANCES

- Blender, high-speed
- Juicer
- Food processor
- Multipurpose pressure cooker and slow cooker (such as an Instant pot) or stand-alone slow cooker

HANDHELD TOOLS

- Can opener
- Garlic press
- Pancake turner (metal spatula)
- Rubber spatulas, 3 (small, medium, and large)
- Slotted spoon
- Soup ladle
- Spring-loaded tongs
- Vegetable peeler
- Vegetable scrub brush

- Whisks, 2 (small and medium)
- Wooden spoons, 2

KNIVES

- Chef's knife (10 inch/25 cm)
- Paring knife

MISCELLANEOUS

- Colander
- Cutting boards, 2 (large and small)
- Food grater
- Funnels, 2 (small and medium)
- Measuring cup set
- Measuring spoon set
- Mixing bowls, 3 (small, medium, and large)
- Silicone baking mats, 2, or parchment paper

STORAGE ITEMS

- Canisters and jars for grains, legumes, and other dry goods
- Glass freezer containers
- Storage containers with lids in many sizes

INFO ON INGREDIENTS

Salty Seasonings and Sodium

People who have diabetes need to limit the amount of sodium in the foods they eat. These recipes have been carefully designed to have moderate or minimal amounts of sodium.

For people who want to further reduce their sodium intake (such as those who have hypertension), the following adjustments can be made:

- Use salt-free or low-sodium vegetable broth or substitute water for vegetable broth.
- When there's a range of salty seasonings (salt, tamari, miso, Bragg Liquid Aminos, or soy sauce) to choose from, select the option with the lowest sodium content or omit it altogether.
- Check labels on jarred and canned foods. Choose salt-free or low-sodium products.
- Omit salty additions and increase the amounts of herbs and other salt-free seasonings. Also add a squeeze of lemon or lime juice just before serving.

Sautéing Liquid

Water is always a good option for sautéing, especially with health-supportive herbs and spices added to it. Be selective with broths, as some instant powders or cubes contain unwelcome fats and are very high in sodium. Check package labels. Some packaged broths sold in shelf-stable cartons are based on only vegetables and seasonings. Miso can replace broth; just add 1–3 teaspoons (5–15 ml) per cup (250 ml) of water. Finally, a splash of wine can add lovely flavor to sauces and gravies.

FIVE SHORTCUTS TO MAKE MEAL PREP A SNAP

1. **Batch cook.** On the weekends, cook one pot of beans and another of grains. Prepare a giant undressed salad, bake some sweet potatoes or squash, steam some veggies, throw together Chia Pudding (page 191), and stew some fruit. With these staples ready to go in your fridge, making your breakfast bowl, full-meal salad, or dinner bowl will be a breeze.

2. **Double or triple recipes.** When you discover favorite recipes, make enough to freeze leftovers for quick meals when life gets busy. This is especially helpful for labor-intensive dishes, such as lasagna or loaves.

3. **Soak beans and grains for faster cooking.** To decrease cooking time and increase the digestibility of beans and grains, soak them in advance.

4. **Prep veggies.** Although you don't need to prep all your veggies in advance of using them (as doing so will hasten their demise), prepping some of them will make mealtime planning go a lot faster. Before putting produce in the refrigerator when you get home from the market (or when your bin arrives on your doorstep), immediately prepare a salad that will last a few days. It helps to have a variety of glass storage bowls with lids. Wash greens and put them in storage containers for quick use in dinner bowls and smoothies. Cut up other veggies that you know you'll use within a day or two.

5. **Organize your kitchen equipment for easy use.** Keep your high-speed blender, food processor, and multipurpose pot within quick reach. Arrange your knives and other kitchen tools in a way that makes them instantly accessible. When getting out the necessary tools is easy, you'll be more apt to use them.

PANTRY BASICS

The following list of pantry basics takes you beyond the obvious perishables you need (see pages 183–184). It provides a convenient resource that itemizes both the staples used in our recipes and the ingredients that may be used only occasionally or for recipe variations. **The ingredients in bold are staples in whole-foods, plant-based diets. Those that are accompanied by an asterisk can also be purchased frozen for convenience.** Be sure that they are unsweetened. Start by purchasing your staples and then buy other ingredients that are specific to the recipes you'd like to try. You will not purchase all of the bolded fruits and vegetables at once, however. For example, one week you may purchase broccoli and another week you might purchase cauliflower. Not all of the items listed are essential, and many can be substituted for similar products depending on availability, your preferences, and price.

You may want to photocopy this list and include additional items of your own. Be open to unfamiliar foods. Buy fresh produce as needed and in season and organic and local produce when you can. Dry ingredients can be purchased in appropriate amounts and stored in sealed containers in a cool, dry place. Most are best used within a year, although many items will keep longer. For the best prices, look for sources that offer grains and legumes in bulk. International grocery stores and the international sections of supermarkets and natural food stores are often good places to find unfamiliar ingredients.

COOKING LEGUMES

It's both practical and economical to cook legumes (beans, peas, and lentils) in quantity so you'll have different types on hand whenever you want them. Freeze individual or meal-sized portions of cooked legumes in labeled containers for up to six months.

One option is to invest in a multipurpose, programmable pressure cooker and follow the manufacturer's instructions for cooking legumes. A regular pressure cooker, slow cooker, or stove top are other good choices. Avoid a slow cooker for kidney beans because temperatures may not be high enough to destroy the lectins in the beans. Kidney beans need about thirty minutes of boiling to destroy these toxins and longer to cook thoroughly. Here are basic guidelines for the preparation of dried beans:

1. **CLEAN THE BEANS.** Spread the beans on a tray so you can easily see any small rocks, twigs, or other debris that might have come through the mechanical cleaning process. Put the beans in a colander or strainer and rinse them under cold water to remove any dirt.

TABLE 11.1. Pantry Staples

VEGETABLES (FRESH OR FROZEN*)			
Arugula	Celery	Mushrooms	Rutabaga
Asparagus	Chiles (jalapeño)	Mustard greens	**Salad greens (prewashed wild or power greens, dark green lettuces)**
Avocados	**Chiles, hot (green, orange, red)**	**Onions (green, red, white, yellow)**	
Beans (green, yellow)*	Chives	**Parsley**	**Spinach***
Beet greens	**Collard greens**	Parsnips	**Sprouts (alfalfa, lentil, mung, pea, sunflower)**
Beets (purple, yellow)	**Corn (fresh or frozen kernels)***	**Peas (green, snow, sugar snap)***	**Sweet potatoes**
Bok choy			
Broccoli*	**Cucumbers**	**Peppers, sweet bell (green, orange, red, yellow)**	**Tomatoes (cherry, salad)**
Broccolini	**Garlic**	Potatoes (purple, red, white)	Turnip greens
Cabbage (Chinese, green, napa, red/purple)	**Ginger**	Pumpkin	Turnips (young)
Carrots (orange, purple, yellow)	Jicama	Radicchio	**Winter squash**
	Kale*	Radishes (red, watermelon)	Yams
Cauliflower	Kohlrabi		**Zucchini**

FRUITS (FRESH OR FROZEN*)			
Apples	Cherries*	Nectarines	Pomegranates
Applesauce	Grapefruit	**Oranges**	**Raspberries***
Apricots	Grapes	Papayas	**Strawberries***
Bananas	**Lemons**	Peaches	
Blackberries	**Limes**	Pineapples*	
Blueberries*	Mangoes*	Plums	

FRUITS (DRIED)			
Apricots	Currants	Pears	
Cherries	**Dates**	Prunes	
Coconut (unsweetened shredded dried)	Mangoes	**Raisins**	
	Peaches		

LEGUMES (DRIED OR CANNED)			
Adzuki beans	Great Northern beans	Mung beans	Red beans
Black beans	**Kidney beans (red, white)**	Navy beans	Split peas (green, yellow)
Cannellini beans	**Lentils (green, red)**	Pink beans	White beans
Chickpeas (garbanzo beans)	Lima beans	**Pinto beans**	

GRAINS AND GRAIN PRODUCTS

Barley (whole-grain hulled, pot, scotch)	**Kamut or spelt berries**	**Oats (old-fashioned rolled)**	Rice (brown, brown basmati)
Cornmeal, coarsely ground	Millet	**Oats, steel cut**	Wild rice
	Oat groats	**Quinoa**	

NONDAIRY ALTERNATIVES

Nondairy milk, unsweetened (almond, cashew, hemp, rice, soy)

Nondairy yogurt, unsweetened

NUTS, SEEDS, BUTTERS

Almond butter	**Chia seeds**	Macadamia nuts	Sesame seeds
Almonds	**Flaxseeds (whole or ground)**	**Peanut butter**	**Sunflower seeds**
Brazil nuts	Hazelnuts	Pecans	**Tahini**
Cashew butter	**Hemp seeds**	Pine nuts	**Walnuts**
Cashews		**Pumpkin seeds**	

HERBS AND SPICES

Allspice (ground)	Cumin (ground)	Nutmeg (ground)	**Rosemary (dried, fresh)**
Basil (dried, fresh)	Curry powder	**Onion (powder, granules, flakes)**	**Sage (dried, fresh)**
Bay leaves	**Dill (dried, fresh)**	**Oregano (dried, fresh)**	Salt
Cardamom (ground)	Garam masala	**Paprika (smoked, sweet)**	**Savory (dried, fresh)**
Cayenne	**Garlic (powder, granules, flakes)**	Parsley (dried, fresh)	Tarragon (dried, fresh)
Celery seeds	**Ginger (fresh, ground)**	**Pepper (ground black)**	**Thyme (dried, fresh)**
Chili powder	Marjoram (dried, fresh)	Poultry seasoning	**Turmeric (ground, fresh)**
Cilantro (dried, fresh)	Mint (dried, fresh)	Pumpkin pie spice	
Cinnamon (ground)	**Mustard powder**	**Red pepper flakes, crushed**	
Cloves (ground, whole)			

MISCELLANEOUS ITEMS

Arrowroot starch	**Curry paste (Patak's mild)**	Red peppers, roasted, jarred	**Tomatoes (crushed, diced)**
Baking powder	Hot sauce	Salsa	**Tomatoes, sun-dried**
Baking soda	**Miso (dark, light)**	**Tamari**	**Vanilla extract**
Bragg Liquid Aminos	**Mustard (Dijon, stone-ground)**	Tempeh	**Vegetable broth (cubes, powder, liquid)**
Cocoa or cacao powder	**Nutritional yeast flakes**	**Tofu (medium, firm, extra-firm)**	**Vinegars (balsamic, apple cider)**
Coconut extract	Olives (black or green)	**Tomato paste**	
Cornstarch			

*May be purchased frozen.

2. **SOAK THE BEANS.** With the exception of lentils and split peas, it's a good idea to soak legumes before cooking them to decrease the cooking time. Even lentils can be soaked to improve digestibility. There are three ways to soak beans: hot soak, traditional soak, and quick soak. The hot soak is recommended for beans cooked on the stove top because it decreases cooking time, has maximum gas-reducing potential, and produces tender beans. However, if you're using a pressure cooker, a traditional soak is best.

    ■ **Hot soak.** Put the beans in a large saucepan and add about 5 cups (1.25 L) of water for each cup (250 ml) of beans. Bring to a boil over medium-high heat, then boil for 2–3 minutes. Remove from the heat, cover, and let stand for 4–24 hours. Drain the beans and discard the soaking water. Rinse the beans with cold water before cooking.

    ■ **Traditional soak.** Put the beans in a large bowl or saucepan and add enough water to cover them by 1–2 inches (3–6 cm) above the beans. Cover and let soak for 8–24 hours or longer. Rinse with cool, clean water every 12 hours if you're soaking the beans for longer periods of time. Drain the beans and discard the soaking water. Rinse the beans with cold water before cooking.

    ■ **Quick soak.** Put the beans in a large saucepan and add 3 cups (750 ml) of water for every cup (250 ml) of beans. Bring to a boil over medium-high heat, then boil for 2–3 minutes. Remove from the heat and let stand for 1 hour. Drain the beans and discard the soaking water. Rinse the beans with cold water before cooking.

3. **COOK THE BEANS.** Once the beans have been soaked (or to cook unsoaked lentils and split peas), drain, rinse, and proceed with cooking. If using a multipurpose or other cooker, follow the manufacturer's instructions. If using a stove top, put the beans in a large saucepan with a tight-fitting lid. Add the amount of water indicated in table 11.2 (page 186). Bring to a boil over medium-high leat, decrease the heat to medium-low, and simmer gently for the time indicated. Because beans expand during cooking, add warm water as needed to ensure that they are always covered. Skim off any foam that rises to the top, as this can also cause flatulence.

If you'd like to flavor the legumes while they cook, add acidic ingredients (such as vinegar, tomatoes, or tomato juice) near the end of the cooking time, when the beans are just tender. If these ingredients are added sooner, they can make the beans tough and slow the cooking process. Herbs and spices (including salt) can be added at the beginning of the cooking process if desired.

Beans are done when you can soften them on the roof of your mouth with your tongue. At this stage, they're the most digestible.

TABLE 11.2. Cooking Legumes

LEGUMES (1 CUP/250 ML)	PRESOAK?	WATER	COOKING TIME FOR SOAKED BEANS*	APPROXIMATE YIELD
Adzuki, black, black-eyed peas, cannellini	Yes	4 cups (1 L)	45–60 minutes	2½ cups (625 ml)
Great Northern, kidney, lima, navy, pink, pinto, red (small)	Yes	3 cups (750 ml)	1½–2 hours	2–2½ cups (500–625 ml)
Chickpeas, red or tan (large)	Yes	4 cups (1 L)	2–3 hours	2½ cups (625 ml)
Lentils, brown, green, or gray	No	3 cups (750 ml)	45 minutes	2¼ cups (550 ml)
Lentils, split, red	No	3 cups (750 ml)	15–25 minutes	2¼ cups (550 ml)
Peas, split, green or yellow	No	3 cups (750 ml)	30–45 minutes	2¼ cups (550 ml)

*Beans that are old, have been stored for long periods of time, or are large will take longer to cook.

COOKING GRAINS

Many people are unfamiliar with cooking intact grains other than brown rice and perhaps quinoa. But they are all prepared in a similar manner by boiling with a specified amount of water (see table 11.3, opposite page). When you are cooking a grain, make a large batch to last for several days. Add cooked whole grains to breakfast bowls, soups, salads, and main dishes. You can freeze individual or meal-sized portions of cooked grains in labeled containers for up to six months.

Cook whole grains in a heavy saucepan with a tight-fitting lid to retain moisture. Bring the amount of recommended water to a boil over medium-high heat. Add the grain and return to a boil. Decrease the heat, cover, and cook for the time indicated in table 11.3. Many whole grains will fluff up if you remove the saucepan from the heat and let the grain sit, covered, for a few minutes after all the water has been absorbed. This will also help the cooked grains separate and not stick together as much when they're stored.

If the cooked grains have stuck to the bottom of the saucepan, remove the pan from the heat, add a very small amount of liquid, cover the pan, and let sit for a few minutes. The grain will loosen, making it easier to serve (and also making it easier to clean the saucepan).

TABLE 11.3. Cooking Grains

GRAIN (1 CUP/250 ML)	WATER	COOKING TIME	APPROXIMATE YIELD
Barley, whole-grain hulled, pot, or Scotch	3½ cups (875 ml)	1 hour	3½ cups (875 ml)
Buckwheat groats	2 cups (500 ml)	20 minutes	3 cups (750 ml)
Kamut berries	3 cups (750 ml)	45–60 minutes (30–40 minutes if soaked for 6–12 hours)	3 cups (750 ml)
Oats, steel cut	4 cups (1 L)	20 minutes	4 cups (1 L)
Quinoa	2 cups (500 ml)	15 minutes (let stand covered for 5 minutes)	3 cups (750 ml)
Rice, brown, brown basmati, long grain, short grain	2 cups (500 ml)	35–40 minutes (let stand covered for 5–10 minutes)	3½ cups (875 ml)
Spelt berries	3 cups (750 ml)	45–60 minutes	2½ cups (625 ml)
Wild rice	3 cups (750 ml)	40–45 minutes (let stand covered for 10 minutes)	3½–4 cups (875 ml–1 L)

Chapter

12

RECIPES

Turmeric Tea Elixir

Many of the turmeric tea beverages available commercially are sweetened with added sugars and enriched with milk, cream, or coconut milk. This homemade version is not only more potent but also a valuable part of your treatment protocol, helping to boost disease-fighting compounds. One cup each morning before your first meal will help maximize the absorption of its protective components while contributing few calories.

6 cups (1.5 L) **water**

1 orange, sliced

½ cup (125 ml) **sliced fresh ginger**

6 whole cardamom pods (optional)

3 cinnamon sticks

12 whole cloves

1½ teaspoons (7 ml) **ground turmeric**

½ teaspoon (2 ml) **ground black pepper**

½ teaspoon (2 ml) **cayenne**

6 lemons (to be used when preparing individual servings)**, or 6 tablespoons** (90 ml) **apple cider vinegar**

Put the water, orange slices, ginger, optional cardamom, cinnamon sticks, and cloves in a large saucepan. Bring to a boil over medium-high heat. Decrease the heat to medium-low and simmer for 15 minutes.

Stir in the turmeric, pepper, and cayenne and simmer for 10 minutes longer. Remove from the heat, cool slightly, and strain. Pour into glass jars or storage containers. Seal tightly and store in the refrigerator. This will be your tea concentrate for the week.

For individual servings, shake the concentrate, then pour ½ cup (125 ml) into a large mug. Add 1 cup (250 ml) boiling water and the juice of ½ lemon or 1 tablespoon (15 ml) apple cider vinegar.

TIPS: If you prefer a milder flavor, dilute with additional water. If the tea is too tart, add a sliced apple along with the orange. For a sweeter taste, add 4 or 5 dates along with the orange or add a few drops of monk fruit sweetener or stevia to the tea just before serving it.

PER SERVING:

calories: 16

Green Giant Juice

MAKES 3 CUPS (750 ML),
2 SERVINGS

This juice is rich in superstars from the bone-building team. The greens supply plenty of vitamin A (as beta-carotene), vitamin K, and folate. As a bonus, the calcium in kale is about twice as available to the body as the calcium in cow's milk.

PER SERVING:
calories: 57
protein: 5 g
fat: 0.4 g
carbohydrate: 8 g
dietary fiber: 3 g
calcium: 155 mg
copper: 110 mcg
iron: 1.4 mg
magnesium: 48 mg
phosphorus: 119 mg
potassium: 835 mg
sodium: 111 mg
zinc: 0.6 mg
vitamin C: 16 mg
omega-6 fatty acids: 0.1 g
omega-3 fatty acids: 0.2 g

1 bunch (8 ounces/240 g) **kale or collard greens, stems removed**

½ head romaine lettuce

1 cucumber, quartered lengthwise

1 carrot, or ½ apple

4 stalks celery

1 piece (1 inch/3 cm) **fresh ginger** (optional)

Juice of ½ lemon or lime

Juice the greens, lettuce, cucumber, carrot, celery, and ginger. Stir in the lemon juice. Serve immediately.

VARIATIONS:

- Replace the kale with bok choy or other dark leafy greens.
- Add other vegetables, such as sprouts, zucchini, broccolini, kohlrabi, or sweet peppers.
- Replace the carrot with 1 beet (although this will change the color).
- Add 1 small piece (1 inch/3 cm) fresh turmeric root, or ⅛ teaspoon (0.5 ml) ground turmeric.

A WORD ABOUT JUICERS

You can process fruits and vegetables in a powerful blender and then strain the mixture to get juice, but a juicer will do the job more efficiently and effectively. There are two basic types of juicers: centrifugal and masticating. Centrifugal juicers use rapidly spinning blades to break down produce, but some juice aficionados believe that the heat they produce can compromise the nutrients in the juice and that the blades don't extract as much juice from the produce as masticators. Masticating juicers use slow-moving augers that do a good job of grinding out the juice while preserving fragile vitamins, but these machines may be more pricey.

Juicing expert Steve Meyerowitz used to say that the best juicer for you is the one you'll use. Consider how easy a particular juicer is to take apart and clean. The size of the feed chute is also important; the larger the chute, the less you'll need to cut down the produce to fit through it.

Juicers can range from slightly under $100 all the way to $1,000. If you've never had experience with a juicer before, you might be more comfortable trying an inexpensive model first, no matter what type. Keep in mind that a used juicer can also be an inexpensive choice. Check out what's available online and at yard sales.

Chia Berry Bowl

This tapioca-like pudding is brimming with omega-3 fatty acids and has no added sweetener.

MAKES 4 SERVINGS

CHIA PUDDING

2 cups (500 ml) **unsweetened soy milk or other nondairy milk**

6 tablespoons (90 ml) **chia seeds**

½ teaspoon (2 ml) **ground cinnamon**

½ teaspoon (2 ml) **vanilla extract**

TOPPINGS (PER SERVING)

½ cup (125 ml) **fresh or thawed frozen berries** (such as blueberries, blackberries, raspberries, or chopped strawberries)

¼ cup (60 ml) **Very Berry Sauce** (page 193)

1–2 tablespoons (15–30 ml) **chopped walnuts**

OPTIONAL TOPPINGS

Pear Cream (page 192) **or unsweetened nondairy yogurt**

Goji berries

Unsweetened shredded dried coconut

Pumpkin seeds

Ground flaxseeds

To make the pudding, put the milk, chia seeds, cinnamon, and vanilla extract in a medium bowl or mason jar and whisk briskly. Let sit for 10 minutes, then whisk again to prevent clumping. Cover and refrigerate for 2–12 hours. Whisk again before serving.

To serve, spoon into bowls, stir in the berries, and top with the sauce and walnuts. Add any optional toppings as desired. Alternatively, layer the pudding with the berries, sauce, and toppings and decorate with any optional toppings as desired. Stored in a sealed container in the refrigerator, the pudding (without toppings) will keep for 5 days.

VARIATIONS:

- Replace the berries with ½ cup (125 ml) chopped fresh fruit.
- Add a small amount of monk fruit sweetener, stevia, or up to 1 tablespoon (15 ml) of chopped dried fruit (prunes, dates, or raisins) until your palate adjusts to less-sweet foods.
- For a thicker pudding, use 7 tablespoons (105 ml) chia seeds.
- For a flavor boost, add ⅛–¼ teaspoon (0.5–1 ml) ground allspice, cardamom, cloves, ginger, or nutmeg.

PER SERVING
(with unsweetened soy milk without optional toppings):
calories: 198
protein: 7 g
fat: 11 g
carbohydrate: 19 g
dietary fiber: 13 g
calcium: 376 mg
iron: 3.9 mg
magnesium: 43 mg
potassium: 163 mg
sodium: 54 mg
zinc: 1.3 mg
thiamin: 0.3 mg
riboflavin: 0.3 mg
niacin: 2.2 mg
folate: 39 mcg
vitamin A: 54 mcg RAE
vitamin C: 5 mg
omega-6 fatty acids: 2.4 g
omega-3 fatty acids: 5.4 g

Pear Cream

MAKES 1¾ CUPS (435 ML)

Use this light, creamy topping to embellish fruit salad, stewed fruit, porridge, pudding, or a fruit crisp. For a more economical version, replace the cashews with raw sunflower seeds. Soaking the cashews or seeds makes this topping extra-creamy. Limit your serving size to 2–4 tablespoons (30–60 ml), as this topping is naturally high in fat and calories.

1 can (14 ounces/398 ml) **pears, packed in water or juice**

½ cup (125 ml) **raw cashew pieces or sunflower seeds, soaked for 2–4 hours and then drained and rinsed**

½ teaspoon (2 ml) **vanilla extract**

Drain the pears but reserve the liquid. Put the pears, cashews, and vanilla extract in a high-speed blender and process until smooth, 1–2 minutes. Add some of the liquid from the pears to achieve the desired consistency. Stored in a sealed container in the refrigerator, the cream will keep for 5–7 days.

PER 2 TABLESPOONS (30 ml):
calories: 39
protein: 1 g
fat: 2 g
carbohydrate: 4 g
dietary fiber: 1 g
calcium: 3 mg
iron: 0.4 mg
magnesium: 17 mg
potassium: 52 mg
sodium: 1.3 mg
zinc: 0.3 mg
thiamin: 0.03 mg
riboflavin: 0.01 mg
niacin: 0.3 mg
folate: 1.6 mcg
vitamin A: 0 mcg RAE
vitamin C: 0.3 mg
omega-6 fatty acids: 0.4 g
omega-3 fatty acids: 0 g

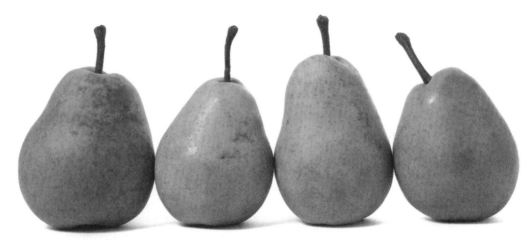

Very Berry Sauce

Use this eye-catching sauce on breakfast bowls, as a sauce to top puddings or other desserts, or as a replacement for jam. Double, triple, or quadruple the recipe to make large batches to freeze for later use.

2 cups (500 ml) **fresh or frozen berries**

¼ cup (60 ml) **water**

2 teaspoons (10 ml) **cornstarch or arrowroot starch mixed with**
2 tablespoons (30 ml) **water**

Put the berries and water in a small saucepan and bring to a simmer over medium heat. Decrease the heat to low and cook, stirring occasionally, for 10 minutes. Stir the cornstarch mixture, then slowly pour it into the berries, stirring constantly, until the sauce thickens, about 1 minute. Serve warm or cold.

VARIATION: This sauce can be made without the cornstarch and with little or no water by stewing the fruit on the lowest temperature until it's covered in its own juice. Although this method takes more time, it works beautifully with other fruits, such as apricots, peaches, nectarines, and Italian prune plums.

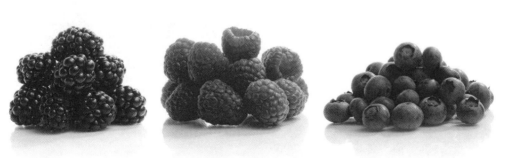

PER SERVING:
calories: 45
protein: 0.3 g
fat: 0.5 g
carbohydrate: 11 g
dietary fiber: 2 g
calcium: 6 mg
iron: 0.2 mg
magnesium: 4 mg
potassium: 42 mg
sodium: 0.9 mg
zinc: 0.06 mg
thiamin: 0.02 mg
riboflavin: 0.03 mg
niacin: 0.4 mg
folate: 5 mcg
vitamin A: 2 mcg RAE
vitamin C: 2 mg
omega-6 fatty acids: 0.13 g
omega-3 fatty acids: 0.09 g

Green Smoothie

MAKES 1 LARGE OR
2 SMALL SERVINGS

Smoothies are popular for breakfast because they are quick and easy to make, nutrient-dense, and super-portable. This one boasts 36 grams of protein and 13 grams of fiber! Frozen peas contribute to the generous protein and fiber content, as well as to the gorgeous fresh-green color. Frozen ingredients are the key to thick, rich-tasting smoothies and smoothie bowls.

2 cups (500 ml) **dark leafy greens** (kale, spinach, broccoli, sunflower sprouts, pea shoots), **firmly packed**

1 cup (250 ml) **unsweetened soy milk or other nondairy milk**

3–4 ounces (90–120 g) **soft organic tofu or unsweetened nondairy yogurt**

¾ cup (185 ml) **frozen peas**

2 tablespoons (30 ml) **hemp seeds**

1 small frozen banana, broken into chunks

½ cup (125 ml) **frozen pineapple or mango pieces** (optional)

Put all the ingredients in a high-speed blender in the order listed and process until smooth, 1–2 minutes. Serve immediately.

PER FULL RECIPE
(with unsweetened soy milk):
calories: 525
protein: 35 g
fat: 21 g
carbohydrate: 60 g
dietary fiber: 12 g
calcium: 373 mg
iron: 9 mg
magnesium: 329 mg
potassium: 1,929 mg
sodium: 193 mg
zinc: 3.4 mg
thiamin: 0.9 mg
riboflavin: 0.6 mg
niacin: 13 mg
folate: 156 mcg
vitamin A: 1,145 mcg RAE
vitamin C: 189 mg
omega-6 fatty acids: 7.5 g
omega-3 fatty acids: 2.7 g

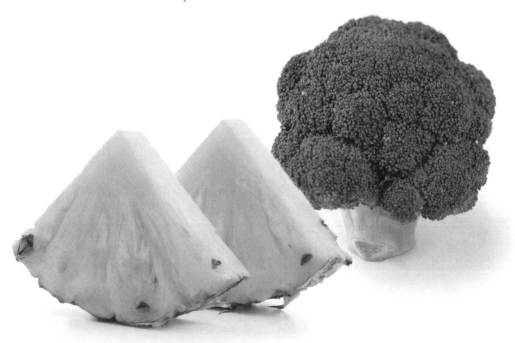

Green Smoothie Bowl

Smoothie bowls need to be extra-thick so the toppings don't sink. Solid toppings add a lot of nutrition and flavor to the meal. Put the berries on top rather than adding them to the smoothie base to preserve the smoothie's vibrant green color.

MAKES 1 LARGE OR
2 SMALL SERVINGS

SMOOTHIE BOWL

2 cups (500 ml) **dark leafy greens** (kale, spinach, broccoli, sunflower sprouts, pea shoots), **firmly packed**

¾ cup (185 ml) **unsweetened soy milk or other nondairy milk, plus more as needed**

3–4 ounces (90–120 g) **soft organic tofu or unsweetened nondairy yogurt**

2 tablespoons (30 ml) **hemp seeds**

¾ cup (185 ml) **frozen peas**

1 small frozen banana, broken into chunks

½ cup (125 ml) **frozen pineapple or mango pieces** (optional)

OPTIONAL TOPPINGS (PER SERVING)

½ cup (125 ml) **berries, pomegranate seeds, goji berries, or chopped fresh fruit**

¼ cup (60 ml) **cooked and cooled or sprouted grain** (barley, oat groats, Kamut, spelt, or quinoa)

1 tablespoon (15 ml) **seeds** (chia, flax, pumpkin, sunflower)

1 tablespoon (15 ml) **chopped walnuts, almonds, or other nuts**

1 tablespoon (15 ml) **cacao nibs or unsweetened shredded dried coconut**

Put all the ingredients in a high-speed blender in the order listed and process until smooth. Add a little more milk only if needed to facilitate processing. Alternatively, put all the ingredients in a food processor and process until smooth. Serve immediately with the optional toppings of your choice.

PER FULL RECIPE
(with unsweetened soy milk without optional toppings):
calories: 496
protein: 32 g
fat: 19 g
carbohydrate: 58 g
dietary fiber: 11 g
calcium: 360 mg
iron: 8 mg
magnesium: 313 mg
potassium: 1,814 mg
sodium: 192 mg
zinc: 3.1 mg
thiamin: 0.8 mg
riboflavin: 0.5 mg
niacin: 13 mg
folate: 156 mcg
vitamin A: 1,145 mcg RAE
vitamin C: 189 mg
omega-6 fatty acids: 7.5 g
omega-3 fatty acids: 2.7 g

Whole-Food Breakfast Bowl

MAKES 1 SERVING

Once you've gathered the ingredients, this filling and delicious breakfast will come together in minutes. Below are suggested layers with amounts and options. Choose one item for each layer. While it's not essential to add legumes, they will help to boost the fiber, protein, iron, zinc, and other nutrients.

Layer 1: Whole Grains and Lentils (½–1 cup/125–250 ml)

Cooked barley, Kamut, spelt, oat groats, or steel-cut oats with lentils

Raw sprouted Kamut, spelt, barley, buckwheat, or lentils

Layer 2: Fruits (1 cup/250 ml fresh or frozen fruit, or ¼–½ cup/60–125 ml stewed fruit)

Berries, chopped fruit, grated apple

Stewed unsweetened fruit or Very Berry Sauce (page 193)

Layer 3: Nuts/Seeds (1 tablespoon/15 ml each of an omega-3-rich option and one other choice)

Omega-3-Rich Seed Mix (page 197)

Omega-3-rich seeds (chia, flax, hemp); other seeds (pumpkin, sunflower)

Chopped walnuts, Brazil nuts, pecans, hazelnuts, or almonds

Layer 4: Optional Creamy Additions (2–4 tablespoons/30–60 ml)

Unsweetened nondairy yogurt

Pear Cream (page 192)

Chia Pudding (page 191)

Fortified Unsweetened Nondairy Milk (1 cup/250 ml)

Optional spices (⅛–¼ teaspoon/1–2 ml)**, such as allspice, cardamom, cinnamon, cloves, nutmeg, or pumpkin pie spice**

TIP: To cook lentils with grains, use ¾ cup (185 ml) grains and ¼ cup (60 ml) lentils and follow the cooking instructions for grains in table 11.3, page 187. Red, green, or small brown lentils will work well.

PER SERVING (using
½ cup/125 ml cooked kamut
½ cup/125 ml berries
½ cup/125 ml chopped apple
¼ cup/60 ml stewed plums
¼ cup/60 ml nondairy yogurt
2 tablespoons/30 ml Omega-3-Rich Seed Mix
1 cup/250 ml unsweetened soy milk):
calories: 376
protein: 12 g
fat: 13 g
carbohydrate: 63 g
dietary fiber: 13 g
calcium: 363 mg
iron: 3.3 mg
magnesium: 92 mg
potassium: 353 mg
sodium: 17 mg
zinc: 1 mg
thiamin: 0.3 mg
riboflavin: 0.1 mg
niacin: 3.6 mg
folate: 31 mcg
vitamin A: 33 mcg RAE
vitamin C: 13 mg
omega-6 fatty acids: 3.3 g
omega-3 fatty acids: 3.6 g

Omega-3-Rich Seed Mix

This seed mix makes it super-simple to enjoy a variety of seeds and Brazil nuts on your breakfast bowl, salads, or power bowls. It includes a blend of the most common omega-3-rich seeds, iron- and zinc-rich pumpkin seeds, and selenium-rich Brazil nuts. For ease, chop the pumpkin seeds and Brazil nuts in a food processor.

MAKES 5 CUPS (1.25 L)

1 cup (250 ml) **ground flaxseeds**

1 cup (250 ml) **chia seeds**

1 cup (250 ml) **hemp seeds**

1 cup (250 ml) **coarsely chopped pumpkin seeds**

1 cup (250 ml) **finely chopped Brazil nuts**

Put all the ingredients in a large bowl and mix well. Transfer to two glass jars. Keep a scoop in the jars for convenience. The jar you will use first may be kept in the refrigerator or freezer; store the second jar in the freezer.

PER 2 TABLESPOONS (30 ml):
calories: 107
protein: 4 g
fat: 9 g
carbohydrate: 4 g
dietary fiber: 3 g
calcium: 42 mg
iron: 1.4 mg
magnesium: 57 mg
potassium: 103 mg
sodium: 3 mg
zinc: 0.4 mg
thiamin: 0.16 mg
riboflavin: 0.02 mg
niacin: 1.6 mg
folate: 13 mcg
vitamin A: 0 mcg RAE
vitamin C: 0.7 mg
omega-6 fatty acids: 2.2 g
omega-3 fatty acids: 1.9 g

Berry Burst Muesli

This breakfast requires no cooking and minimal preparation time. It provides an excellent balance of protein, fat, and carbohydrate. Soaking the grains and nuts enhances their digestibility and increases mineral absorption. Leftovers can be enjoyed the following day.

> **1½ cups** (375 ml) **rolled oats or other rolled grains**
>
> **¼ cup** (60 ml) **nuts and/or seeds** (such as walnuts, almonds, chia seeds, hemp seeds, or pumpkin seeds)
>
> **½ teaspoon** (2 ml) **ground cinnamon**
>
> **2 cups** (500 ml) **unsweetened soy milk or other nondairy milk, plus more for serving**
>
> **2 cups** (500 ml) **fresh or frozen berries**
>
> **Ground flaxseeds** (optional)

Put the oats, nuts, and cinnamon in a medium bowl. Stir in the milk and berries. Refrigerate for 8–12 hours. Serve with additional milk and sprinkle with the optional ground flaxseeds.

VARIATION: Replace some of the nondairy milk with nondairy yogurt. Replace the fresh berries with frozen berries, chopped fresh fruit, or grated apples. Frozen berries and fruits that discolor quickly are best added just before serving.

PER SERVING
(made with walnuts):
calories: 279
protein: 11 g
fat: 9 g
carbohydrate: 40 g
dietary fiber: 9 g
calcium: 69 mg
iron: 3.2 mg
magnesium: 15 mg
potassium: 217 mg
sodium: 18 mg
zinc: 2.7 mg
thiamin: 1 mg
riboflavin: 0.12 mg
niacin: 1 mg
folate: 44.7 mcg
vitamin A: 2.3 mcg RAE
vitamin C: 7 mg
omega-6 fatty acids: 2.3 g
omega-3 fatty acids: 1 g

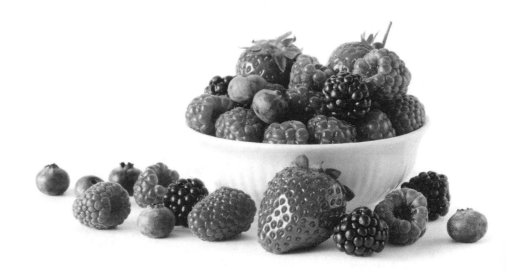

Spiced Creamy Barley Bowl

Keep a supply of cooked barley on hand for this low GI breakfast. Enjoy it at home or spoon it into a mason jar and take it to work. Use fresh or frozen berries, or replace the berries with chopped peach, nectarine, or mango.

MAKES 2½ CUPS (625 ML), 1 LARGE OR 2 SMALLER SERVINGS

1 banana

1 cup (250 ml) **cooked barley**

¼ **cup** (60 ml) **unsweetened nondairy yogurt or Pear Cream** (page 192)

¾ **cup** (185 ml) **unsweetened soy milk or other nondairy milk**

1 tablespoon (15 ml) **chia seeds**

½ **teaspoon** (2 ml) **ground cinnamon**

⅛ **teaspoon** (½ ml) **ground nutmeg**

⅛ **teaspoon** (½ ml) **ground ginger**

⅛ **teaspoon** (½ ml) **ground cardamom**

1 cup (250 ml) **fresh or frozen berries, or** ½ **cup** (125 ml) **Very Berry Sauce** (page 193)

2 tablespoons (30 ml) **chopped walnuts**

Mash the banana in a small bowl. Add the barley, yogurt, milk, chia seeds, cinnamon, nutmeg, ginger, and cardamom and stir to combine. Let stand for at least 15 minutes. Stir well to break up any clumps. Top with the berries and walnuts.

TIP: To boost the health benefits even more, decrease the barley to ¾ cup (185 ml) and add ¼ cup (60 ml) cooked lentils.

PER 1 LARGE SERVING (full recipe):
calories: 445
protein: 14 g
fat: 16 g
carbohydrate: 69 g
dietary fiber: 16 g
calcium: 377 mg
iron: 3.8 mg
magnesium: 36 mg
potassium: 585 mg
sodium: 38 mg
zinc: 1 mg
thiamin: 0.2 mg
riboflavin: 0.1 mg
niacin: 2.8 mg
folate: 32 mcg
vitamin A: 5 mcg RAE
vitamin C: 25 mg
omega-6 fatty acids: 5.5 g
omega-3 fatty acids: 3 g

Apple Pie Oats

MAKES 5 CUPS (1.25 L),
5 SERVINGS

This oat-based breakfast provides a delicious, nourishing start to the day. See the variations below to use steel-cut oats or oat groats in place of rolled oats. Leftovers keep well in the refrigerator and can be reheated or enjoyed cold.

OATS

1½ cups (375 ml) **rolled oats**

2 apples, chopped

2 cups (500 ml) **unsweetened soy milk or other nondairy milk**

2 teaspoons (10 ml) **ground cinnamon**

¾ teaspoon (4 ml) **ground nutmeg**

½ teaspoon (2 ml) **ground allspice**

¼ teaspoon (1 ml) **salt** (optional)

1 tablespoon (15 ml) **Omega-3-Rich Seed Mix** (page 197) **or chia, flax, or hemp seeds**

OPTIONAL TOPPINGS (PER SERVING)

¼ cup (60 ml) Very Berry Sauce (page 193)

1–2 tablespoons (15–30 ml) **Pear Cream** (page 192) **or unsweetened nondairy yogurt**

1 tablespoon (15 ml) **chopped walnuts**

PER SERVING (without
toppings or salt):
calories: 249
protein: 11 g
fat: 6 g
carbohydrate: 44 g
dietary fiber: 9 g
calcium: 274 mg
iron: 3.3 mg
magnesium: 4 mg
potassium: 76 mg
sodium: 13 mg
zinc: 1.5 mg
thiamin: 0.03 mg
riboflavin: 0.04 mg
niacin: 0.7 mg
folate: 3 mcg
vitamin A: 40 mcg RAE
vitamin C: 2 mg
omega-6 fatty acids: 0.2 g
omega-3 fatty acids: 0.5 g

Put the oats, apples, milk, cinnamon, nutmeg, allspice, and optional salt in a medium saucepan and stir to combine. Bring to a boil over medium heat, then decrease the heat to low and cook, stirring occasionally, for 15–20 minutes. To serve, spoon into individual bowls. Sprinkle with the seed mix and any optional toppings as desired. Stored in a sealed container in the refrigerator, leftover oats will keep for 5 days.

VARIATIONS: Replace the rolled oats with 1 cup (250 ml) steel-cut oats soaked in 3 cups (750 ml) water for 8–12 hours, then drained and rinsed. Alternatively, replace the rolled oats with 1 cup (250 ml) oat groats soaked in 3 cups (750 ml) boiling water for 8–12 hours, then drained and rinsed. To further boost fiber and nutrition, replace ¼ cup (60 ml) of the steel-cut oats or oat groats with dried red lentils.

Indian Breakfast Lentils

MAKES 2 SERVINGS

In many regions of the world, legumes are a part of breakfast every day. Lentils and other legumes served for breakfast can be made with savory seasonings or with sweet-tasting spices, as they are in this recipe. Having lentils for breakfast can help to stabilize blood sugar and augment nutrients that some people may fall short on. Legumes have a lower glycemic index than grains and are more concentrated sources of fiber, protein, iron, and zinc.

LENTILS

¾ **cup** (185 ml) **dried lentils**

1 apple, finely chopped

¼ **cup** (60 ml) **raisins**

1 tablespoon (15 ml) **ground cinnamon**

2 teaspoons (10 ml) **ground cardamom**

2 teaspoons (10 ml) **ground coriander**

¾ **teaspoon** (4 ml) **ground cloves**

¼ **teaspoon** (1 ml) **salt** (optional)

2 cups (500 ml) **water**

TOPPINGS (PER SERVING)

1 cup (250 ml) **fresh fruit** (such as apples, bananas, pears, or berries)

2 tablespoons (30 ml) **Pear Cream** (page 192) **or unsweetened nondairy yogurt** (optional)

1 tablespoon (15 ml) **walnuts**

1 tablespoon (15 ml) **Omega-3-Rich Seed Mix** (page 197)**, ground flaxseeds, or chia seeds**

Put the lentils, apple, raisins, cinnamon, cardamom, coriander, cloves, and optional salt in a medium saucepan and bring to a boil over medium-high heat. Decrease the heat to medium and cook, stirring occasionally, until the lentils are soft, 20–40 minutes. To warm the fruit, stir it into the lentils during the last 2 minutes of cooking. Stir in the optional Pear Cream and top with the walnuts and seed mix.

TIP: When reheating leftover breakfast lentils, add a little unsweetened soy milk or other nondairy milk.

PER SERVING (without toppings or added salt):
calories: 355
protein: 19 g
fat: 0.9 g
carbohydrate: 70 g
dietary fiber: 26 g
calcium: 46 mg
iron: 6.2 mg
magnesium: 94 mg
potassium: 340 mg
sodium: 10 mg
zinc: 3.5mg
thiamin: 0.9 mg
riboflavin: 0.2 mg
niacin: 5.2 mg
folate: 350 mcg
vitamin A: 4 mcg RAE
vitamin C: 7 mg
omega-6 fatty acids: 0.3 g
omega-3 fatty acids: 0.09 g

Ezekiel Nut Butter and Banana Wrap

MAKES 1 SERVING

Ezekiel breads are among the most healthful breads available, as they are made with sprouted grains and legumes. Their glycemic index (GI) is about 36 or lower (compared to over 70 for many whole-grain breads). The taco-sized tortilla has 80 calories (equal to one slice of bread), and the full-sized tortilla has 150 calories (equal to about two slices of bread). This is a super-simple recipe for days when you just don't feel like cooking.

1 Ezekiel whole–grain tortilla (taco-sized or ½ full-sized)

2 tablespoons (30 ml) **nut butter** (almond, cashew, peanut)

⅓ cup (85 ml) berries (optional)

1–2 tablespoons (15–30 ml) **Omega-3-Rich Seed Mix** (page 197)**, chia seeds, or chopped walnuts**

½ teaspoon (2 ml) **ground cinnamon**

1 banana

PER SERVING (with peanut butter, raspberries, and 1 tablespoon/15 ml chia seeds):

calories: 455

protein: 13 g

fat: 21 g

carbohydrate: 57 g

dietary fiber: 14 g

calcium: 99 mg

iron: 3.4 mg

magnesium: 72 mg

potassium: 570 mg

sodium: 84 mg

zinc: 1.3 mg

thiamin: 0.14 mg

riboflavin: 0.15 mg

niacin: 3.4 mg

folate: 44 mcg

vitamin A: 4.4 mcg RAE

vitamin C: 23 mg

omega-6 fatty acids: 0.7 g

omega-3 fatty acids: 1.8 g

Lay the tortilla on a large cutting board. Spread the nut butter down the center and out toward the edges. If using the optional berries, distribute them over the nut butter and mash. Sprinkle with the seed mix and cinnamon. Place the banana on one side of the tortilla and roll. Slice in half to serve if desired.

TIPS: For a softer tortilla, steam it for about 15 seconds or microwave it in a clean, damp tea towel or brown paper bag for 45 seconds. Ezekiel tortillas can also be used as savory wraps stuffed with hummus, grated vegetables, slivered kale, and sprouts.

Better Broth Base

Commercial liquid vegetable broths work well for all the soup recipes in this book, but they can be expensive and high in sodium. More economical broth cubes and powders are often based on palm oil or other hard fats and sugar. This fast and easy homemade substitute is based on nutritional yeast and seasonings. It provides a healthy and low-cost alternative to commercial products. When mixed with boiling water, it can be used instead of liquid vegetable broth in soups and stews. Adjust the herbs and spices to suit your palate.

MAKES 2 CUPS (500 ML), **32 SERVINGS**

1 cup (250 ml) **nutritional yeast flakes**

½ cup (125 ml) **dried onion flakes, or 3 tablespoons** (45 ml) **onion powder**

2 tablespoons (30 ml) **dried garlic flakes, or 1 tablespoon** (15 ml) **garlic powder**

1 tablespoon (15 ml) **salt**

1 tablespoon (15 ml) **dried oregano**

1 tablespoon (15 ml) **dried parsley flakes**

2 teaspoons (10 ml) **dried thyme**

1 teaspoon (5 ml) **ground black pepper**

1 teaspoon (5 ml) **ground turmeric**

1 teaspoon (5 ml) **paprika**

1 teaspoon (5 ml) **whole celery seeds**

Put all the ingredients in a medium bowl and stir until well combined. Stored in a sealed container at room temperature, the broth base will keep for about 3 months. To make 1 cup (250 ml) of broth, combine 1 tablespoon (15 ml) of the broth base with 1 cup (250 ml) of boiling water.

TIP: For a low- or no-sodium version, decrease or omit the salt.

PER TABLESPOON (15 ml) dry broth mix:
calories: 13
protein: 1.1 g
fat: 0.1 g
carbohydrate: 1.9 g
dietary fiber: 0.7 g
calcium: 8 mg
iron: 0.4 mg
magnesium: 5 mg
potassium: 24 mg
sodium: 222 mg
zinc: 0.04 mg
thiamin: 1.5 mg
riboflavin: 1.2 mg
niacin: 5.8 mg
vitamin B_{12}: 2.2 mcg
folate: 2 mcg
vitamin A: 2.5 mcg RAE
vitamin C: 1 mg
omega-6 fatty acids: 0.01 g
omega-3 fatty acids: 0 g

Healing Greens, Beans, and Vegetable Soup

MAKES 12 CUPS (3 L),
4–6 SERVINGS

Turmeric, garlic, and ginger are legendary for their healing powers, and kale and broccoli are cancer-fighting, bone-building superstars. Beans add fiber and protein to this recipe; use your favorites. A squeeze of lime juice on each serving adds a burst of flavor, which reduces the need for salt.

6 cups (1.5 L) **vegetable broth**

3 cups (750 ml) **sliced mushrooms**

1 large red or white onion, chopped

1 cup (250 ml) **chopped carrots**

1½–3 teaspoons (7–15 ml) **peeled and grated fresh ginger**

3 cloves garlic, minced

1–2 bay leaves

2 teaspoons (10 ml) **ground cumin**

1 teaspoon (5 ml) **ground turmeric**

⅛ teaspoon (0.5 ml) **ground cinnamon**

3 cups (750 ml) **chopped broccoli florets**

1½ cups (375 ml) **cooked or canned beans, drained and rinsed**

4 cups (1 L) **stemmed and thinly sliced kale or other dark leafy greens, packed**

½ teaspoon (2 ml) **salt** (optional)

Ground black pepper

Juice of 1 lime or lemon

PER ¼ RECIPE (3 cups/750 ml):
calories: 195
protein: 12 g
fat: 1 g
carbohydrate: 37 g
dietary fiber: 9 g
calcium: 194 mg
iron: 3.5 mg
magnesium: 83 mg
potassium: 284 mg
sodium: 438 mg
zinc: 2 mg
thiamin: 0.3 mg
riboflavin: 0.5 mg
niacin: 6.8 mg
folate: 146 mcg
vitamin A: 864 mcg RAE
vitamin C: 136 mg
omega-6 fatty acids: 0.25 g
omega-3 fatty acids: 0.25 g

Put the broth, mushrooms, onion, carrots, ginger, garlic, bay leaves, cumin, turmeric, and cinnamon in a large soup pot and bring to a boil over medium-high heat. Decrease the heat to medium-low and simmer until the vegetables are soft, about 15 minutes. Add the broccoli and beans and simmer until the broccoli is tender, about 10 minutes. Add the kale and simmer until it has wilted, 2–3 minutes. Add the salt and season with pepper to taste. Stir in the lime juice just before serving. Serve hot.

VARIATION: Instead of stirring the lime juice into the soup, serve a lime wedge with each portion.

Smokin' Lentil Soup

This is a beautifully spiced soup using lentils, which provide an excellent source of protein and iron. Omit the hot chile or cayenne if you prefer a milder soup.

MAKES 6 CUPS (1.5 L),
3 SERVINGS

5 cups (1.25 L) **vegetable broth**

1 cup (250 ml) **dried lentils**

2 cups (500 ml) **chopped onions**

2 cloves garlic, minced

2 teaspoons (10 ml) **chili powder**

1 small hot chile, diced, or ¼ teaspoon (1 ml) **cayenne**

1¼ teaspoons (6 ml) **ground cumin**

½ teaspoon (2 ml) **ground coriander**

½ teaspoon (2 ml) **smoked paprika**

3 cups (750 ml) **stemmed and thinly sliced kale, packed**

2–3 diced tomatoes, or 1 can (14 ounces/398 ml) **diced tomatoes**

Ground black pepper

Lemon wedges

Put the broth, lentils, onions, garlic, chili powder, chile, cumin, coriander, and paprika in a large soup pot. Bring to a boil over medium-high heat. Decrease the heat to medium-low and cook, stirring occasionally, until the lentils are soft, 45–60 minutes. (If you use red lentils, the cooking time will be cut in half.) Add the kale and tomatoes and bring to a boil over medium-high heat. Decrease the heat to medium-low and cook, stirring occasionally, until the kale has wilted, about 3 minutes. Season with pepper to taste. Serve hot, with lemon wedges on the side.

VARIATION: For a Mediterranean flavor, replace the cumin, chili, coriander, paprika, and chile with 1 cup (250 ml) fresh herbs (such as basil, oregano, parsley, rosemary, and thyme), coarsely chopped and lightly packed, or 3 tablespoons (45 ml) dried Italian herb mix.

PER SERVING:
calories: 388
protein: 22 g
fat: 2 g
carbohydrate: 74 g
dietary fiber: 25 g
calcium: 174 mg
iron: 7.4 mg
magnesium: 138 mg
potassium: 1,618 mg
sodium: 1,037 mg
zinc: 3.9 mg
thiamin: 0.8 mg
riboflavin: 0.4 mg
niacin: 7.6 mg
folate: 383 mcg
vitamin A: 651 mcg RAE
vitamin C: 112 mg
omega-6 fatty acids: 0.7 g
omega-3 fatty acids: 0.2 g

Old-Fashioned Split Pea Soup

This nutritious comfort food easily satisfies the heartiest appetites.

1 large onion, diced

3 stalks celery, minced

9 cups (2.25 L) **vegetable broth**

3 cups (750 ml) **dried green or yellow split peas**

2 carrots, minced

1 medium potato, diced

4 cloves garlic, minced

3 bay leaves

1 tablespoon (15 ml) **dried thyme**

1½ teaspoons (7 ml) **salt** (optional)

1½ teaspoons (7 ml) **smoked paprika** (optional)

½ teaspoon (2 ml) **ground black pepper**

2 tablespoons (30 ml) **apple cider vinegar**

¼ cup (60 ml) **chopped fresh parsley or dill, lightly packed** (optional)

PER SERVING (without
optional salt):
calories: 386
protein: 19 g
fat: 1 g
carbohydrate: 60 g
dietary fiber: 20 g
calcium: 65 mg
iron: 3.5 mg
magnesium: 95 mg
potassium: 931 mg
sodium: 352 mg
zinc: 2.4 mg
thiamin: 0.6 mg
riboflavin: 0.2 mg
niacin: 6.2 mg
folate: 220 mcg
vitamin A: 163 mcg RAE
vitamin C: 6 mg
omega-6 fatty acids: 0.4 g
omega-3 fatty acids: 0.1 g

Put the onion and celery in a large soup pot. Add 3 tablespoons (45 ml) of the broth and sauté until the vegetables are tender, about 5 minutes. Add more broth if needed to keep the vegetables from sticking to the pot.

Stir in the remaining broth. Add the split peas, carrots, potato, garlic, bay leaves, thyme, optional salt, optional paprika, and pepper. Bring to a boil over medium-high heat. Decrease the heat to medium-low, cover, and cook, stirring occasionally, until the split peas are very soft, 60–90 minutes. Remove the bay leaves and stir in the vinegar. Garnish with the optional parsley.

TIPS: Soaking the peas in water to cover for at least 2 hours will speed the cooking time and increase digestibility.

VARIATIONS: For a heartier meal, replace the potato with ½ cup (125 ml) uncooked barley; add it at the same time as the peas. For even greater nutrition, serve the soup over spinach, which will wilt as soon as the hot soup is poured over it. If you prefer to include tougher greens (such as kale or collard greens), add them the last 3–5 minutes of cooking. Add greens only to the soup you will be eating right away as they tend to discolor quickly.

Queen of Greens Soup

This is a delicious and incredibly healthy dish. Get creative with the seasonings if you like—fresh ginger, mint, thyme, rosemary, and other herbs will all work well.

MAKES 10 CUPS (2.5 L), 5 SERVINGS

6 cups (1.5 L) **vegetable broth**

1 white onion, coarsely chopped

4 cloves garlic, coarsely chopped

8 cups (2 L) **stemmed and coarsely chopped kale, spinach, or collard greens, packed**

3 cups (750 ml) **coarsely chopped broccoli**

2 cups (500 ml) **frozen peas**

1½ cups (375 ml) **cooked or canned cannellini beans or other white beans, drained and rinsed**

½ cup (125 ml) **coarsely chopped fresh parsley, lightly packed**

¼ cup (60 ml) **coarsely chopped fresh basil, lightly packed, or 1 tablespoon** (15 ml) **dried basil**

2 cups (500 ml) **unsweetened soy milk or other nondairy milk**

1 ripe avocado, or ½ cup (125 ml) **cashews, soaked for 2–4 hours and then drained and rinsed**

Juice of 1 lemon

½ teaspoon (2 ml) **salt** (optional)

Ground black pepper

Put the broth, onion, and garlic in a large soup pot and bring to a boil over medium-high heat. Decrease the heat to medium-low and simmer for 20 minutes. Add the kale, broccoli, peas, beans, parsley, and basil and cook, stirring occasionally, until the vegetables are just tender, about 10 minutes. Do not overcook the vegetables or the greens will discolor. Add the milk and avocado and stir to combine. Transfer to a high-speed blender in batches and process until smooth. Add the lemon juice and optional salt. Season with pepper to taste.

VARIATION: To make this soup extra-special, steam 4 cups (1 L) of additional green vegetables (such as chopped Brussels sprouts, small broccoli florets, coarsely chopped leafy greens, chopped green beans, or thinly sliced leeks) and put about ½ cup (125 ml) on the top of each bowl before serving. Decorate with dehydrated colored peppers and pumpkin seeds.

PER SERVING:
calories: 342
protein: 18.3 g
fat: 10 g
carbohydrate: 49 g
dietary fiber: 14 g
calcium: 273 mg
iron: 6 mg
magnesium: 107 mg
potassium: 1,190 mg
sodium: 424 mg
zinc: 2 mg
thiamin: 0.4 mg
riboflavin: 0.4 mg
niacin: 5.9 mg
folate: 139 mcg
vitamin A: 930 mcg RAE
vitamin C: 198 mg
omega-6 fatty acids: 0.93 g
omega-3 fatty acids: 0.28 g

Curry in a Hurry Soup

MAKES 6 CUPS (1.5 L), **6 SERVINGS**

This tasty soup is incredibly easy to make. Red lentils cook very quickly. Other types of lentils may be used, but the cooking time will need to be extended to an hour. Curry paste is the secret ingredient in this dish; my favorite is Patak's mild curry paste. It's available at grocery stores and online.

> **4 cups** (1 L) **vegetable broth or water**
>
> **1 cup** (250 ml) **dried red lentils**
>
> **1 onion, diced**
>
> **1 tablespoon** (15 ml) **peeled and grated fresh ginger**
>
> **1 tablespoon** (15 ml) **minced garlic**
>
> **2 cups** (500 ml) **stemmed and chopped kale or spinach, lightly packed**
>
> **14 ounces** (398 g) **canned stewed or crushed tomatoes**
>
> **1½ tablespoons** (22 ml) **mild Indian curry paste**
>
> **½ teaspoon** (2 ml) **salt** (optional)
>
> **Juice of 1 lime** (optional)

Put the water, lentils, onion, ginger, and garlic in a large soup pot and bring to a boil over medium-high heat. Decrease the heat to medium-low and cook, stirring occasionally, until the lentils are soft, about 20 minutes. Add the kale, tomatoes, curry paste, and optional salt and cook, stirring occasionally, until the greens are tender, about 5 minutes. Stir in the optional lime juice just before serving.

VARIATIONS: Add other vegetables, such as cauliflower or other greens, or additional seasonings, such as ground black pepper, ground turmeric, or cayenne.

PER SERVING:
calories: 147
protein: 10 g
fat: 1 g
carbohydrate: 26 g
dietary fiber: 6.6 g
calcium: 71 mg
iron: 2.9 mg
magnesium: 18 mg
potassium: 546 mg
sodium: 305 mg
zinc: 0.24 mg
thiamin: 0.14 mg
riboflavin: 0.07 mg
niacin: 0.72 mg
folate: 16 mcg
vitamin A: 299 mcg RAE
vitamin C: 26 mg
omega-6 fatty acids: 0.07 g
omega-3 fatty acids: 0.05 g

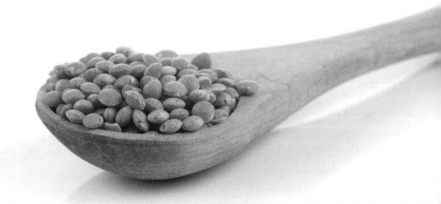

Full-Meal Rainbow Salad

A full-meal salad is a balanced and complete meal. One of the best ways to pull this dish together quickly is to prepare a giant salad and store it in a tightly covered glass bowl in the refrigerator. The ingredients should keep for four or five days. All the vegetables except those that need to be cut at the last minute should be in the salad bowl. Keep the toppings handy and have a dressing as well as cooked beans and grains in the refrigerator. At mealtime, assembly will take under five minutes!

MAKES 1 SERVING

LEAFY GREENS: Begin with 4 cups (1 L) or more of dark leafy greens. To make this super-fast, purchase prewashed greens that require no preparation. Otherwise, use dark lettuces, arugula, thinly sliced kale, spinach, or other favorite greens.

VEGETABLES: Add 2 cups (500 ml) of colorful veggies, and include something from every color of the rainbow. For example, green sprouts and snow peas, red cherry tomatoes or red pepper slices, grated or sliced orange carrots, thinly sliced or grated purple cabbage, and white kohlrabi or cauliflower. For a flavor boost, mix in ½ cup (125 ml) chopped fresh basil, cilantro, dill, parsley, or other fresh herbs.

FRUIT: Fruit is optional, but it can be a delightful addition. Add berries; chopped apples, mangoes or pears; or sliced citrus segments (oranges, tangerines, or grapefruit).

PROTEIN SOURCES: Top your salad with two protein-rich choices. Your best bets are ½–1 cup (125–250 ml) cooked beans (such as chickpeas, edamame, or lentils), 2–3 ounces (60–90 g) tofu (baked or smoked) or tempeh, ¼–⅓ cup (60–85 ml) hummus or other bean-based dip, and ½–1 ounce (15–30 g) seeds or nuts (such as chia, hemp, pumpkin, or sunflower seeds, or almonds or walnuts).

HEALTHY STARCHES: Add ¼–½ cup (60–125 ml) cooked intact whole grains (such as Kamut or spelt berries, quinoa, wild rice, or barley) or ½ cup (125 ml) cooked starchy vegetable (such as steamed and cooled corn, purple potato, sweet potato, or squash cubes). Refrigerating the grain or starchy vegetable after cooking will lower the GI.

SALAD DRESSING: Use 3–4 tablespoons (45–60 ml) of dressing from the options on pages 217–221. Alternatively, use balsamic vinegar instead of a dressing.

Select a medium-sized bowl or plate to assemble your full-meal salad. If you have the basic greens and vegetable salad prepped and ready to go, simply scoop up about 6 cups (1.5 L) in total and put it in your bowl or on your plate. Top with protein and starch choices, optional fruit, and dressing. Enjoy!

Power Greens Salad

You can find prewashed, ready-to-eat salad mixes containing kale, collard greens, spinach, arugula, and other nutrient-dense greens in almost any grocery store. These make salads almost instant. Other no-work additions include cherry tomatoes, bagged shredded carrots, packaged broccoli or cauliflower florets, snap peas, or snow peas. Serve the salad with your favorite dressing (see pages 217–221).

9–10 ounces (270–300 g) **packaged, prewashed power greens** (including baby kale, spinach, arugula, and other dark leafy greens)

1–2 cups (250–500 ml) **sliced or chopped vegetables**

1 cup (250 ml) **berries or other chopped fruit**

2½ ounces (75 g) **microgreens or sprouts**

Put the power greens in a large bowl. Top with the vegetables, berries, and microgreens. Stored in a sealed container (without dressing) in the refrigerator, the salad will keep for about 5 days.

VARIATION: Sprinkle with Omega-3-Rich Seed Mix (page 197), ground flaxseeds, or hemp seeds just before serving.

PER SERVING WITHOUT DRESSING (greens, 1 cup/250 ml mixed-color bell peppers, blueberries, microgreens):
calories: 88
protein: 5 g
fat: g
carbohydrate: 19 g
dietary fiber: 4 g
calcium: 87 mg
iron: 2 mg
magnesium: mg
potassium: 445 mg
sodium: 48 mg
zinc: 0.7 mg
thiamin: 0.16 mg
riboflavin: 0.15 mg
niacin: 2.15 mg
folate: 120 mcg
vitamin A: 280 mcg RAE
vitamin C: 74 mg
omega-6 fatty acids: 0.19 g
omega-3 fatty acids: 0.14 g

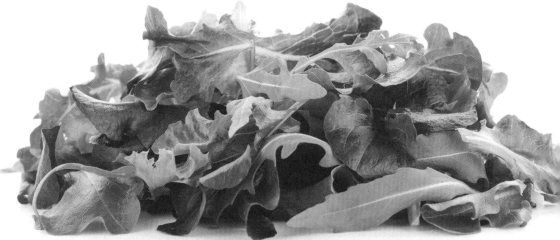

Cauliflower and Red Quinoa Salad

Raisins, curry paste, cauliflower florets, and red quinoa join forces in this delicious and colorful salad. For an attractive presentation and wholesome finish, garnish the salad with a sprinkle of slivered almonds or chia seeds.

MAKES 4 CUPS (1 L), 4 SERVINGS

3 cups (750 ml) **small cauliflower florets**

1 cup (250 ml) **cooked red quinoa**

1 large red bell pepper, diced

1 cup (250 ml) **chopped fresh parsley or cilantro, lightly packed**

¼ cup (60 ml) **raisins, soaked in hot water for 30 minutes, then drained**

2 tablespoons (30 ml) **mild Indian curry paste** (such as Patak's)

3 tablespoons (45 ml) **lemon or lime juice**

Steam the cauliflower for 5 minutes. Transfer to a medium bowl and add the quinoa, bell pepper, parsley, and raisins.

Put the curry paste in a small bowl. Add the lemon juice and stir until well combined. Add to the quinoa mixture and gently stir with a fork until evenly distributed. Stored in a sealed container in the refrigerator, leftover salad will keep for 4 days.

VARIATIONS: Use black or white quinoa instead of red. For even more flavor, add ¼ teaspoon (1 ml) ground turmeric and 1 teaspoon (5 ml) ground coriander along with the curry paste, and/or replace one-third of the parsley with chopped fresh mint or basil. To turn this salad into a main dish, add 1½ cups (375 ml) cooked or canned chickpeas, drained and rinsed.

PER SERVING:

calories: 129

protein: 5 g

fat: 3 g

carbohydrate: 26 g

dietary fiber: 8 g

calcium: 55 mg

iron: 3 mg

magnesium: 47 mg

potassium: 477 mg

sodium: 184 mg

zinc: 1.1 mg

thiamin: 0.1 mg

riboflavin: 0.2 mg

niacin: 1 mg

folate: 83 mcg

vitamin A: 94 mcg RAE

vitamin C: 98 mg

omega-6 fatty acids: 0.16 g

omega-3 fatty acids: 0.19 g

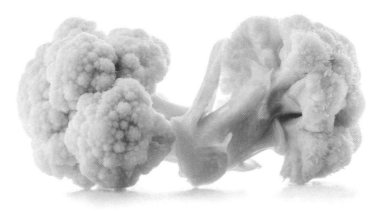

Chickpea Salad in Endive or Radicchio Cups

MAKES ABOUT 2 CUPS
(500 ML), 3 SERVINGS

This chickpea mixture is reminiscent of tuna salad. It's stuffed into cup-shaped endive or radicchio leaves. For a beautiful finish, decorate the tops with fresh herbs or a few sprouts. This makes a fun appetizer for company.

9–12 endive or radicchio cups

1½ cups (375 ml) cooked or canned chickpeas, drained and rinsed

1 large dill pickle, diced

⅓ cup (85 ml) finely diced celery

¼ cup (60 ml) minced red onion

2 tablespoons (30 ml) raw sunflower seeds

1 tablespoon (15 ml) chopped fresh parsley

1 tablespoon (15 ml) chopped fresh dill, or 1 teaspoon dried dill weed

3 tablespoons (45 ml) tahini

2 tablespoons (30 ml) lemon juice or apple cider vinegar

2 teaspoons (10 ml) Dijon mustard

1 teaspoon (5 ml) tamari

¼–½ teaspoon (1–2 ml) kelp powder (optional)

1 tablespoon (15 ml) nutritional yeast flakes

Ground black pepper

PER SERVING:

calories: 295

protein: 11 g

fat: 12 g

carbohydrate: 36 g

dietary fiber: 7.7 g

calcium: 91 mg

iron: 3 mg

magnesium: 59 mg

potassium: 482 mg

sodium: 530 mg

zinc: 2.2 mg

thiamin: 0.3 mg

riboflavin: 0.09 mg

niacin: 2.7 mg

folate: 121 mcg

vitamin A: 13 mcg RAE

vitamin C: 15 mg

omega-6 fatty acids: 4 g

omega-3 fatty acids: 0.09 g

Prepare the endive or radicchio cups by trimming, separating, washing, and drying the leaves. Select medium-sized leaves for this dish and reserve the remaining leaves to add to salads. Refrigerate until you're ready to fill the cups.

Put the chickpeas in a medium bowl and mash. Stir in the pickle, celery, onion, sunflower seeds, parsley, and dill. Put the tahini, lemon juice, mustard, tamari, optional kelp powder, and nutritional yeast in a small bowl and stir to combine. Season with pepper to taste. Add to the chickpea mixture and stir until well combined. Cover and refrigerate until serving time. Spoon into the lettuce cups just before serving.

VARIATIONS: For a hearty meal, roll the chickpea salad in a wrap (such as a raw or Ezekiel tortilla) or spread it on heavy pumpernickel bread for an open-faced sandwich. The chickpea salad also works nicely as a protein option on a Full-Meal Rainbow Salad (page 209).

Carrot-Raisin Salad

This classic duo is dressed with a delicious peanut sauce. The combination of flavors works remarkably well. For a lovely finish, garnish with chopped peanuts.

MAKES 4 SERVINGS

2 tablespoons (30 ml) **organic peanut butter**

2 tablespoons (30 ml) **lemon or lime juice or apple cider vinegar**

1 tablespoon (15 ml) **water**

1 tablespoon (15 ml) **peeled and grated fresh ginger** (optional)

1 teaspoon (5 ml) **tamari**

Pinch crushed red pepper flakes

2 cups (500 ml) **grated carrots, packed**

½ cup (125 ml) **chopped fresh cilantro or parsley, lightly packed**

⅓ cup (85 ml) **raisins**

Put the peanut butter, lemon juice, water, optional ginger, tamari, and red pepper flakes in a small bowl and stir until well combined. Put the carrots, cilantro, and raisins in a medium bowl and toss until well combined. Add the peanut sauce and stir until evenly distributed. Serve immediately or cover and refrigerate until serving time.

TIP: If your peanut butter is very thick, add a little extra water to the dressing, 1 teaspoon at a time, until the desired consistency is achieved.

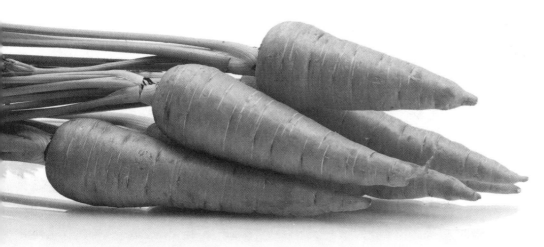

PER SERVING:
calories: 117
protein: 3 g
fat: 4 g
carbohydrate: 18 g
dietary fiber: 2.8 g
calcium: 36 mg
iron: 1 mg
magnesium: 0.14 mg
potassium: 323 mg
sodium: 157 mg
zinc: 0.25 mg
thiamin: 0.06 mg
riboflavin: 0.06 mg
niacin: 1 mg
folate: 23 mcg
vitamin A: 494 mcg RAE
vitamin C: 14 mg
omega-6 fatty acids: 0.08 g
omega-3 fatty acids: 0 g

Whole-Food Caesar Salad

MAKES 8 SERVINGS

Caesar salad is traditionally made with oil, eggs, and Parmesan cheese, and topped with fried croutons. This recipe is full of flavor but free of those unhealthy ingredients. Croutons are replaced with crispy baked tempeh or tofu, and although romaine lettuce is typically the only green used, this version includes kale for both nutrition and visual appeal.

1 head romaine lettuce, torn into bite-sized pieces

3 cups (750 ml) **stemmed and finely chopped or thinly sliced kale, packed**

1 cup (250 ml) **Caesar Salad Dressing** (page 217)

½ cup (125 ml) **Nut Parmesan** (page 216)

8 ounces (240 g) **Tempeh or Tofu Croutons** (page 215)

Put the lettuce and kale in a large bowl. Add the dressing and Nut Parmesan and toss until the greens are evenly coated. Top with the tempeh croutons.

PER SERVING:
calories: 189
protein: 12 g
fat: 11 g
carbohydrate: 16 g
dietary fiber: 5 g
calcium: 134 mg
iron: 3.4 mg
magnesium: 83 mg
potassium: 595 mg
sodium: 292 mg
zinc: 1.4 mg
thiamin: 0.2 mg
riboflavin: 0.2 mg
niacin: 3.4 mg
folate: 102 mcg
vitamin A: 541 mcg RAE
vitamin C: 76 mg
omega-6 fatty acids: 2.9 g
omega-3 fatty acids: 0.2 g

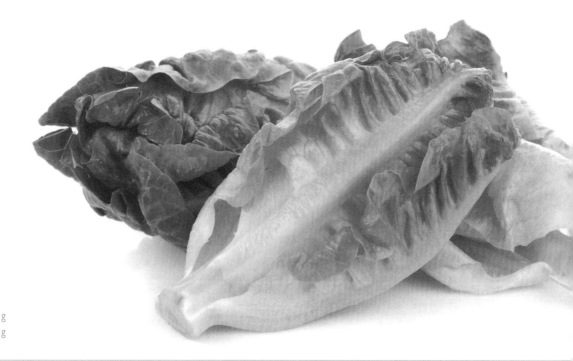

Tempeh or Tofu Croutons

These tasty nuggets are terrific on Caesar Salad (page 214) as well as on any other salad. Also use them hot from the oven to top dinner bowls or pasta.

MAKES 8 OUNCES (240 G), 8 SERVINGS

1 tablespoon (15 ml) **tamari**

1 teaspoon (5 ml) **Italian seasoning or mixed herbs and spices of your choice**

1 teaspoon (5 ml) **balsamic vinegar**

¼ teaspoon (1 ml) **ground turmeric**

8 ounces (240 g) **tempeh or firm or extra-firm tofu, cut into ½-inch** (1¼-cm) **cubes**

1 tablespoon (15 ml) **nutritional yeast flakes**

Preheat the oven to 350 degrees F (177 degrees C). Line a baking sheet with a silicone mat or parchment paper.

Put the tamari, Italian seasoning, vinegar, and turmeric in a small bowl and stir to combine. Add the tempeh and gently stir until evenly coated. Sprinkle with the nutritional yeast and gently stir again.

Arrange the tempeh in a single layer on the lined baking sheet. Bake until crispy, 25–30 minutes.

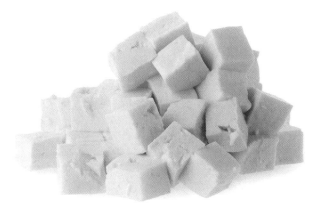

PER SERVING:

calories: 58

protein: 6 g

fat: 3 g

carbohydrate: 3 g

dietary fiber: 2 g

calcium: 32 mg

iron: 1 mg

magnesium: 24 mg

potassium: 124 mg

sodium: 128 mg

zinc: 0.3 mg

thiamin: 0.02 mg

riboflavin: 0.1 mg

niacin: 1.8 mg

folate: 7 mcg

vitamin A: 0 mcg RAE

vitamin C: 0 mg

omega-6 fatty acids: 1 g

omega-3 fatty acids: 0.06 g

Nut Parmesan

MAKES ABOUT 1¼ CUPS (310 ML), 20 SERVINGS

This great-tasting, dairy-free Parmesan should be a staple in your fridge. This one is made with nuts and seeds, which provide a crumbly texture, and nutritional yeast, which adds an irresistible cheesy flavor. Use it just as you would dairy-based Parmesan.

½ **cup** (125 ml) **raw cashews**

¼ **cup** (60 ml) **raw almonds**

¼ **cup** (60 ml) **raw sunflower seeds**

3 **heaping tablespoons** (45 ml) **nutritional yeast flakes**

1 **heaping teaspoon** (5 ml) **onion granules**

1 **heaping teaspoon** (5 ml) **garlic powder**

¼ **teaspoon** (1 ml) **salt**

Put the cashews, almonds, and sunflower seeds in a food processor and pulse just until crumbly. Add the nutritional yeast, onion granules, garlic powder, and salt and pulse just until combined. Store in a sealed container in the refrigerator.

PER TABLESPOON (15 ml):
calories: 39
protein: 2 g
fat: 3 g
carbohydrate: 2 g
dietary fiber: 0.6 g
calcium: 8 mg
iron: 0.4 mg
magnesium: 14 mg
potassium: 48 mg
sodium: 30 mg
zinc: 0.25 mg
thiamin: 0.02 mg
riboflavin: 0.02 mg
niacin: 0.16 mg
folate: 1.5 mcg
vitamin A: 0 mcg RAE
vitamin C: 0.12 mg
omega-6 fatty acids: 0.5 g
omega-3 fatty acids: 0 g

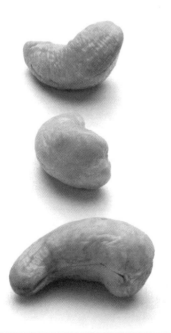
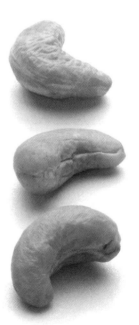
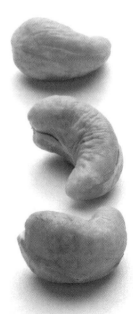

Caesar Salad Dressing

Of course this is perfect for Caesar Salad (page 214), but give it a try on other salads or on full-meal bowls.

MAKES ABOUT 1 CUP (250 ML), 8 SERVINGS

- ⅓ **cup** (85 ml) **raw cashews, rinsed, or soaked for 4–8 hours and then drained and rinsed**
- ⅓ **cup** (85 ml) **water**
- 3 **tablespoons** (45 ml) **lemon juice**
- 2 **tablespoons** (30 ml) **nutritional yeast flakes**
- 2 **tablespoons** (30 ml) **tahini**
- 2 **teaspoons** (10 ml) **capers**
- 1 **teaspoon** (5 ml) **caper brine**
- 1 **teaspoon** (5 ml) **Dijon mustard**
- 1 **teaspoon** (5 ml) **vegan Worcestershire sauce (optional)**
- 1 **large garlic clove**
- ¼ **teaspoon** (1 ml) **salt**
- ¼ **teaspoon** (1 ml) **ground black pepper**

Put all the ingredients in a high-speed blender and process until smooth and creamy.

PER 2 TABLESPOONS (30 ml):
calories: 58
protein: 2 g
fat: 4 g
carbohydrate: 4 g
dietary fiber: 0.6 g
calcium: 9 mg
iron: 0.6 mg
magnesium: 20 mg
potassium: 67 mg
sodium: 108 mg
zinc: 0.5 mg
thiamin: 0.09 mg
riboflavin: 0.01 mg
niacin: 0.3 mg
folate: 6 mcg
vitamin A: 0.3 mcg RAE
vitamin C: 3 mg
omega-6 fatty acids: 1.3 g
omega-3 fatty acids: 0.02 g

Creamy Dill Dip

MAKES 1½ CUPS (375 ML), **6 SERVINGS**

Fresh dill is the magic ingredient in this dip. Serve it with raw veggies or swirl it into soup to add flavor and creaminess.

- **¾ cup** (185 ml) **cashews, rinsed, or soaked for 4–8 hours and then drained and rinsed**
- **½ cup** (125 ml) **unsweetened soy milk or other nondairy milk**
- **1 tablespoon** (15 ml) **lemon juice**
- **1 tablespoon** (15 ml) **apple cider vinegar**
- **1 clove garlic, minced**
- **½ teaspoon** (2 ml) **salt**
- **½ teaspoon** (2 ml) **onion powder**
- **¼ cup** (60 ml) **finely chopped fresh dill**

Put the cashews, milk, lemon juice, vinegar, garlic, salt, and onion powder in a high-speed blender and process until smooth. Transfer to a bowl or storage container and stir in the dill. Stored in a sealed container in the refrigerator, the dip will keep for 3–4 days.

CREAMY DILL DRESSING: Increase the nondairy milk to 1¼ cups (310 ml), the lemon juice to 3 tablespoons (45 ml), the apple cider vinegar to 2 tablespoons (30 ml), the onion powder to 1 teaspoon (5 ml), and the fresh dill to ⅓ cup (85 ml). Serve over a green salad or a potato- or pasta-based salad. Makes 2⅓ cups (585 ml).

PER ¼ CUP (60 ml):
calories: 96
protein: 3 g
fat: 7 g
carbohydrate: 6 g
dietary fiber: 0.7 g
calcium: 26 mg
iron: 1.2 mg
magnesium: 0.28 mg
potassium: 129 mg
sodium: 209 mg
zinc: 1 mg
thiamin: 0.1 mg
riboflavin: 0.04 mg
niacin: 0.9 mg
folate: 5 mcg
vitamin A: 1.5 mcg RAE
vitamin C: 2 mg
omega-6 fatty acids: 1.2 g
omega-3 fatty acids: 0.01 g

Lemon-Tahini Dressing

Tahini can be used to flavor sauces and soups or to make salad dressings creamy. If the oil in your tahini rises to the top, just give it a good stir before using. This dressing can also be used as a sauce for full-meal bowls, steamed broccoli and other vegetables, baked potatoes, or beans. Freshly squeezed lemon juice provides better flavor than bottled, along with more vitamin C and no sulfites.

MAKES 2⅓ CUPS (585 ML), ABOUT 12 SERVINGS

1 cup (250 ml) **water**

⅔ cup (165 ml) **tahini**

⅔ cup (165 ml) **lemon juice**

1½ tablespoons (22 ml) **tamari**

1 pitted medjool date, or 2 small pitted soft dates

4 cloves garlic, crushed

Pinch cayenne (optional)

Put all the ingredients in a high-speed blender and process until smooth. Stored in a sealed container in the refrigerator, the dressing will keep for 3 weeks.

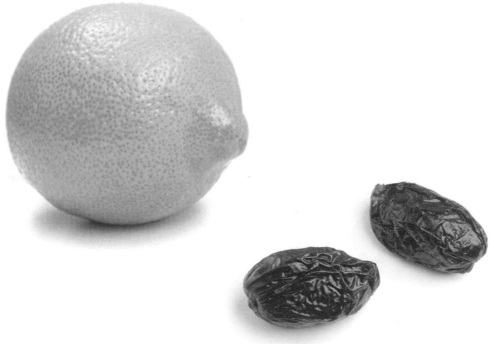

PER 3 TABLESPOONS (45 ml):

calories: 87

protein: 3 g

fat: 7 g

carbohydrate: 6 g

dietary fiber: 1.4 g

calcium: 58 mg

iron: 1.2 mg

magnesium: 0.2 mg

potassium: 89 mg

sodium: 136 mg

zinc: 0.6 mg

thiamin: 0.2 mg

riboflavin: 0.07 mg

niacin: 0.8 mg

folate: 15 mcg

vitamin A: 0.5 mcg RAE

vitamin C: 6 mg

omega-6 fatty acids: 3 g

omega-3 fatty acids: 0.05 g

Cheezy Roasted Red Pepper Dressing

MAKES 2 CUPS (500 ML),
16 SERVINGS

This dressing is reminiscent of cheese sauce. It's spectacular as a topping for vegetables, potatoes, and pasta. Serve it cold, room temperature, or heated. The dressing will thicken when stored in the refrigerator.

1 cup (250 ml) **unsweetened nondairy milk or water**

¾ cup (185 ml) **roasted red peppers** (about 2 large)**, homemade or jarred**

½ cup (125 ml) **cashews, rinsed, or soaked for 4–8 hours and then drained and rinsed**

½ cup (125 ml) **hemp seeds**

3 tablespoons (45 ml) **nutritional yeast flakes**

2 tablespoons (30 ml) **tamari**

2 tablespoons (30 ml) **lemon juice or apple cider vinegar**

2 cloves garlic, peeled

Ground black pepper

Pinch cayenne, optional

PER 2 TABLESPOONS (30 ml):
calories: 82
protein: 4 g
fat: 5 g
carbohydrate: 6 g
dietary fiber: 0.8 g
calcium: 15 mg
iron: 1 mg
magnesium: 48 mg
potassium: 95 mg
sodium: 305 mg
zinc: 0.3 mg
thiamin: 0.08 mg
riboflavin: 0.02 mg
niacin: 0.9 mg
folate: 7.2 mcg
vitamin A: 16 mcg RAE
vitamin C: 2 mg
omega-6 fatty acids: 1.9 g
omega-3 fatty acids: 0.5 g

Put the milk, red peppers, cashews, hemp seeds, nutritional yeast, tamari, lemon juice, and garlic in a high-speed blender and process until smooth and creamy. Season with pepper and optional cayenne to taste. Stored in a sealed container in the refrigerator, the dressing will keep for 3–4 days.

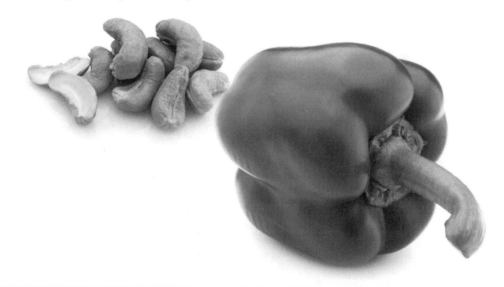

Liquid Gold Dressing

This dressing supplies omega-3 fatty acids and is packed with B vitamins. When it's made with nutritional yeast that is grown on a medium enriched with vitamin B12, you'll obtain that vitamin when you eat the yeast. The zucchini creates a dressing that's relatively low in fat but still has body. If you opt not to peel the zucchini, the dressing will have a green tinge.

MAKES 2 CUPS (500 ML), **8 SERVINGS**

2 cups (500 ml) **peeled and chopped zucchini**

¾ cup (185 ml) **hemp seeds**

½ cup (125 ml) **lemon juice, lime juice, or apple cider vinegar**

½ cup (125 ml) **nutritional yeast flakes**

2 tablespoons (30 ml) **tamari**

4 teaspoons (20 ml) **ground golden flaxseeds**

2 cloves garlic, crushed

1 teaspoon (5 ml) **Dijon mustard**

1 teaspoon (5 ml) **ground cumin**

1 teaspoon (5 ml) **ground turmeric**

Put all the ingredients in a high-speed blender and process until smooth. Stored in a sealed container in the refrigerator, the dressing will keep for 4 days.

PER ¼ CUP (60 ml):
calories: 34
protein: 3 g
fat: 1 g
carbohydrate: 5 g
dietary fiber: 1.7 g
calcium: 14 mg
iron: 0.7 mg
magnesium: 14 mg
potassium: 131 mg
sodium: 270 mg
zinc: 0.2 mg
thiamin: 0.05 mg
riboflavin: 0.06 mg
niacin: 0.7 mg
folate: 13 mcg
vitamin A: 3 mcg RAE
vitamin C: 13 mg
omega-6 fatty acids: 0.1 g
omega-3 fatty acids: 0.33 g

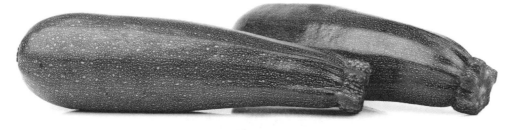

Gado Gado Sauce

MAKES ABOUT 1½ CUPS
(375 ML)

This spicy peanut sauce can also be used on salads or power bowls. It's also an excellent dip for collard wraps. Tahini replaces the more traditional sesame oil used in peanut sauce, and dates replace the sugar. Although tamarind paste is optional, it is a traditional part of gado gado sauce. If refrigerated, the sauce may thicken too much. Add a little water or unsweetened nondairy milk to thin to the desired consistency.

½ **cup** (125 ml) **organic peanut butter**

2 **tablespoons** (30 ml) **tahini**

2 **tablespoons** (30 ml) **lime juice**

¾ **cup** (185 ml) **boiling water**

1 **tablespoon** (15 ml) **tamari**

1 **teaspoon** (5 ml) **tamarind paste** (optional)

2 **pitted medjool dates**

½ **inch** (1.25 cm) **piece ginger, peeled**

2 **cloves garlic**

1–3 **small hot peppers, or ½ teaspoon hot sauce**

PER SERVING:

PER 3 TABLESPOONS (45 ml):

calories: 148

protein: 5 g

fat: 10 g

carbohydrate: 11 g

dietary fiber: 2 g

calcium: 15 mg

iron: 0.8 mg

magnesium: 12 mg

potassium: 114 mg

sodium: 129 mg

zinc: 0.3 mg

thiamin: 0.07 mg

riboflavin: 0.02 mg

niacin: 0.7 mg

folate: 8 mcg

vitamin A: 12 mcg; RAE

vitamin C: 18 mg

omega-6 fatty acids: 0.9 g

omega-3 fatty acids: 0.2 g

Put all the ingredients in high-speed blender and process on high until smooth. Refrigerate until ready to use.

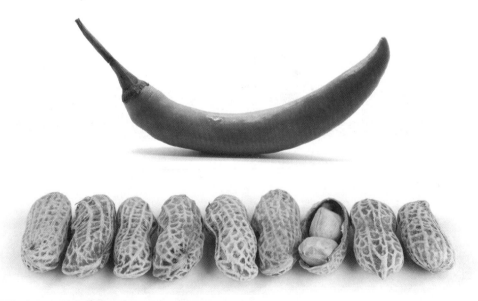

Cheezy Kale Chips

Kale chips make a fun addition to a light lunch and are a perfect treat for guests. They are best made in a dehydrator, but if you don't have a one, an oven will do the trick.

MAKES 8 SERVINGS

6 cups (1.5 L) **stemmed and coarsely torn kale leaves, packed**

½ cup (125 ml) **Cheezy Roasted Red Pepper Dressing** (page 220)

Put the kale and dressing in a large bowl and massage until the leaves are evenly coated with the dressing.

If using an oven, preheat the oven to 250 degrees F (121 degrees C). Lightly mist two baking sheets with nonstick cooking spray. Arrange the kale in a single layer on the lined baking sheets, making sure the pieces don't overlap. Bake until crispy, 45–60 minutes. Watch closely to ensure they don't burn.

If using a dehydrator, arrange the kale in a single layer on dehydrator trays, making sure the leaves don't overlap. Dehydrate at 130 degrees F (50 degrees C) until crispy, 10–12 hours.

Stored in a sealed container in the freezer, the chips will keep for 24 hours.

TIP: To prepare the kale, wash it thoroughly, remove the stems, and tear the leaves into bite-sized pieces. Dry them with a salad spinner or clean tea towel.

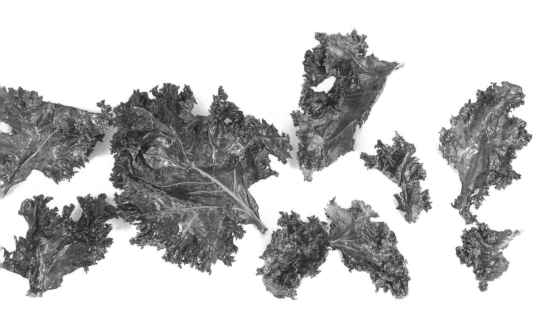

PER SERVING:
calories: 69
protein: 4 g
fat: 3 g
carbohydrate: 9 g
dietary fiber: 1.5 g
calcium: 84 mg
iron: 1.5 mg
magnesium: 43 mg
potassium: 301 mg
sodium: 177 mg
zinc: 0.4 mg
thiamin: 0.1 mg
riboflavin: 0.08 mg
niacin: 1.5 mg
folate: 20 mcg
vitamin A: 444 mcg RAE
vitamin C: 69 mg
omega-6 fatty acids: 0.9 g
omega-3 fatty acids: 0.4 g

Big Green Power Bowl

MAKES 2 SERVINGS

Power bowls make the perfect meal—they're satisfying, gorgeous, and super-nutritious. Black grains are suggested here for added phytochemicals, but you can substitute regular grains if you wish. Edamame is the protein addition in this dish, but other choices, such as lentils, chickpeas, tempeh, or tofu, can be used. Vary the veggies to suit your taste; asparagus, beets, broccolini, green beans, mushrooms, onions, and squash are excellent choices.

1 cup (250 ml) **finely cubed beets or winter squash**

10 Brussels sprouts, sliced in half

2 cups (500 ml) **trimmed and chopped broccoli**

2 cups (500 ml) **stemmed and thinly sliced kale or collard greens, firmly packed**

1 cup (250 ml) **snap peas or green beans**

1 cup (250 ml) **shelled frozen edamame**

1 cup (250 ml) **cooked black quinoa, black barley, black rice, or wild rice, kept warm**

1 small red bell pepper, chopped

1 cup (250 ml) **sunflower sprouts or other sprouts** (optional)

2 tablespoons (30 ml) **raw pumpkin seeds**

2 tablespoons (30 ml) **chia seeds**

6 tablespoons (90 ml) **Cheezy Roasted Red Pepper Dressing** (page 220), **Liquid Gold Dressing** (page 221), **or Lemon-Tahini Dressing** (page 219)

PER SERVING:
calories: 531
protein: 29 g
fat: 15 g
carbohydrate: 78 g
dietary fiber: 25 g
calcium: 398 mg
iron: 11.5 mg
magnesium: 167 mg
potassium: 1,694 mg
sodium: 231 mg
zinc: 3 mg
thiamin: 0.5 mg
riboflavin: 0.6 mg
niacin: 8.2 mg
folate: 377 mcg
vitamin A: 791 mcg RAE
vitamin C: 336 mg
omega-6 fatty acids: 1.5 g
omega-3 fatty acids: 2.2 g

Steam the beets for 5 minutes. Add the Brussels sprouts to the beets in the steamer and steam for 5 minutes. Add the broccoli and steam for 2 minutes. Add the kale and snap peas and steam for 3 minutes.

Boil the edamame until tender, 3–4 minutes. Drain.

Put the warm grain in two wide serving bowls. Add the steamed vegetables, bell pepper, and edamame. Top with the optional sprouts and the pumpkin and chia seeds. Drizzle with the dressing. Serve warm.

Black Bean Stuffed Sweet Potato

This dish requires minimal preparation. The dressing is optional but amps up the flavor factor. For a well-rounded meal, serve it with a green salad or steamed green vegetables.

MAKES 4 SERVINGS

4 medium sweet potatoes

2 cups (500 ml) **salsa**

1½ cups (375 ml) **cooked or canned black beans, drained and rinsed**

1 cup (250 ml) **frozen corn**

1 avocado, cubed or sliced

½ cup (125 ml) **Cheezy Roasted Red Pepper Dressing** (page 220; optional)

Preheat the oven to 350 F (175 C). Line a baking sheet with a silicone mat or parchment paper.

Pierce each potato several times with a knife or fork. Put on the lined baking sheet and bake until soft (a fork should easily pierce them), 50–60 minutes.

About 10 minutes before the potatoes are finished cooking, put the salsa, beans, and corn in a medium saucepan. Cook on medium-low heat, stirring occasionally, until hot.

Slice the cooked potatoes lengthwise down the center. Scoop out about half the flesh, leaving enough so the shell holds its shape. Add the flesh to the bean mixture and stir to combine. Spoon the bean mixture into the sweet potato shells. Top with the avocado and optional dressing.

TIP: You can stuff sweet potatoes with a variety of fillings. Chili is always a great choice.

PER SERVING
(without dressing):
calories: 379
protein: 10 g
fat: 8 g
carbohydrate: 68 g
dietary fiber: 14 g
calcium: 45 mg
iron: 4 mg
magnesium: 71 mg
potassium: 908 mg
sodium: 550 mg
zinc: 1.3 mg
thiamin: 0.2 mg
riboflavin: 0.1 mg
niacin: 3.3 mg
folate: 151 mcg
vitamin A: 1,108 mcg RAE
vitamin C: 44 mg
omega-6 fatty acids: 1 g
omega-3 fatty acids: 0.1 g

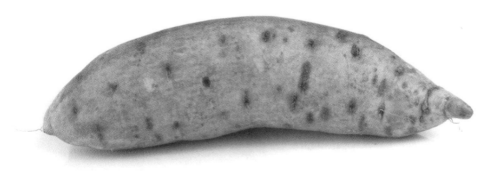

Gado Gado

MAKES 4 SERVINGS

Gado Gado is one of the five national dishes of Indonesia. It consists of steamed and raw vegetables and fried tofu or tempeh, and is topped with a spicy peanut sauce. We give the dish a health lift by baking rather than frying the tofu or tempeh and leaving oil out of the sauce. Get creative with the vegetables and vary them to include local, seasonal choices. If you are serving company, put all the items on a buffet and let your guests assemble their own plates. The toppings are optional, but they will make the meal more fun and flavorful.

SAUCE AND VEGETABLES

1½ cups (375 ml) **Gado Gado Sauce** (page 222)

4 cups (1 L) **stemmed and finely chopped kale or collard greens, packed and steamed**

2 **sweet potatoes, cubed and steamed**

2 cups (500 ml) **cut green beans, steamed**

2 cups (500 ml) **small broccoli florets and pieces, steamed**

2 cups (500 ml) **bean sprouts, lightly steamed**

2 cups (500 ml) **finely shredded red or purple cabbage**

2 **carrots, shredded**

1 **cucumber, thinly sliced**

1 **red bell pepper, sliced into strips**

TOFU OR TEMPEH

12 ounces (360 g) **firm tofu or tempeh, cut into ¾-inch (2-cm) cubes**

1 tablespoon (15 ml) **tamari**

1 teaspoon (5 ml) **salt-free seasoning blend of your choice**

½ teaspoon (2 ml) **ground turmeric**

OPTIONAL TOPPINGS

½ cup (125 ml) **sliced green onions**

½ cup (125 ml) **chopped fresh cilantro, lightly packed**

¼ cup (60 ml) **crushed organic peanuts**

1–2 **limes cut into wedges**

Hot sauce

PER SERVING

(with ¼ cup/60 ml sauce):

calories: 536

protein: 33 g

fat: 22 g

carbohydrate: 64 g

dietary fiber: 20 g

calcium: 902 mg

iron: 11 mg

magnesium: 296 mg

potassium: 2,287 mg

sodium: 693 mg

zinc: 4 mg

thiamin: 0.6 mg

riboflavin: 0.8 mg

niacin: 11 mg

folate: 448 mcg

vitamin A: 1,574 mcg RAE

vitamin C: 198 mg

omega-6 fatty acids: 5 g

omega-3 fatty acids: 0.9 g

Prepare the sauce and vegetables and set aside. See table 8.2, page 132, for steaming times.

To make the tofu, preheat the oven to 350 degrees F (177 degrees C). Line a baking sheet with a silicone mat or parchment paper. Put the tofu in a medium bowl. Add the tamari, seasoning blend, and turmeric and toss until the tofu is evenly coated. Arrange in a single layer on the lined baking sheet. Bake until crispy, about 30 minutes.

For each serving, arrange one-quarter of the vegetables on a plate. Top with one-quarter of the tofu, sauce, and optional toppings.

Moroccan Stew

The combination of spices in this one-pot meal is delicious. To switch things up, you can replace the squash with cubed sweet potatoes and the cauliflower with other vegetables, such as eggplant, broccoli, or carrots.

1 large onion, sliced into thin strips

4 cloves garlic, minced

2 cups (500 ml) **vegetable broth**

1 hot chile, minced

1 teaspoon (5 ml) **ground cumin**

1 teaspoon (5 ml) **ground coriander**

1 teaspoon (5 ml) **paprika**

1 teaspoon (5 ml) **ground turmeric**

½ teaspoon (2 ml) **ground cinnamon**

28 ounces (828 ml) **canned diced tomatoes**

3 cups (750 ml) **peeled and cubed butternut squash**

2 cups (500 ml) **cooked or canned chickpeas, drained and rinsed**

10 dried apricots, cut in half (optional)

3 cups (750 ml) **cauliflower florets**

6 cups (1.5 L) **spinach, lightly packed and coarsely chopped**

1 teaspoon (5 ml) **grated lime or lemon zest**

½ teaspoon (2 ml) **salt**

Ground black pepper

2 tablespoons (30 ml) **lime or lemon juice**

½ cup (125 ml) **chopped fresh cilantro, lightly packed** (optional)

¼ cup (60 ml) **slivered almonds** (optional)

Put the onion and garlic in a large soup pot. Add 2–3 tablespoons (30–45 ml) of the broth and cook over medium heat, stirring occasionally, until the onion is soft, about 5 minutes. Stir in the chile, cumin, coriander, paprika, turmeric, and cinnamon and cook for 1 minute. Add the remaining broth and the tomatoes, squash, chickpeas, and apricots and cook, stirring occasionally, for 20 minutes. Add the cauliflower and cook, stirring occasionally, until tender, about 15 minutes. Add the spinach and lime zest and stir to combine. Cook just until the spinach is wilted, 2–3 minutes. Add the salt and season with pepper to taste. Stir in the lime juice just before serving. Garnish with the optional cilantro and slivered almonds.

PER SERVING:

calories: 370;

protein: 15 g

fat: 3 g

carbohydrate: 78 g

dietary fiber: 18 g

calcium: 246 mg

iron: 6.2 mg

magnesium: 149 mg

potassium: 1,226 mg

sodium: 385 mg

zinc: 2.1 mg

thiamin: 0.4 mg

riboflavin: 0.3 mg

niacin: 6 mg

folate: 254 mcg

vitamin A: 1,241 mcg RAE

vitamin C: 142 mg

omega-6 fatty acids: 1 g

omega-3 fatty acids: 0.3 g

Fettuccine Alfredo

MAKES ABOUT 6 CUPS
(1.5 L), 6 SERVINGS

Pasta with a creamy sauce is arguably the ultimate comfort food. Fettuccine Alfredo is traditionally prepared with cream, butter, and cheese, but this surprisingly healthy variation uses cauliflower as a base for the sauce. Serve it over edamame fettuccine or your favorite nutritious legume or whole-grain pasta, and garnish it with Nut Parmesan (page 216).

3 cups (750 ml) **chopped wild or other mushrooms**

1 **white onion, chopped**

⅓ **cup** (85 ml) **white wine, or 3 tablespoons** (45 ml) **vegetable broth and 2 tablespoons** (30 ml) **white wine vinegar**

3 **cloves garlic, minced**

1 **tablespoon** (15 ml) **tamari**

2 **heaping cups** (500 ml) **cauliflower florets**

2½ **cups** (625 ml) **unsweetened cashew milk or other nondairy milk**

½ **cup** (125 ml) **raw cashews, rinsed, or soaked for 4–8 hours and then drained and rinsed**

3 **tablespoons** (45 ml) **nutritional yeast flakes**

2 **tablespoons** (30 ml) **arrowroot starch or cornstarch**

¼ **cup** (60 ml) **chopped fresh basil or parsley, lightly packed**

½ **teaspoon** (2 ml) **salt**

Ground nutmeg (optional)

Ground black pepper

PER SERVING
with 2 ounces (60 g)
edamame pasta:
calories: 327
protein: 30 g
fat: 9.6 g
carbohydrate: 37 g
dietary fiber: 16 g
calcium: 260 mg
iron: 8.6 mg
magnesium: 47 mg
potassium: 1,783 mg
sodium: 443 mg
zinc: 1.3 mg
thiamin: 0.12 mg
riboflavin: 0.3 mg
niacin: 2.1 mg
folate: 34 mcg
vitamin A: 5 mcg RAE
vitamin C: 22 mg
omega-6 fatty acids: 0.9 g
omega-3 fatty acids: 0.03 g

Put the mushrooms, onion, wine, garlic, and tamari in a large skillet and cook over medium-high heat, stirring frequently, until the vegetables are tender and slightly browned and the liquid has evaporated, 5–10 minutes.

Steam the cauliflower until tender, 5–7 minutes. Transfer to a high-speed blender. Add the milk, cashews, nutritional yeast, and arrowroot and process on high until smooth. Pour into the skillet with the mushrooms. Cook over medium heat, stirring frequently, until the mixture begins to thicken, about 5 minutes. Stir in the basil and salt. Season with optional nutmeg and pepper to taste.

TIP: For a complete meal, serve it with a Whole-Food Caesar Salad (page 214) topped with Tempeh or Tofu Croutons (page 215) for extra protein.

VARIATION: Add other vegetables, such as spinach, asparagus, artichoke hearts, or peas.

Old-Fashioned Bean and Vegetable Stew

Stew is a perennial favorite. This one features beans instead of beef, boosting the fiber and phytochemical content. You can use any beans, such as white and red kidney (or try half of each), great Northern, pinto, red, or adzuki.

MAKES 18 CUPS,
6 SERVINGS

2 cups (500 ml) **chopped or sliced mushrooms**

1 large onion, **diced**

2 stalks celery, **diced**

3 cloves garlic, **minced**

½ **cup** (125 ml) **white or red wine, or**
    ¼ **cup** (60 ml) **vegetable broth and**
    ¼ **cup** (60 ml) **wine vinegar**

4 cups (1 L) **vegetable broth**

3 tablespoons (45 ml) **tamari**

2 bay leaves

1 tablespoon (15 ml) **dried thyme**

1 teaspoon (5 ml) **dried savory**

1 teaspoon (5 ml) **dried rosemary**

½ teaspoon (2 ml) **ground turmeric**

3 potatoes (sweet, white, red, or purple), **chopped**

4 cups (1 L) **chopped cabbage**

2 medium carrots, **sliced**

1 small turnip, **cubed**

3 cups (750 ml) **cooked or canned beans, drained and rinsed**

2 cups (500 ml) **cut green beans, steamed until tender**

2 cups (500 ml) **unsweetened soy milk or other nondairy milk**

6 tablespoons (90 ml) **cornstarch mixed with 6 tablespoons** (90 ml) **water**

Ground black pepper

Put the mushrooms, onion, celery, and garlic in a large saucepan. Add the wine and cook over medium heat, stirring frequently, until the vegetables are soft, about 10 minutes. Add the broth, tamari, bay leaves, thyme, savory, rosemary, and turmeric and stir to combine. Add the potatoes, cabbage, carrots, and turnip and cook, stirring occasionally, until the vegetables are tender, about 45 minutes. Stir in the beans and cook, stirring occasionally, for 15 minutes. Add the green beans, milk, and cornstarch mixture. Cook, stirring constantly, until the gravy thickens. Remove the bay leaves. Season with pepper to taste. Serve hot.

TIP: To increase the nutritional value of the meal, add 4 cups (1 L) chopped dark leafy greens, lightly packed, 2–5 minutes before serving.

PER SERVING:
calories: 333
protein: 17 g
fat: 2 g
carbohydrate: 65 g
dietary fiber: 15 g
calcium: 160 mg
iron: 3.9 mg
magnesium: 83 mg
potassium: 936 mg
sodium: 508 mg
zinc: 1.6 mg
thiamin: 0.3 mg
riboflavin: 0.3 mg
niacin: 5 mg
folate: 212 mcg
vitamin A: 247 mcg RAE
vitamin C: 67 mg
omega-6 fatty acids: 0.14 g
omega-3 fatty acids: 0.15 g

Swiss-Style Tofu

MAKES 4 SERVINGS

This recipe was inspired by Ron Pickarski, seven-time medalist in the Culinary Olympics. This variation is oil-free and makes a wonderful dish for company. Serve it with baked sweet or regular potatoes or baked squash and a steamed green vegetable or salad.

12 ounces (360 g) **firm tofu cut into four equal pieces**

4 teaspoons (20 ml) **tamari**

2 cups (500 ml) **sliced mushrooms**

2 cups (500 ml) **thinly sliced onions**

1 green bell pepper, diced

3 cloves garlic, minced

¼ cup (60 ml) **red wine, or 2 tablespoons** (30 ml) **vegetable broth and 2 tablespoons** (30 ml) **red wine vinegar**

2 cups (500 ml) **canned crushed tomatoes**

3 fresh tomatoes, seeded if desired and chopped

2 tablespoons (30 ml) **miso dissolved in 2 tablespoons** (30 ml) **hot water**

2 tablespoons (30 ml) **tomato paste**

2 tablespoons (30 ml) **minced fresh basil**

PER SERVING:

calories: 286

protein: 23 g

fat: 8 g

carbohydrate: 33 g

dietary fiber: 8 g

calcium: 672 mg

iron: 5.2 mg

magnesium: 112 mg

potassium: 1,363 mg

sodium: 744 mg

zinc: 2.7 mg

thiamin: 0.4 mg

riboflavin: 0.5 mg

niacin: 9.8 mg

folate: 85 mcg

vitamin A: 124 mcg RAE

vitamin C: 69 mg

omega-6 fatty acids: 4 g

omega-3 fatty acids: 0.5 g

Preheat the oven to 350 F (175 C). Line a baking sheet with a silicone mat or parchment paper.

To make the tofu, put the tamari on a plate. Dip the tofu into the tamari and arrange it in a single layer on the lined baking sheet. Bake for 30 minutes.

To make the sauce, put the mushrooms, onions, bell pepper, and garlic in a medium saucepan. Add the wine and cook over medium-high heat, stirring frequently, until the vegetables are soft, 5–8 minutes. Stir in the crushed tomatoes, fresh tomatoes, dissolved miso, tomato paste, and basil. Decrease the heat to low and cook, stirring occasionally, for 10 minutes.

Spoon half the sauce into an 8-inch (20-cm) square glass baking dish. Arrange the tofu in a single layer on top of the sauce, then pour the remaining sauce evenly over the tofu. Cover and bake until hot and bubbly, 20–25 minutes.

Resources

Support Programs

Diabetes Undone	diabetesundone.com
E4 Diabetes Solutions	e4balance.org/ds
iThrive	go.ithriveseries.com
Mastering Diabetes	masteringdiabetes.org
PCRM Program for Reversing Diabetes	pcrm.org/reversingdiabetes

Informational Websites

Dr. Joel Fuhrman	drfuhrman.com
Dr. McDougall's Health & Medical Center	drmcdougall.com
Food Revolution Network	foodrevolution.org
Forks Over Knives	forksoverknives.com
Kick Diabetes Cookbook	kickdiabetescookbook.com
NutritionFacts.org	nutritionfacts.org
Ornish Lifestyle Medicine	ornish.com
The Plantrician Project	plantricianproject.org

References

CHAPTER 1

1. Centers for Disease Control and Prevention. 2017 Diabetes Report Card. 2017;TTY:232-4636. www.cdc.gov/diabetes/library/reports/congress.html.

2. Franz MJ, MacLeod J, Evert A, et al. Academy of Nutrition and Dietetics Nutrition Practice Guideline for Type 1 and Type 2 Diabetes in Adults: Systematic Review of Evidence for Medical Nutrition Therapy Effectiveness and Recommendations for Integration into the Nutrition Care Process. *J Acad Nutr Diet*. 2017;117(10):1659-1679.

3. Chia JSJ, McRae JL, Kukuljan S, et al. A1 beta-casein milk protein and other environmental pre-disposing factors for type 1 diabetes. *Nutr Diabetes*. 2017;7(5):e274.

4. Pozzilli P, Pieralice S. Latent Autoimmune Diabetes in Adults: Current Status and New Horizons. *Endocrinol Metab*. 2018;33(2):147.

5. Taylor R. Banting Memorial Lecture 2012 Reversing the twin cycles of Type 2 diabetes. *Diabet Med*. 2013;30(3):267-275.

6. Accili D, Talchai SC, Kim-Muller JY, et al. When b-cells fail: lessons from dedifferentiation. *Diabetes, Obes Metab*. 2016;18(April):117-122.

7. Dabelea D, Mayer-Davis EJ, Saydah S, et al. Prevalence of Type 1 and Type 2 Diabetes Among Children and Adolescents From 2001 to 2009. *JAMA*. 2014;311(17):1778.

8. Rodrigo N, Glastras S. The emerging role of biomarkers in the diagnosis of gestational diabetes mellitus. *J Clin Med 2018, Vol 7, Page 120*. 2018;7(6):120.

9. CDC. Gestational Diabetes | Basics | Diabetes | CDC. *Cdc*. 2017. https://www.cdc.gov/diabetes/basics/gestational.html.

10. American Diabetes Association. Classification and diagnosis of diabetes: Standards of medical care in Diabetes-2018. *Diabetes Care*. 2018;41(January):S13-S27.

11. Rosenquist KJ, Fox CS. Chapter 36: Mortality Trends in Type 2 Diabetes. *Diabetes Am*. 2009:1-14. https://www.niddk.nih.gov/about-niddk/strategic-plans-reports/Documents/Diabetes in America 3rd Edition/DIA_Ch36.pdf.

12. American Heart Association. Cardiovascular Disease and Diabetes | American Heart Association. http://www.heart.org/en/health-topics/diabetes/why-diabetes-matters/cardiovascular-disease--diabetes. Published 2015. Accessed August 31, 2018.

13. Chen H-F, Ho C-A, Li C-Y. Risk of heart failure in type 2 diabetes population: Comparison with non-diabetes subjects with and without coronary heart diseases. *Diabetes, Obes Metab*. 2019;1:12-119.

14. Boyko EJ, Monteiro-Soares M, Wheeler SGB. Chapter 20: Peripheral Arterial Disease, Foot Ulcers, Lower Extremity Amputations, and Diabetes. Cowie CC, Casagrande SS, Menke A, et al. eds. *Diabetes in America*. 3rd ed. Bethesda, MD: National Institues of Health, NIH Pb No. 17-1468; 2017. Chap. 20.

15. Cannon A, Handelsman Y, Heile M, Shannon M. Burden of Illness in Type 2 Diabetes Mellitus. *J Manag Care Spec Pharm*. 2018;24(9-a Suppl):S5-S13.

16. Yeh H, Golozar A, Brancati FL. *Cancer and diabetes.* Cowie CC, Casagrande SS, Menke A, et al. eds. *Diabetes in America.* 3rd ed. Bethesda, MD: National Institutes of Health, NIH Pb No. 17-1468; 2017. Chap. 29.

17. Restifo D, Williams JS, Garacci E, et al. Differential relationship between colorectal cancer and diabetes in a nationally representative sample of adults. *J Diabetes Complications.* 2018;32(9):819-823.

18. Zhang J, Chen C, Hua S, et al. An updated meta-analysis of cohort studies: Diabetes and risk of Alzheimer's disease. *Diabetes Res Clin Pract.* 2017;124:41-47.

19. Willis JR, Doan QV, Gleeson M, et al. Vision-Related Functional Burden of Diabetic Retinopathy Across Severity Levels in the United States. *JAMA Ophthalmol.* 2017;135(9):926-932.

20. Xu Y, Zhang Y, Yang Y, et al. Prevalence and correlates of erectile dysfunction in type 2 diabetic men: a population-based cross-sectional study in Chinese men. *Int J Impot Res.* 2019;31(1):9-14.

21. Semenkovich K, Brown ME, Svrakic DM, Lustman PJ. Depression in type 2 diabetes mellitus: prevalence, impact, and treatment. *Drugs.* 2015;75(6):577-587.

22. World Health Organization. *Waist Circumference and Waist-Hip Ratio: Report of a WHO Expert Consultation.* 2008; Geneva 8-11.

23. Johnson AMF, Olefsky JM. The origins and drivers of insulin resistance. *Cell.* 2013;152(4):673-684.

24. Nicholson T, Church C, Baker DJ, Jones SW. The role of adipokines in skeletal muscle inflammation and insulin sensitivity. *J Inflamm (United Kingdom).* 2018;15(1):1-11.

25. Chen L, Chen R, Wang H, Liang F. Mechanisms Linking Inflammation to Insulin Resistance. *In J Endocrinol.* 2015;2015:508409.

26. Agrawal NK. Targeting inflammation in diabetes: Newer therapeutic options. *World J Diabetes.* 2014;5(5):697.

27. Odegaard AO, Jacobs DR, Sanchez OA, et al. Oxidative stress, inflammation, endothelial dysfunction and incidence of type 2 diabetes. *Cardiovasc Diabetol.* 2016;15(1):1-12.

28. Nowotny K, Jung T, Höhn A, et al. Advanced glycation end products and oxidative stress in type 2 diabetes mellitus. *Biomolecules.* 2015;5(1):194-222.

29. Morales PE, Bucarey JL, Espinosa A. Muscle lipid metabolism: Role of lipid droplets and perilipins. *J Diabetes Res.* 2017;2017:1789395.

30. Li Y, Xu S, Zhang X, Yi Z, Cichello S. Skeletal intramyocellular lipid metabolism and insulin resistance. *Biophys Reports.* 2015;1(2):90-98.

31. Yazıcı D, Sezer H. Insulin Resistance, Obesity and Lipotoxicity. *Adv Exp Med Biol.* 2017;960:277-304.

32. Mota M, Banini BA, Cazanave SC, Sanyal AJ. Molecular mechanisms of lipotoxicity and glucotoxicity in nonalcoholic fatty liver disease. *Metabolism.* 2016;65(8):1049-1061.

33. Roseman HM. Progression from obesity to type 2 diabetes: lipotoxicity, glucotoxicity, and implications for management. *J Manag Care Pharm.* 2005;11(6 Suppl B):S3-11.

34. Del Turco S, Gaggini M, Daniele G, et al. Insulin resistance and endothelial dysfunction: a mutual relationship in cardiometabolic risk. *Curr Pharm Des.* 2013;19(13):2420-2431.

35. Neves AL, Coelho J, Couto L, Leite-Moreira A, Roncon-Albuquerque R. Metabolic endotoxemia: A molecular link between obesity and cardiovascular risk. *J Mol Endocrinol.* 2013;51(2).

36. Caricilli A, Saad M. The Role of Gut Microbiota on Insulin Resistance. *Nutrients.* 2013;5(3):829-851.

37. Scheithauer TPM, Dallinga-Thie GM, de Vos WM, et al. Causality of small and large intestinal microbiota in weight regulation and insulin resistance. *Mol Metab.* 2016;5(9):759-770.

38. Martínez Steele E, Popkin BM, Swinburn B, Monteiro CA. The share of ultra-processed foods and the overall nutritional quality of diets in the US: evidence from a nationally representative cross-sectional study. *Popul Health Metr.* 2017;15(1):6.

39. Gibney MJ, Forde CG, Mullally D, Gibney ER. Ultra-processed foods in human health: a critical appraisal. *Am J Clin Nutr*. 2017;106(3):ajcn160440.

40. Blumenthal DM, Gold MS. Neurobiology of food addiction. *Curr Opin Clin Nutr Metab Care*. 2010;13(4):359-365.

41. Daily Mail Reporter. How the size of an average restaurant meal has QUADRUPLED since the 1950s - with U.S. burgers now three times as big | Daily Mail Online. Daily Mail. http://www.dailymail.co.uk/news/article-2148970/How-size-average-restaurant-meal-QUADRUPLED-1950s-U-S-burgers-times-big.html. Published 2012. Accessed July 14, 2018.

42. Avena NM, Rada P, Hoebel BG. Evidence for sugar addiction: behavioral and neurochemical effects of intermittent, excessive sugar intake. *Neurosci Biobehav Rev*. 2008;32(1):20-39.

43. U.S. Dept of Health and Human Services. CDC. *Health, United States, 2016*. W.S. Government Printing Office. Washington DC. 2017. https://www.cdc.gov/nchs/data/hus/hus16.pdf#053. Accessed July 14, 2018.

CHAPTER 2

1. Brown A, Guess N, Dornhorst A, Taheri S, Frost G. Insulin-associated weight gain in obese type 2 diabetes mellitus patients: What can be done? *Diabetes, Obes Metab*. 2017;19(12):1655-1668.

2. Waugh N, Cummins E, Royle P, et al. Newer agents for blood glucose control in type 2 diabetes: Systematic review and economic evaluation. *Health Technol Assess (Rockv)*. 2010;14(36):3-247.

3. Buse JB, Caprio S, Cefalu WT, et al. How do we define cure of diabetes? *Diabetes Care*. 2009;32(11):2133-2135.

4. Cummings DE, Rubino F. Metabolic surgery for the treatment of type 2 diabetes in obese individuals. *Diabetologia*. 2018;61(2):257-264.

5. Steven S, Carey PE, Small PK, Taylor R. Reversal of Type 2 diabetes after bariatric surgery is determined by the degree of achieved weight loss in both short- and long-duration diabetes. *Diabet Med*. 2015;32(1):47-53.

6. Lim EL, Hollingsworth KG, Aribisala BS, et al. Reversal of type 2 diabetes: Normalisation of beta cell function in association with decreased pancreas and liver triacylglycerol. *Diabetologia*. 2011;54(10):2506-2514.

7. Bhatt AA, Choudhari PK, Mahajan RR, et al. Effect of a Low-Calorie Diet on Restoration of Normoglycemia in Obese subjects with Type 2 Diabetes. *Indian J Endocrinol Metab*. 2017;21(5):776-780.

8. Lean ME, Leslie WS, Barnes AC, et al. Primary care-led weight management for remission of type 2 diabetes (DiRECT): an open-label, cluster-randomised trial. *Lancet (London, England)*. 2018;391(10120):541-551.

9. Dunaief DM, Fuhrman J, Dunaief JL, Ying G. Glycemic and cardiovascular parameters improved in type 2 diabetes with the high nutrient density (HND) diet. *Open J Prev Med*. 2012;2(3):364-371.

10. Eddy JV. E4 Alive Diabetes Solutions. http://www.e4balance.org/ds/. Accessed August 18, 2018.

11. Kiehm TG, Anderson JW, Ward K. Beneficial effects of a high carbohydrate, high fiber diet on hyperglycemic diabetic men. *Am J Clin Nutr*. 1976;29(8):895-899.

12. Anderson JW. Effect of carbohydrate restriction and high carbohydrate diets on men with chemical diabetes. *Am J Clin Nutr*. 1977;30(3):402-408.

13. Anderson JW, Ward K. Long-term effects of high-carbohydrate, high-fiber diets on glucose and lipid metabolism: a preliminary report on patients with diabetes. *Diabetes Care*. 1978;1(2):77-82.

14. Anderson JW. High carbohydrate, high fiber diets for patients with diabetes. *Adv Exp Med Biol*. 1979;119:263-273.

15. Anderson JW. High-fibre diets for diabetic and hypertriglyceridemic patients. *Can Med Assoc J*. 1980;123(10):975-979.

16. Story L, Anderson JW, Chen WJ, Karounos D, Jefferson B. Adherence to high-carbohydrate, high-fiber diets: long-term studies of non-obese diabetic men. *J Am Diet Assoc*. 1985;85(9):1105-1110.

17. Anderson JW, Zeigler JA, Deakins DA, et al. Metabolic effects of high-carbohydrate, high-fiber diets for insulin-dependent diabetic individuals. *Am J Clin Nutr*. 1991;54(5):936-943.

18. Anderson JW, Hamilton CC, Brinkman-Kaplan V. Benefits and risks of an intensive very-low-calorie diet program for severe obesity. *Am J Gastroenterol*. 1992;87(1):6-15.

19. Anderson JW, Brinkman-Kaplan V, Hamilton CC, et al. Food-containing hypocaloric diets are as effective as liquid-supplement diets for obese individuals with NIDDM. *Diabetes Care*. 1994;17(6):602-604.

20. Collins RW, Anderson JW. Medication cost savings associated with weight-loss for obese non-insulin-dependent diabetic men and women. *Prev Med (Baltim)*. 1995;24(4):369-374.

21. Geil PB, Anderson JW. Nutrition and health implications of dry beans: a review. *J Am Coll Nutr*. 1994;13(6):549-558.

22. Anderson JW, Major AW. Pulses and lipaemia, short- and long-term effect: Potential in the prevention of cardiovascular disease. *Br J Nutr*. 2002;88(S3):263.

23. Anderson JW, Allgood LD, Turner J, et al. Effects of psyllium on glucose and serum lipid responses in men with type 2 diabetes and hypercholesterolemia. *Am J Clin Nutr*. 1999;70(4):466-473.

24. Anderson JW. Whole grains protect against atherosclerotic cardiovascular disease. *Proc Nutr Soc*. 2003;62(01):135-142.

25. Anderson JW, Waters AR. Raisin Consumption by Humans: Effects on Glycemia and Insulinemia and Cardiovascular Risk Factors. *J Food Sci*. 2013;78(s1):A11-A17.

26. Stephenson TJ, Setchell KDR, Kendall CWC, et al. Effect of soy protein-rich diet on renal function in young adults with insulin-dependent diabetes mellitus. *Clin Nephrol*. 2005;64(1):1-11.

27. Anderson JW, Smith BM, Washnock CS. Cardiovascular and renal benefits of dry bean and soybean intake. *Am J Clin Nutr*. 1999;70(3):464s-474s.

28. Keith M, Kuliszewski MA, Liao C, et al. A modified portfolio diet complements medical management to reduce cardiovascular risk factors in diabetic patients with coronary artery disease. *Clin Nutr*. 2015;34(3):541-548.

29. Jenkins D, Kendall C, Marchie A, et al. Type 2 diabetes and the vegetarian diet. *Am J Clin Nutr*. 2003;78(3):610S-616S.

30. Jenkins DJA, Kendall CWC, Faulkner DA, et al. Long-term effects of a plant-based dietary portfolio of cholesterol-lowering foods on blood pressure. *Eur J Clin Nutr*. 2008;62(6):781-788.

31. Jenkins DJA, Kendall CWC, McKeown-Eyssen G, et al. Effect of a Low–Glycemic Index or a High–Cereal Fiber Diet on Type 2 Diabetes. *JAMA*. 2008;300(23):2742.

32. Jenkins DJA, Kendall CWC, Banach MS, et al. Nuts as a Replacement for Carbohydrates in the Diabetic Diet. *Diabetes*. 2011;34(August):1706-1711.

33. Viguiliouk E, Stewart SE, Jayalath VH, et al. Effect of replacing animal protein with plant protein on glycemic control in diabetes: A systematic review and meta-analysis of randomized controlled trials. *Nutrients*. 2015;7(12):9804-9824.

34. Jenkins DJA, Hu FB, Tapsell LC, et al. Possible benefit of nuts in type 2 diabetes. *J Nutr*. 2008;138(9):1752S-1756S.

35. Jenkins DJA, Kendall CWC, Marchie, A, et al. The Garden of Eden - plant based diets, the genetic drive to conserve cholesterol and its implications for heart disease in the 21st century. Comparative Biochemistry and Physiology - Part A Molecular and Integrative Physiology. 2003;136(1):141-151.

36. Nishi SK, Kendall CWC, Bazinet RP, et al. Nut consumption, serum fatty acid profile and estimated coronary heart disease risk in type 2 diabetes. *Nutr Metab Cardiovasc Dis.* 2014;24(8):845-852.

37. Jenkins DJA, Kendall CWC, Augustin LSA, et al. Effect of legumes as part of a low glycemic index diet on glycemic control and cardiovascular risk factors in type 2 diabetes mellitus. *Arch Intern Med.* 2012;172(21):1653.

38. Viguiliouk E, Kendall CW, Kahleová H, et al. Effect of vegetarian dietary patterns on cardio-metabolic risk factors in diabetes: A systematic review and meta-analysis of randomized controlled trials. *Clin Nutr.* June 2018.

39. Nicholson AS, Sklar M, Barnard ND, et al. Toward improved management of NIDDM: A randomized, controlled, pilot intervention using a lowfat, vegetarian diet. *Prev Med.* 1999;29(2):87-91.

40. Barnard ND, Cohen J, Jenkins DJA, et al. A low-fat vegan diet improves glycemic control and cardiovascular risk factors in a randomized clinical trial in individuals with type 2 diabetes. *Diabetes Care.* 2006;29(8):1777-1783.

41. Barnard ND, Cohen J, Jenkins DJ, et al. A low-fat vegan diet and a conventional diabetes diet in the treatment of type 2 diabetes: a randomized, controlled, 74-wk clinical trial. *Am J Clin Nutr.* 2009;89(5):1588S-1596S.

42. Barnard ND, Gloede L, Cohen J, et al. A Low-Fat Vegan Diet Elicits Greater Macronutrient Changes, but Is Comparable in Adherence and Acceptability, Compared with a More Conventional Diabetes Diet among Individuals with Type 2 Diabetes. *J Am Diet Assoc.* 2009;109(2):263-272.

43. Yokoyama Y, Barnard ND, Levin SM, Watanabe M. Vegetarian diets and glycemic control in diabetes: a systematic review and meta-analysis. *Cardiovasc Diagn Ther.* 2014;4(5):373-382.

44. Bunner AE, Wells CL, Gonzales J, et al. A dietary intervention for chronic diabetic neuropathy pain: a randomized controlled pilot study. *Nutr Diabetes.* 2015;5(5):e158-e158.

45. Kahleova H, Tura A, Hill M, et al. A plant-based dietary intervention improves beta-cell function and insulin resistance in overweight adults: A 16-week randomized clinical trial. *Nutrients.* 2018;10(2).

46. Kahleova H, Matoulek M, Malinska H, et al. Vegetarian diet improves insulin resistance and oxidative stress markers more than conventional diet in subjects with Type2 diabetes. *Diabet Med.* 2011;28(5):549-559.

47. Kahleova H, Hrachovinova T, Hill M, Pelikanova T. Vegetarian diet in type 2 diabetes - improvement in quality of life, mood and eating behaviour. *Diabet Med.* 2013;30(1):127-129.

48. Belinova L, Kahleova H, Malinska H, et al. Differential acute postprandial effects of processed meat and isocaloric vegan meals on the gastrointestinal hormone response in subjects suffering from type 2 diabetes and healthy controls: A randomized crossover study. *PLoS One.* 2014;9(9):1-10.

49. Veleba J, Matoulek M, Hill M, et al. A Vegetarian vs. Conventional Hypocaloric Diet: The Effect on Physical Fitness in Response to Aerobic Exercise in Patients with Type 2 Diabetes. A Parallel Randomized Study. *Nutrients.* 2016;8(11).

50. Kahleova H, Klementova M, Herynek V, et al. The effect of a vegetarian vs conventional hypocaloric diabetic diet on thigh adipose tissue distribution in subjects with type 2 diabetes: A randomized study. *J Am Coll Nutr.* 2017;36(5):364-369.

51. Klementova M, Thieme L, Haluzik M, et al. A plant-based meal increases gastrointestinal hormones and satiety more than an energy- and macronutrient-matched processed-meat meal in T2D, obese, and healthy men: A three-group randomized crossover study. *Nutrients.* 2019;11(1):157.

52. Lee YM, Kim SA, Lee IK, et al. Effect of a brown rice based vegan diet and conventional diabetic diet on glycemic control of patients with type 2 diabetes: A 12-week randomized clinical trial. *PLoS One*. 2016;11(6):1-14.

53. Rinaldi S, Campbell EE, Fournier J, O'Connor C, Madill J. A Comprehensive Review of the Literature Supporting Recommendations From the Canadian Diabetes Association for the Use of a Plant-Based Diet for Management of Type 2 Diabetes. *Can J Diabetes*. 2016;40(5):471-477.

54. McMacken M, Shah S. A plant-based diet for the prevention and treatment of type 2 diabetes. *J Geriatr Cardiol*. 2017;14(5):342-354.

55. Olfert MD, Wattick RA. Vegetarian Diets and the Risk of Diabetes. *Curr Diab Rep*. 2018;18(11):1-6.

56. Utami DB, Findyartini A. Plant-based Diet for HbA1c Reduction in Type 2 Diabetes Mellitus: an Evidence-based Case Report. *Acta Med Indones*. 2018;50(3):260-267.

57. Toumpanakis A, Turnbull T, Alba-Barba I. Effectiveness of plant-based diets in promoting well-being in the management of type 2 diabetes: a systematic review. *BMJ Open Diabetes Res Care*. 2018;6(1):e000534.

58. International Diabetes Federation. IDF. *IDF Diabetes Atlas, 8th Edn*. Brussels, Belgium; 2017. http://www.diabetesatlas.org/.

59. Korsmo-Haugen H-K, Brurberg KG, Mann J, Aas A-M. Carbohydrate quantity in the dietary management of type 2 diabetes - a systematic review and meta-analysis. *Diabetes, Obes Metab*. 2019;21(1):15-27.

60. Sainsbury E, Kizirian N V, Partridge SR, Gill T, Colagiuri S, Gibson AA. Effect of dietary carbohydrate restriction on glycemic control in adults with diabetes: A systematic review and meta-analysis. *Diabetes Res Clin Pract*. 2018;139:239-252.

61. van Zuuren EJ, Fedorowicz Z, Kuijpers T, Pijl H. Effects of low-carbohydrate- compared with low-fat-diet interventions on metabolic control in people with type 2 diabetes: a systematic review including GRADE assessments. *Am J Clin Nutr*. 2018;(August):300-331.

62. Huntriss R, Campbell M, Bedwell C. The interpretation and effect of a low-carbohydrate diet in the management of type 2 diabetes: A systematic review and meta-analysis of randomised controlled trials. *Eur J Clin Nutr*. 2018;72(3):311-325.

63. Meng Y, Bai H, Wang S, et al. Efficacy of low carbohydrate diet for type 2 diabetes mellitus management: A systematic review and meta-analysis of randomized controlled trials. *Diabetes Res Clin Pract*. 2017;131:124-131.

64. Czyzewska-Majchrzak Ł, Grzelak T, Kramkowska M, Czyzewska K, Witmanowski H. The use of low-carbohydrate diet in type 2 diabetes-benefits and risks. *Ann Agric Environ Med*. 2014;21(2):320-326.

65. Kephart W, Pledge C, Roberson P, et al. The three-month effects of a ketogenic diet on body composition, blood parameters, and performance metrics in crossfit trainees: A pilot study. *Sports*. 2018;6(1):1.

66. Urbain P, Singler F, Ihorst G, et al. Bioavailability of vitamin D 2 from UV-B-irradiated button mushrooms in healthy adults deficient in serum 25-hydroxyvitamin D: A randomized controlled trial. *Eur J Clin Nutr*. 2011;65(8):965-971.

67. Numao S, Kawano H, Endo N, et al. Short-term high-fat diet alters postprandial glucose metabolism and circulating vascular cell adhesion molecule-1 in healthy males. *Appl Physiol Nutr Metab*. 2016;41(8):895-902.

68. Seidelmann SB, Claggett B, Cheng S, et al. Articles Dietary carbohydrate intake and mortality: a prospective cohort study and meta-analysis. *Lancet Public Heal*. 2018;2667(18):1-10.

69. Noto H, Goto A, Tsujimoto T, Noda M. Low-Carbohydrate Diets and All-Cause Mortality : A Systematic Review and Meta-Analysis of Observational Studies. *PLoS One.* 2013;8(1): e55030.

70. Li S, Flint A, Pai JK, et al. Low carbohydrate diet from plant or animal sources and mortality among myocardial infarction survivors. *J Am Heart Assoc.* 2014;3(5):1-12.

71. Ruzzin J. Public health concern behind the exposure to persistent organic pollutants and the risk of metabolic diseases. *BMC Public Health.* 2012;12(1):1.

72. Desrosiers TA, Siega-Riz AM, Mosley BS, Meyer RE. National Birth Defects Prevention Study. Low carbohydrate diets may increase risk of neural tube defects. *Birth defects Res.* 2018;110(11):901-909.

73. Schwingshackl L, Hoffmann G. Low-carbohydrate diets impair flow-mediated dilatation: evidence from a systematic review and meta-analysis. *Br J Nutr.* 2013;110(5):969-970.

74. Pan P, Yu J, Wang L-S. Colon Cancer. *Surg Oncol Clin N Am.* 2018;27(2):243-267.

75. David Katz. Toasting 2017 Goodbye With Ketogenic Kool-aid. Linked in. https://www.linkedin.com/pulse/toasting-2017-goodbye-ketogenic-kool-aid-david/?trackingId=6dLhnaaA0h72KLpsr DZVEQ%3D%3D. Published 2017.

76. Salas-Salvadó J, Martinez-González MÁ, Bulló M, Ros E. The role of diet in the prevention of type 2 diabetes. *Nutr Metab Cardiovasc Dis.* 2011;21(SUPPL. 2).

77. Sylvia H. Ley, Osama Hamdy, V. Mohan FBH. Prevention and Management of Type 2 Diabetes: Dietary Components and Nutritional Strategies. *Lancet.* 2014;383(9933):1999-2007.

78. Sievenpiper JL, Chan CB, Dworatzek PD, et al. Diabetes Canada Clinical Practice Guidelines Expert Committee - 2018 Clinical Practice Guidelines, Nutrition Therapy. *Can J Diabetes.* 2018;42:S64-S79.

79. Satija A, Bhupathiraju SN, Rimm EB, et al. Plant-Based Dietary Patterns and Incidence of Type 2 Diabetes in US Men and Women: Results from Three Prospective Cohort Studies. *PLoS Med.* 2016;13(6).

80. Tonstad S, Butler T, Ru Y, Fraser GE. Type of vegetarian diet, body weight, and prevalence of type 2 diabetes. *Diabetes Care.* 2009;32(5):791-796.

81. Chiu THT, Huang HY, Chiu YF, et al. Taiwanese vegetarians and omnivores: Dietary composition, prevalence of diabetes and IFG. *PLoS One.* 2014;9(2):1-7.

82. Chiu THT, Pan W-H, Lin M-N, Lin C-L. Vegetarian diet, change in dietary patterns, and diabetes risk: a prospective study. *Nutr Diabetes.* 2018;8(1):12.

83. Vang A, Singh PN, Lee JW, Haddad EH, Brinegar CH. Meats, processed meats, obesity, weight gain and occurrence of diabetes among adults: Findings from adventist health studies. *Ann Nutr Metab.* 2008;52(2):96-104.

CHAPTER 3

1. Ornish D, Magbanua MJM, Weidner G, et al. Changes in prostate gene expression in men undergoing an intensive nutrition and lifestyle intervention. *Proc Natl Acad Sci.* 2008;105(24):8369-8374.

2. Willett WC. Balancing Life-Style and Genomics Research for Disease Prevention. *Science.* 2002;296(5568):695-698.

3. Taylor R, Leslie WS, Barnes AC, et al. Clinical and metabolic features of the randomised controlled Diabetes Remission Clinical Trial (DiRECT) cohort. *Diabetologia.* 2018;61(3):589-598.

4. Lean ME, Leslie WS, Barnes AC, et al. Primary care-led weight management for remission of type 2 diabetes (DiRECT): an open-label, cluster-randomised trial. *Lancet.* 2018;391(10120):541-551.

5. Dunaief DM, Fuhrman J, Dunaief JL, Ying G. Glycemic and cardiovascular parameters improved in type 2 diabetes with the high nutrient density (HND) diet. *Open J Prev Med*. 2012;2(3):364-371.

6. Fraser GE. Vegetarian diets: what do we know of their effects on common chronic diseases? *Am J Clin Nutr*. 2009;89(5):1607S-1612S.

7. Tonstad S, Stewart K, Oda K, et al. Vegetarian diets and incidence of diabetes in the Adventist Health Study-2. *Nutr Metab Cardiovasc Dis*. 2013;23(4):292-299.

8. Bradbury KE, Crowe FL, Appleby PN, et al. Serum concentrations of cholesterol, apolipoprotein A-I and apolipoprotein B in a total of 1694 meat-eaters, fish-eaters, vegetarians and vegans. *Eur J Clin Nutr*. 2014;68(2):178-183.

9. Yao B, Fang H, Xu W, et al. Dietary fiber intake and risk of type 2 diabetes: a dose–response analysis of prospective studies. *Eur J Epidemiol*. 2014;29(2):79-88.

10. InterAct Consortium. Dietary fibre and incidence of type 2 diabetes in eight European countries: the EPIC-InterAct Study and a meta-analysis of prospective studies. *Diabetologia*. 2015;58(7):1394-1408.

11. Krishnan S, Rosenberg L, Singer M, et al. Glycemic Index, Glycemic Load, and Cereal Fiber Intake and Risk of Type 2 Diabetes in US Black Women. *Arch Intern Med*. 2007;167(21):2304.

12. Schulze MB, Schulz M, Heidemann C, et al. Fiber and Magnesium Intake and Incidence of Type 2 Diabetes. *Arch Intern Med*. 2007;167(9):956.

13. Bozzetto L, Costabile G, Pepa G Della, et al. Dietary Fibre as a Unifying Remedy for the Whole Spectrum of Obesity-Associated Cardiovascular Risk. *Nutrients*. 2018;10:943.

14. Silva FM, Kramer CK, de Almeida JC, et al. Fiber intake and glycemic control in patients with type 2 diabetes mellitus: a systematic review with meta-analysis of randomized controlled trials. *Nutr Rev*. 2013;71(12):790-801.

15. McIntosh M, Miller C. A diet containing food rich in soluble and insoluble fiber improves glycemic control and reduces hyperlipidemia among patients with type 2 diabetes mellitus. *Nutr Rev*. 2001;59(2):52-55.

16. Aydin Ö, Nieuwdorp M, Gerdes V. The Gut Microbiome as a Target for the Treatment of Type 2 Diabetes. *Genetics*. 2018;18(8):55.

17. Islam MA, Alam F, Solayman M, et al. Dietary Phytochemicals: Natural Swords Combating Inflammation and Oxidation-Mediated Degenerative Diseases. *Oxid Med Cell Longev*. 2016;2016:5137431.

18. Aryaeian N, Sedehi SK, Arablou T. Polyphenols and their effects on diabetes management: A review. *Med J Islam Repub Iran*. 2017;31:134.

19. Silveira AC, Dias JP, Santos VM, et al. The action of polyphenols in Diabetes Mellitus and Alzheimer's disease: a common agent for overlapping pathologies. *Curr Neuropharmacol*. 2018;16.

20. Singh H, Venkatesan V. Treatment of 'Diabesity': Beyond Pharmacotherapy. *Curr Drug Targets*. 2018;19(14):1672-1682.

21. Carrera-Quintanar L, López Roa RI, Quintero-Fabián S, et al. Phytochemicals That Influence Gut Microbiota as Prophylactics and for the Treatment of Obesity and Inflammatory Diseases. *Mediators Inflamm*. 2018;2018:9734845.

22. Ahangarpour A, Sayahi M, Sayahi M. The antidiabetic and antioxidant properties of some phenolic phytochemicals: A review study. *Diabetes Metab Syndr Clin Res Rev*. 2019;13(1):854-857.

23. Silva B, Oliveira P, Casal S, et al. Promising Potential of Dietary (Poly)Phenolic Compounds in the Prevention and Treatment of Diabetes Mellitus. *Curr Med Chem*. 2017;24(4):334-354.

24. Leiherer A, Mündlein A, Drexel H. Phytochemicals and their impact on adipose tissue inflammation and diabetes. *Vascul Pharmacol.* 2013;58(1-2):3-20.

25. Zhang D-W, Fu M, Gao S-H, Liu J-L. Curcumin and Diabetes: A Systematic Review. *Evidence-Based Complement Altern Med.* 2013;2013:16.

26. Sanati S, Razavi BM, Hosseinzadeh H. A review of the effects of Capsicum annuum L. and its constituent, capsaicin, in metabolic syndrome. *Iran J Basic Med Sci.* 2018;21(5):439-448.

27. Zhu J, Chen H, Song Z, et al. Effects of Ginger (Zingiber officinale Roscoe) on Type 2 Diabetes Mellitus and Components of the Metabolic Syndrome: A Systematic Review and Meta-Analysis of Randomized Controlled Trials. *Evid Based Complement Alternat Med.* 2018;2018:5692962.

28. Fernando WMADB, Somaratne G, Goozee KG, et al. Diabetes and Alzheimer's Disease: Can Tea Phytochemicals Play a Role in Prevention? *J Alzheimer's Dis.* 2017;59(2):481-501.

29. Fu Q-Y, Li Q-S, Lin X-M, et al. Antidiabetic Effects of Tea. *Molecules.* 2017;22(5):849.

30. Szkudelski T, Szkudelska K. Resveratrol and diabetes: from animal to human studies. *Biochim Biophys Acta - Mol Basis Dis.* 2015;1852(6):1145-1154.

31. Öztürk E, Arslan AKK, Yerer MB, Bishayee A. Resveratrol and diabetes: A critical review of clinical studies. *Biomed Pharmacother.* 2017;95:230-234.

32. Behloul N, Wu G. Genistein: A promising therapeutic agent for obesity and diabetes treatment. *Eur J Pharmacol.* 2013;698(1-3):31-38.

33. Chen S, Jiang H, Wu X, Fang J. Therapeutic Effects of Quercetin on Inflammation, Obesity, and Type 2 Diabetes. *Mediators Inflamm.* 2016;2016:9340637.

34. Link LB, Potter JD. Raw versus cooked vegetables and cancer risk. *Cancer Epidemiol Biomarkers Prev.* 2004;13(9):1422-1435.

35. Roohbakhsh A, Karimi G, Iranshahi M. Carotenoids in the treatment of diabetes mellitus and its complications: A mechanistic review. *Biomed Pharmacother.* 2017;91:31-42.

36. Manna P, Jain SK. Obesity, Oxidative Stress, Adipose Tissue Dysfunction, and the Associated Health Risks: Causes and Therapeutic Strategies. *Metab Syndr Relat Disord.* 2015;13(10):423-444.

37. Yoo JY, Kim SS. Probiotics and Prebiotics: Present Status and Future Perspectives on Metabolic Disorders. *Nutrients.* 2016;8(3):173.

38. Barengolts E. Gut microbiota, prebiotics, probiotics, and synbiotics in management of obesity and prediabetes: review of randomized controlled trials. *Endocr Pract.* 2016;22(10):1224-1234.

39. Sáez-Lara MJ, Robles-Sanchez C, Ruiz-Ojeda FJ, et al. Effects of probiotics and synbiotics on obesity, insulin resistance syndrome, type 2 diabetes and non-alcoholic fatty liver disease: A review of human clinical trials. *Int J Mol Sci.* 2016;17(6).

40. Baker EJ, Miles EA, Burdge GC, et al. Metabolism and functional effects of plant-derived omega-3 fatty acids in humans. *Prog Lipid Res.* 2016;64:30-56.

41. Molfino A, Amabile MI, Monti M, Muscaritoli M. Omega-3 Polyunsaturated Fatty Acids in Critical Illness: Anti-Inflammatory, Proresolving, or Both? *Oxid Med Cell Longev.* 2017;2017:5987082.

42. Bhaswant M, Poudyal H, Brown L. Mechanisms of enhanced insulin secretion and sensitivity with n-3 unsaturated fatty acids. *J Nutr Biochem.* 2015;26(6):571-584.

43. Trautwein EA, Koppenol WP, De Jong A, et al. Plant sterols lower LDL-cholesterol and triglycerides in dyslipidemic individuals with or at risk of developing type 2 diabetes; a randomized, double-blind, placebo-controlled study. *Nutr Diabetes.* 2018;8:30.

44. Vilahur G, Ben-Aicha S, Diaz E, et al. Phytosterols and inflammation. *Curr Med Chem.* 2018; June 22 (e-pub ahead of print).

45. Derdemezis CS, Filippatos TD, Mikhailidis DP, Elisaf MS. Review Article: Effects of Plant Sterols and Stanols Beyond Low-Density Lipoprotein Cholesterol Lowering. *J Cardiovasc Pharmacol Ther*. 2010;15(2):120-134.

46. Cooper AJM, Sharp SJ, Luben RN, et al. The association between a biomarker score for fruit and vegetable intake and incident type 2 diabetes: the EPIC-Norfolk study. *Eur J Clin Nutr*. 2015;69(4):449-454.

47. Liang J, Zhang Y, Xue A, et al. Association between fruit, vegetable, seafood, and dairy intake and a reduction in the prevalence of type 2 diabetes in Qingdao, China. *Asia Pac J Clin Nutr*. 2017;26(2):255-261.

48. Li M, Fan Y, Zhang X, et al. Fruit and vegetable intake and risk of type 2 diabetes mellitus: meta-analysis of prospective cohort studies. *BMJ Open*. 2014;4(11):e005497.

49. Schwingshackl L, Hoffmann G, Lampousi A-M, et al. Food groups and risk of type 2 diabetes mellitus: a systematic review and meta-analysis of prospective studies. *Eur J Epidemiol*. 2017;32(5):363-375.

50. Clark JL, Taylor CG, Zahradka P. Rebelling against the (Insulin) Resistance: A Review of the Proposed Insulin-Sensitizing Actions of Soybeans, Chickpeas, and Their Bioactive Compounds. *Nutrients*. 2018;10(4).

51. Agrawal S, Ebrahim S. Association between legume intake and self-reported diabetes among adult men and women in India. *BMC Public Health*. 2013;13(1):1.

52. Villegas R, Gao Y-T, Yang G, et al. Legume and soy food intake and the incidence of type 2 diabetes in the Shanghai Women's Health Study. *Am J Clin Nutr*. 2008;87(1):162-167.

53. Tian S, Xu Q, Jiang R, Het al. Dietary Protein Consumption and the Risk of Type 2 Diabetes: A Systematic Review and Meta-Analysis of Cohort Studies. *Nutrients*. 2017;9(9).

54. Aune D, Norat T, Romundstad P, Vatten LJ. Whole grain and refined grain consumption and the risk of type 2 diabetes: a systematic review and dose–response meta-analysis of cohort studies. *Eur J Epidemiol*. 2013;28(11):845-858.

55. Ye EQ, Chacko SA, Chou EL, et al. Greater whole-grain intake is associated with lower risk of type 2 diabetes, cardiovascular disease, and weight gain. *J Nutr*. 2012;142(7):1304-1313.

56. Kyrø C, Tjønneland A, Overvad K, et al. Higher whole-grain intake is associated with lower risk of type 2 diabetes among middle-aged men and women: The Danish Diet, Cancer, and Health Cohort. *J Nutr*. 2018;148(9):1434-1444.

57. Asghari G, Ghorbani Z, Mirmiran P, Azizi F. Nut consumption is associated with lower incidence of type 2 diabetes: The Tehran Lipid and Glucose Study. *Diabetes Metab*. 2017;43(1):18-24.

58. Luo C, Zhang Y, Ding Y, et al. Nut consumption and risk of type 2 diabetes, cardiovascular disease, and all-cause mortality: a systematic review and meta-analysis. *Am J Clin Nutr*. 2014;100(1):256-269.

59. Vuksan V, Choleva L, Jovanovski E, et al. Comparison of flax (Linum usitatissimum) and Salba-chia (Salvia hispanica L.) seeds on postprandial glycemia and satiety in healthy individuals: a randomized, controlled, crossover study. *Eur J Clin Nutr*. 2017;71(2):234-238.

60. Sylvia H. Ley, Osama Hamdy, V. Mohan FBH. Prevention and management of type 2 diabetes: dietary components and nutritional strategies. *Lancet*. 2014;383(9933):1999-2007.

61. Dam RM Van, Seidell JC. Carbohydrate intake and obesity. *Eur J Clin Nutr*. 2007;61. Suppl 1:S75-99.

62. Buyken AE, Flood V, Empson M, et al. Carbohydrate nutrition and inflammatory disease mortality in older adults. *Am J Clin Nutr*. 2010;3:634-643.

63. Myles IA. Fast Food Fever: Reviewing the impacts of the western diet on immunity. *Nutrition Journal*. 2014:13;61.

64. DiNicolantonio JJ, Mehta V, Onkaramurthy N, O'Keefe JH. Fructose-induced inflammation and increased cortisol: A new mechanism for how sugar induces visceral adiposity. *Prog Cardiovasc Dis*. 2018;61(1):3-9.

65. Stanhope KL. Sugar consumption, metabolic disease and obesity: The state of the controversy HHS Public Access. *Crit Rev Clin Lab Sci*. 2016;53(1):52-67.

66. Bhardwaj B, O'keefe EL, O'keefe JH. Death by Carbs: Added sugars and refined carbohydrates cause diabetes and cardiovascular disease in asian indians. *Mo Med*. 2016;113(5):395-400.

67. Asgari-Taee F, Zerafati-Shoae N, Dehghani M, Sadeghi M, Baradaran HR, Jazayeri S. Association of sugar sweetened beverages consumption with non-alcoholic fatty liver disease: a systematic review and meta-analysis. *Eur J Nutr*. 2018. (e-pub ahead of print)

68. Liu B, Sun Y, Snetselaar LG, et al. Association between plasma trans-fatty acid concentrations and diabetes in a nationally representative sample of US adults. *J Diabetes*. 2018;10(8):653-664.

69. Dorfman SE, Laurent D, Gounarides JS, et al. Metabolic implications of dietary trans-fatty acids. *Obesity*. 2009;17(6):1200-1207.

70. Tsutsui W, Fujioka Y. Is the association between dietary trans fatty acids and insulin resistance remarkable in Japan? *J Atheroscler Thromb*. 2017;24:1199-1201.

71. Liu B, Sun Y, Snetselaar LG, et al. Association between plasma trans-fatty acid concentrations and diabetes in a nationally representative sample of US adults. *J Diabetes*. 2018;10(8):653-664.

72. Zhang Q, Yang Y, Hu M, et al. Relationship between plasma trans-fatty acid isomer concentrations and self-reported cardiovascular disease risk in US adults. *Int J Food Sci Nutr*. 2018;69(8):976-984.

73. U.S. Department of Health and Human Services and U.S. Department of Agriculture. *2015-2020 Dietary Guidelines for Americans*. 8th Edition. December 2015. http://health.gov/dietaryguidelines/2015/guidelines/. Accessed October 29, 2018.

74. Eckel RH, Jakicic JM, Miller NH, et al. 2013 AHA / ACC Guideline on Lifestyle Management to Reduce Cardiovascular Risk A Report of the American College of Cardiology / American Heart Association Task Force on Practice Guidelines. *Circulation*. 2013:1-46.

75. Koska J, Ozias MK, Deer J, et al. A human model of dietary saturated fatty acid induced insulin resistance. *Metabolism*. 2016;65(11):1621-1628.

76. Fritsche KL. The Science of Fatty Acids and Inflammation. *Adv Nutr*. 2015;6(3):293S-301S.

77. Newsholme P, Keane D, Welters HJ, Morgan NG. Life and death decisions of the pancreatic b-cell: the role of fatty acids. *Clin Sci*. 2007;112(1):27-42.

78. Sacks FM, Lichtenstein AH, Wu JHY, et al. Dietary fats and cardiovascular disease: A presidential advisory from the American Heart Association. *Circulation*. 2017;136(3):e1-e23.

79. U.S. Deparment of Agriculture. Agriculture Research Service. Nutrient Data Library. USDA National Nutrition Database for Standard Reference, Legacy Version Current: April 2018. https://ndb.nal.usda.gov/ndb/search/list.

80. Fabricio G, Malta A, Chango A, De Freitas Mathias PC. Environmental Contaminants and Pancreatic Beta-Cells. *J Clin Res Pediatr Endocrinol*. 2016;8(3):257-263.

81. Magliano DJ, Loh VHY, Harding JL, et al. Persistent organic pollutants and diabetes: A review of the epidemiological evidence. *Diabetes Metab*. 2014;40(1):1-14.

82. EFSA. Cadmium dietary exposure. *EFSA Journal*. 2012;10(1):1-37.

83. Evangelou E, Ntritsos G, Chondrogiorgi M, et al. Exposure to pesticides and diabetes: A systematic review and meta-analysis. *Environ Int*. 2016;91:60-68.

84. Liu G, Zong G, Wu K, et al. Meat cooking methods and risk of type 2 diabetes: Results from three prospective cohort studies. *Diabetes Care*. 2018;41(5):1049-1060.

85. Stallings-Smith S, Mease A, Johnson TM, Arikawa AY. Exploring the association between polycyclic aromatic hydrocarbons and diabetes among adults in the United States. *Environ Res*. 2018;166:588-594.

86. Abdel-Shafy HI, Mansour MSM. A review on polycyclic aromatic hydrocarbons: Source, environmental impact, effect on human health and remediation. *Egypt J Pet*. 2016;25(1):107-123.

87. Vlassara H, Uribarri J. Advanced Glycation End Products (AGE) and Diabetes: Cause, Effect, or Both? *Curr Diab Rep*. 2014;14(1):453.

88. Nowotny K, Jung T, Höhn A, Weber D, Grune T. Advanced glycation end products and oxidative stress in type 2 diabetes mellitus. *Biomolecules*. 2015;5(1):194-222.

89. Velasquez MT, Ramezani A, Manal A, Raj DS. Trimethylamine N-Oxide: The Good, the Bad and the Unknown. *Toxins (Basel)*. 2016;8(11).

90. Janeiro M, Ramírez M, Milagro F, et al. Implication of trimethylamine n-oxide (tmao) in disease: potential biomarker or new therapeutic target. *Nutrients*. 2018;10(10):1398.

91. Samraj AN, Pearce OMT, Läubli H, et al. A red meat-derived glycan promotes inflammation and cancer progression. *Proc Natl Acad Sci*. 2015;112(2):542-547.

92. Alisson-Silva F, Kawanishi K, Varki A. Human risk of diseases associated with red meat intake: Analysis of current theories and proposed role for metabolic incorporation of a non-human sialic acid. *Mol Aspects Med*. 2016;51:16-30.

93. Erridge C. The capacity of foodstuffs to induce innate immune activation of human monocytes in vitro is dependent on food content of stimulants of Toll-like receptors 2 and 4. *Br J Nutr*. 2011;105(01):15-23.

94. Piya MK, Harte AL, McTernan PG. Metabolic endotoxaemia: is it more than just a gut feeling? *Curr Opin Lipidol*. 2013;24(1):78-85.

95. Fei N, Zhao L. An opportunistic pathogen isolated from the gut of an obese human causes obesity in germfree mice. *ISME J*. 2013;7(4):880-884.

96. White D, Collinson A. Red meat , dietary heme iron , and risk of type 2 diabetes : the involvement of advanced lipoxidation endproducts. *Adv Nutr*. 2013;4:403-411.

97. Radzeviciene L, Ostrauskas R. Adding salt to meals as a risk factor of type 2 diabetes mellitus: a case–control study. *Nutrients*. 2017;9(1):67.

98. Horikawa C, Yoshimura Y, Kamada C, et al. Dietary sodium intake and incidence of diabetes complications in Japanese patients with type 2 diabetes: analysis of the Japan Diabetes Complications Study (JDCS). *J Clin Endocrinol Metab*. 2014;99(10):3635-3643.

99. Colosia AD, Palencia R, Khan S. Prevalence of hypertension and obesity in patients with type 2 diabetes mellitus in observational studies: a systematic literature review. *Diabetes Metab Syndr Obes*. 2013;6:327-338.

100. Suckling RJ, He FJ, Markandu ND, MacGregor GA. Modest Salt Reduction Lowers Blood Pressure and Albumin Excretion in Impaired Glucose Tolerance and Type 2 Diabetes Mellitus. *Hypertension*. 2016;67(6):1189-1195.

101. Purohit V, Mishra S. The truth about artificial sweeteners – Are they good for diabetics? *Indian Heart J*. 2018;70(1):197-199.

102. Fagherazzi G, Gusto G, Affret A, et al. Chronic consumption of artificial sweetener in packets or tablets and type 2 diabetes risk: evidence from the E3N-European Prospective Investigation into Cancer and Nutrition Study. *Ann Nutr Metab*. 2017;70(1):51-58.

103. Suez J, Korem T, Zeevi D, et al. Artificial sweeteners induce glucose intolerance by altering the gut microbiota. *Nature.* 2014;514(7521):181-186.

104. Talaei M, Wang Y-L, Yuan J-M, Pan A, Koh W-P. Meat, dietary heme iron, and risk of type 2 diabetes mellitus: The Singapore Chinese Health Study. *Am J Epidemiol.* 2017;186(7):824-833.

105. Osorio-Yáñez C, Gelaye B, Qiu C, et al. Maternal intake of fried foods and risk of gestational diabetes mellitus. *Ann Epidemiol.* 2017;27(6):384-390.e1.

106. Schumacher L, Abbott LC. Effects of methyl mercury exposure on pancreatic beta cell development and function. *J Appl Toxicol.* 2017;37(1):4-12.

107. Brouwer-Brolsma EM, Sluik D, Singh-Povel CM, Feskens EJM. Dairy product consumption is associated with pre-diabetes and newly diagnosed type 2 diabetes in the Lifelines Cohort Study. *Br J Nutr.* 2018;119(04):442-455.

108. Drouin-Chartier J-P, Brassard D, Tessier-Grenier M, et al. Systematic review of the association between dairy product consumption and risk of cardiovascular-related clinical outcomes. *Adv Nutr.* 2016;7(6):1026-1040.

109. Virtanen JK, Mursu J, Tuomainen T-P, et al. Egg consumption and risk of incident type 2 diabetes in men: the Kuopio Ischaemic Heart Disease Risk Factor Study. *Am J Clin Nutr.* 2015;101(5):1088-1096.

110. Djoussé L, Petrone AB, Hickson DA, et al. Egg consumption and risk of type 2 diabetes among African Americans: The Jackson Heart Study. *Clin Nutr.* 2016;35(3):679-684.

111. Jang J, Shin M-J, Kim OY, Park K. Longitudinal association between egg consumption and the risk of cardiovascular disease: interaction with type 2 diabetes mellitus. *Nutr Diabetes.* 2018;8(1):20.

112. Hu EA, Pan A, Malik V, Sun Q. White rice consumption and risk of type 2 diabetes: meta-analysis and systematic review. *BMJ.* 2012;344:e1454.

113. Zhou J, Sheng J, Fan Y, et al. Dietary patterns, dietary intakes and the risk of type 2 diabetes: results from the Hefei Nutrition and Health Study. Int J Food Sci Nutr. 2018:1-9. (epub ahead of print).

114. AlEssa HB, Bhupathiraju SN, Malik VS, et al. Carbohydrate quality and quantity and risk of type 2 diabetes in US women. *Am J Clin Nutr.* 2015;102(6):1543-1553.

115. Malik VS, Popkin BM, Bray GA, et al. Sugar-sweetened beverages and risk of metabolic syndrome and type 2 diabetes: a meta-analysis. *Diabetes Care.* 2010;33(11):2477-2483.

116. Medina-Remón A, Kirwan R, Lamuela-Raventós RM, Estruch R. Dietary patterns and the risk of obesity, type 2 diabetes mellitus, cardiovascular diseases, asthma, and neurodegenerative diseases. *Crit Rev Food Sci Nutr.* 2018;58(2):262-296.

117. Schwingshackl L, Hoffmann G. Diet Quality as Assessed by the Healthy Eating Index, the Alternate Healthy Eating Index, the Dietary Approaches to Stop Hypertension Score, and Health Outcomes: A Systematic Review and Meta-Analysis of Cohort Studies. *J Acad Nutr Diet.* 2015;115(5):780-800.e5.

118. Odegaard AO, Koh WP, Yuan J-M, Gross MD, Pereira MA. Western-style fast food intake and cardiometabolic risk in an Eastern country. *Circulation.* 2012;126(2):182-188.

119. Mezuk B, Li X, Cederin K, et al. Beyond Access: characteristics of the food environment and risk of diabetes. *Am J Epidemiol.* 2016;183(12):1129-1137.

120. Bao W, Tobias DK, Olsen SF, Zhang C. Pre-pregnancy fried food consumption and the risk of gestational diabetes mellitus: a prospective cohort study. *Diabetologia.* 2014;57(12):2485-2491.

CHAPTER 4

1. World Health Organization. Obesity and Overweight Factsheet. 2003. https://www.who.int/dietphysicalactivity/media/en/gsfs_obesity.pdf. Accessed January 21, 2019.

2. Clifton P. Assessing the evidence for weight loss strategies in people with and without type 2 diabetes. *World J Diabetes*. 2017;8(10):440-454.

3. Rehackova L, Araújo-Soares V, Adamson AJ, et al. Acceptability of a very-low-energy diet in Type 2 diabetes: patient experiences and behaviour regulation. *Diabet Med*. 2017;34(11):1554-1567.

4. Tonstad S, Butler T, Yan R, Fraser GE. Type of Vegetarian Diet, Body Weight, and Prevalence of Type 2 Diabetes. *Diabetes Care*. 2009;32(5):791-796.

5. Spencer EA, Appleby PN, Davey GK, Key TJ. Diet and body mass index in 38 000 EPIC-Oxford meat-eaters, fish-eaters, vegetarians and vegans. *Int J Obes*. 2003;27(6):728-734.

6. Jackson AS, Ellis KJ, McFarlin BK, Sailors MH, Bray MS. Body mass index bias in defining obesity of diverse young adults: the Training Intervention and Genetics of Exercise Response (TIGER) Study. *Br J Nutr*. 2009;102(07):1084.

7. Campbell MC, Tishkoff SA. African genetic diversity: implications for human demographic history, modern human origins, and complex disease mapping. *Annu Rev Genomics Hum Genet*. 2008;9(1):403-433.

8. Shiwaku K, Anuurad E, Enkhmaa B, et al. Overweight Japanese with body mass indexes of 23.0-24.9 have higher risks for obesity-associated disorders: a comparison of Japanese and Mongolians. *Int J Obes Relat Metab Disord*. 2004;28(1):152-158.

9. Gray LJ, Yates T, Davies MJ, et al. Defining Obesity Cut-Off Points for Migrant South Asians. *PLoS One*. 2011;6(10):4-10.

10. Nishida C. Appropriate Body-Mass Index for Asian Populations and Its Implications for Policy and Intervention Strategies. *Lancet*. 2004;363(9403):157-63.

11. Center for Health Statistics N. Table 53. Selected Health Conditions and Risk Factors, by Age: United States, Selected Years 1988–1994 through 2015–2016; 2017. https://www.cdc.gov/nchs/hus/contents2017.htm#053. Accessed January 21, 2019.

12. Corsica JA, Pelchat ML. Food addiction: true or false? *Curr Opin Gastroenterol*. 2010;26(2):165-169.

13. Ifland JR, Preuss HG, Marcus MT, et al. Refined food addiction: a classic substance use disorder. *Med Hypotheses*. 2009;72(5):518-526.

14. Liu Y, von Deneen KM, Kobeissy FH, Gold MS. Food addiction and obesity: evidence from bench to bedside. *J Psychoactive Drugs*. 2010;42(2):133-145.

15. Holtcamp W. Obesogens: an environmental link to obesity. *Environ Health Perspect*. 2012;120(2):a62-8.

16. Grün F, Blumberg B. Minireview: the case for obesogens. *Mol Endocrinol*. 2009;23(8):1127-1134.

17. Janesick A, Blumberg B. Endocrine disrupting chemicals and the developmental programming of adipogenesis and obesity. *Birth Defects Res C Embryo Today*. 2011;93(1):34-50.

18. Darbre PD. Endocrine Disruptors and Obesity. *Curr Obes Rep*. 2017;6(1):18-27.

19. Chao A, Grey M, Whittemore R, et al. Examining the mediating roles of binge eating and emotional eating in the relationships between stress and metabolic abnormalities. *J Behav Med*. 2016;39(2):320-332.

20. Guerdjikova AI, Mori N, Casuto LS, McElroy SL. Binge Eating Disorder. *Psychiatr Clin North Am*. 2017;40(2):255-266.

21. Lim EL, Hollingsworth KG, Aribisala BS, et al. Reversal of type 2 diabetes: Normalisation of beta cell function in association with decreased pancreas and liver triacylglycerol. *Diabetologia*. 2011;54(10):2506-2514.

22. Lean MEJ, Leslie WS, Barnes AC, et al. Primary care-led weight management for remission of type 2 diabetes (DiRECT): An open-label, cluster-randomised trial. *Lancet*. 2017;391(10120):541-551.

23. Bhatt AA, Choudhari PK, Mahajan RR, et al. Effect of a low-calorie diet on restoration of normo-glycemia in obese subjects with type 2 diabetes. *Indian J Endocrinol Metab*. 2017;21(5):776-780.

24. Cheng C-W, Villani V, Buono R, et al. Fasting-mimicking diet promotes Ngn3-driven b-Cell regeneration to reverse diabetes. *Cell*. 2017;168(5):775-788.e12.

25. Patterson RE, Sears DD. Metabolic effects of intermittent fasting. *Annu Rev Nutr*. 2017;37(1):371-393.

26. Jane L, Atkinson G, Jaime V, et al. Intermittent fasting interventions for the treatment of over-weight and obesity in adults aged 18 years and over: a systematic review protocol. *JBI Database Syst Rev Implement Reports*. 2015;13(10):60-68.

27. Rothschild J, Hoddy KK, Jambazian P, Varady KA. Time-restricted feeding and risk of metabolic disease: a review of human and animal studies. *Nutr Rev*. 2014;72(5):308-318.

28. Longo VD, Panda S. Fasting, circadian rhythms, and time-restricted feeding in healthy lifespan. *Cell Metab*. 2016;23(6):1048-1059.

29. Mattson MP, Longo VD, Harvie M. Impact of intermittent fasting on health and disease processes. *Ageing Res Rev*. 2017;39:46-58.

30. Harvie M, Howell A. Potential benefits and harms of intermittent energy restriction and inter-mittent fasting amongst obese, overweight and normal weight subjects—A narrative review of human and animal evidence. *Behav Sci (Basel)*. 2017;7(4):4.

31. Brandhorst S, Choi IY, Wei M, et al. A periodic diet that mimics fasting promotes multi-system regeneration, enhanced cognitive performance, and healthspan. *Cell Metab*. 2015;22(1):86-99.

32. Ouchi N, Higuchi A, Ohashi K, et al. Sfrp5 Is an anti-inflammatory adipokine that modulates metabolic dysfunction in obesity. *Science (80-)*. 2010;329(5990):454-457.

33. Karczewski J, ledzi ska E, Baturo A, et al. Obesity and inflammation. *Eur Cytokine Netw*. 2018;29(3):83-94.

34. Sato J, Kanazawa A, Watada H. Type 2 Diabetes and Bacteremia. *Ann Nutr Metab*. 2017;71(1):17-22.

35. Teixeira TFS, Collado MC, Ferreira CLLF, Bressan J, Peluzio M do CG. Potential mecha-nisms for the emerging link between obesity and increased intestinal permeability. *Nutr Res*. 2012;32(9):637-647.

36. Genser L, Aguanno D, Soula HA, et al. Increased jejunal permeability in human obesity is revealed by a lipid challenge and is linked to inflammation and type 2 diabetes. *J Pathol*. 2018;246(2):217-230.

37. Rapin JR, Wiernsperger N. Possible links between intestinal permeability and food processing: A potential therapeutic niche for glutamine. *Clinics (Sao Paulo)*. 2010;65(6):635-643.

38. Catalioto R-M, Maggi CA, Giuliani S. Intestinal epithelial barrier dysfunction in disease and possible therapeutical interventions. *Curr Med Chem*. 2011;18(3):398-426.

39. Fasano A. Zonulin and its regulation of intestinal barrier function : The biological door to inflam-mation , autoimmunity, and cancer. *Physiol Rev*. 2011;91(1):151-175.

40. Fasano A. Leaky gut and autoimmune diseases. *Clin Rev Allergy Immunol*. 2012;42(1):71-78.

41. Kort S De, Keszthelyi D, Masclee AAM. Leaky gut and diabetes mellitus : what is the link? *Obes Rev*. 2011;12(6):449-458.

42. Midura-Kiela MT, Radhakrishnan VM, Larmonier CB, et al. Curcumin inhibits interferon-g signaling in colonic epithelial cells. *Am J Physiol Liver Physiol*. 2012;302(1):G85-G96.

43. Kirkley AG, Sargis RM. Environmental endocrine disruption of energy metabolism and cardiovascular risk. *Curr Diab Rep*. 2014;14(6):494.

44. Roca-Saavedra P, Mendez-Vilabrille V, Miranda JM, et al. Food additives, contaminants and other minor components: effects on human gut microbiota—a review. *J Physiol Biochem*. 2018;74(1):69-83.

45. Liontiris MI, Mazokopakis EE. A concise review of Hashimoto thyroiditis (HT) and the importance of iodine, selenium, vitamin D and gluten on the autoimmunity and dietary management of HT patients.Points that need more investigation. *Hell J Nucl Med*. 20(1):51-56.

46. Ferrari SM, Fallahi P, Antonelli A, Benvenga S. Environmental issues in thyroid diseases. *Front Endocrinol (Lausanne)*. 2017;8:50.

47. Hirschberg AL, Naessén S, Stridsberg M, Byström B, Holtet J. Impaired cholecystokinin secretion and disturbed appetite regulation in women with polycystic ovary syndrome. *Gynecol Endocrinol*. 2004;19(2):79-87.

48. Jones A, McMillan MR, Jones RW, et al. Adiposity is associated with blunted cardiovascular, neuroendocrine and cognitive responses to acute mental stress. Lipinski M, ed. *PLoS One*. 2012;7(6):e39143.

49. Joel Fuhrman. ANDI Food Scores: Rating the Nutrient Density of Foods | DrFuhrman.com. https://www.drfuhrman.com/library/eat-to-live-blog/128/andi-food-scores-rating-the-nutrient-density-of-foods. Accessed January 22, 2019.

50. Clifton P. Assessing the evidence for weight loss strategies in people with and without type 2 diabetes. *World J Diabetes*. 2017;8(10):440-454.

CHAPTER 5

1. Food and Agriculture Organization of the United Nations., *Carbohydrates in Human Nutrition: Report of a Joint FAO/WHO Expert Consultation, Rome, 14-18 April 1997*. World Health Organization; 1998.

2. Craig WJ. Phytochemicals: Guardians of our Health. *J Am Diet Assoc*. 1997;97(10):S199-S204.

3. Sievenpiper JL, Chan CB, Dworatzek PD, Freeze C, L WS. Diabetes Canada Clinical Practice Guidelines Expert Committee - 2018 Clinical Practice Guidelines, Nutrition Therapy. *Can J Diabetes*. 2018;42:S64-S79.

4. Johnson RK, Appel LJ, Brands M, et al. Dietary sugars intake and cardiovascular health a scientific statement from the american heart association. *Circulation*. 2009;120(11):1011-1020.

5. Welsh JA, Sharma AJ, Grellinger L, Vos MB. Consumption of added sugars is decreasing in the United States. *Am J Clin Nutr*. 2011;94(3):726-734.

6. Powell ES, Smith-Taillie LP, Popkin BM. Added sugars intake across the distribution of us children and adult consumers: 1977-2012. *J Acad Nutr Diet*. 2016;116(10):1543-1550.e1.

7. Kim Y, Je Y. Prospective association of sugar-sweetened and artificially sweetened beverage intake with risk of hypertension. *Arch Cardiovasc Dis*. 2016;109(4):242-253.

8. Institute of Medicine. *Dietary Reference Intakes for Energy, Carbohydrate, Fiber, Fat, Fatty Acids, Cholesterol, Protein, and Amino Acids (Macronutrients)*. Washington, D.C.: National Academies Press; 2005.

9. Mann J. Dietary carbohydrate: relationship to cardiovascular disease and disorders of carbohydrate metabolism. *Eur J Clin Nutr*. 2007;61(S1):S100-S111.

10. DiNicolantonio JJ, Lucan SC, O'Keefe JH. The evidence for saturated fat and for sugar related to coronary heart disease. *Prog Cardiovasc Dis.* 2016;58(5):464-472.

11. Vreman RA, Goodell AJ, Rodriguez LA, Porco TC, Lustig RH, Kahn JG. Health and economic benefits of reducing sugar intake in the USA, including effects via non-alcoholic fatty liver disease: a microsimulation model. *BMJ Open.* 2017;7(8):e013543.

12. Stanhope KL. Sugar consumption, metabolic disease and obesity: The state of the controversy HHS Public Access. *Crit Rev Clin Lab Sci.* 2016;53(1):52-67.

13. World Cancer Research Fund, American Institute for Cancer Research. *Food, Nutrition, Physical Activity and the Prevention of Cancer: A Global Perspective.* Washington, D.C.; 2007.

14. Key TJ, Spencer EA. Carbohydrates and cancer: an overview of the epidemiological evidence. *Eur J Clin Nutr.* 2007;61(S1):S112-S121.

15. Kabat GC, Kim MY, Strickler HD, et al. A longitudinal study of serum insulin and glucose levels in relation to colorectal cancer risk among postmenopausal women. *Br J Cancer.* 2012;106(1):227-232.

16. Romanos-Nanclares A, Toledo E, Gardeazabal I, Jiménez-Moleón JJ, Martínez-González MA, Gea A. Sugar-sweetened beverage consumption and incidence of breast cancer: the Seguimiento Universidad de Navarra (SUN) Project. *Eur J Nutr.* October 2018.

17. Institute of Medicine. *Dietary Reference Intakes for Energy, Carbohydrate, Fiber, Fat, Fatty Acids, Cholesterol, Protein, and Amino Acids.* Washington, D.C.: National Academies Press. 2002.

18. van Dam RM, Seidell JC. Carbohydrate intake and obesity. *Eur J Clin Nutr.* 2007;61(S1):S75-S99.

19. Ruanpeng D, Thongprayoon C, Cheungpasitporn W, Harindhanavudhi T. Sugar and artificially sweetened beverages linked to obesity: a systematic review and meta-analysis. *QJM An Int J Med.* 2017;110(8):513-520.

20. Paschos P, Paletas K. Non alcoholic fatty liver disease and metabolic syndrome. *Hippokratia.* 2009;13(1):9-19.

21. Vreman RA, Goodell AJ, Rodriguez LA, et al. Health and economic benefits of reducing sugar intake in the USA, including effects via non-alcoholic fatty liver disease: a microsimulation model. *BMJ Open.* 2017;7(8):e013543.

22. Nier A, Brandt A, Conzelmann I, et al. Non-alcoholic fatty liver disease in overweight children: role of fructose intake and dietary pattern. *Nutrients.* 2018;10(9):1329.

23. Nseir W, Nassar F, Assy N. Soft drinks consumption and nonalcoholic fatty liver disease. *World J Gastroenterol.* 2010;16(21):2579-2588.

24. Ter Horst KW, Serlie MJ. Fructose consumption, lipogenesis, and non-alcoholic fatty liver disease. *Nutrients.* 2017;9(9).

25. Jamnik J, Rehman S, Blanco Mejia S, et al. Fructose intake and risk of gout and hyperuricemia: a systematic review and meta-analysis of prospective cohort studies. *BMJ Open.* 2016;6(10):e013191.

26. Ebrahimpour-koujan S, Saneei P, Larijani B, Esmaillzadeh A. Consumption of sugar sweetened beverages and dietary fructose in relation to risk of gout and hyperuricemia: a systematic review and meta-analysis. *Crit Rev Food Sci Nutr.* October 2018:1-10.

27. O'Connor L, Imamura F, Brage S, Griffin SJ, Wareham NJ, Forouhi NG. Intakes and sources of dietary sugars and their association with metabolic and inflammatory markers. *Clin Nutr.* 2018;37(4):1313-1322.

28. Stegenga ME, Crabben SN van der, Dessing MC, et al. Effect of acute hyperglycaemia and/or hyperinsulinaemia on proinflammatory gene expression, cytokine production and neutrophil function in humans. *Diabet Med.* 2008;25(2):157-164.

29. Della Corte K, Perrar I, Penczynski K, et al. Effect of dietary sugar intake on biomarkers of sub-clinical inflammation: A systematic review and meta-analysis of intervention studies. *Nutrients.* 2018;10(5):606.

30. Takeuchi M, Iwaki M, Takino J, et al. Immunological detection of fructose-derived advanced glycation end-products. *Lab Invest.* 2010;90(7):1117-1127.

31. Gugliucci A. Formation of fructose-mediated advanced glycation end products and their roles in metabolic and inflammatory diseases. *Adv Nutr An Int Rev J.* 2017;8(1):54-62.

32. Jang C, Hui S, Lu W, et al. The small intestine converts dietary fructose into glucose and organic acids. *Cell Metab.* 2018;27(2):351-361.e3.

33. Schwarz J-M, Noworolski SM, Erkin-Cakmak A, et al. Effects of dietary fructose restriction on liver fat, de novo lipogenesis, and insulin kinetics in children with obesity. *Gastroenterology.* 2017;153(3):743-752.

34. Schwarz J-M, Noworolski SM, Wen MJ, et al. Effect of a high-fructose weight-maintaining diet on lipogenesis and liver fat. *J Clin Endocrinol Metab.* 2015;100(6):2434-2442.

35. Wells HF, Buzby JC. Economic Information Bulletin Number 33 Dietary Assessment of Major Trends in U.S.; 2008. www.ers.usda.gov. Accessed January 22, 2019.

36. Tappy L, Lê K-A. Metabolic Effects of Fructose and the Worldwide Increase in Obesity. *Physiol Rev.* 2010;90(1):23-46.

37. U.S. Deparment of Agriculture. Agriculture Research Service. Nutrient Data Library. USDA National Nutrition Database for Standard Reference, Legacy Version Current: April 2018. https://ndb.nal.usda.gov/ndb/search/list.

38. White JS. Straight talk about high-fructose corn syrup : what it is and what it. 2008;88:1716-1721.

39. Le MT, Frye RF, Rivard CJ, et al. Effects of high-fructose corn syrup and sucrose on the phar-macokinetics of fructose and acute metabolic and hemodynamic responses in healthy subjects. *Metabolism.* 2012;61(5):641-651.

40. Wikipedia contributors. Fructose: Carbohydrate Content of Commercial Sweeteners.Wikipedia, The Free Encyclopedia. https://en.wikipedia.org/wiki/Fructose. Accessed Jan. 21, 2019.

41. Wise PM, Nattress L, Flammer LJ, Beauchamp GK. Reduced dietary intake of simple sug-ars alters perceived sweet taste intensity but not perceived pleasantness. *Am J Clin Nutr.* 2016;103(1):50-60.

42. U.S. Department of Health and Human Services and U.S. Department of Agriculture. *2015 – 2020 Dietary Guidelines for Americans. 8th Edition. December 2015. Available at Https://Health. Gov/Dietaryguidelines/2015/Guidelines/.* 8th ed. USDA; 2015. https://health.gov/dietaryguide-lines/2015/guidelines/. Accessed Jan. 21, 2019.

43. Imamura F, O'Connor L, Ye Z, et al. Consumption of sugar sweetened beverages, artificially sweet-ened beverages, and fruit juice and incidence of type 2 diabetes: systematic review, meta-analysis, and estimation of population attributable fraction. *Br J Sports Med.* 2016;50(8):496-504.

44. Park A. Processed Foods a Big Source of Added Sugar | Time. Time Magazine. http://time.com/4252515/calories-processed-food/. Published 2016. Accessed January 22, 2019.

45. Lenhart A, Chey WD. A Systematic Review of the Effects of Polyols on Gastrointestinal Health and Irritable Bowel Syndrome. *Adv Nutr.* 2017;8(4):587-596.

46. Arrigoni E, Brouns F, Amadò R. Human gut microbiota does not ferment erythritol. *Br J Nutr.* 2005;94(5):643-646.

47. U.S. Food and Drug Administration. Food additives and ingredients; Additional Information about High-Intensity Sweeteners Permitted for Use in Food in the United States. 2018. https://

www.fda.gov/Food/IngredientsPackagingLabeling/FoodAdditivesIngredients/ucm397725.htm. Accessed January 22, 2019.

48. Zhang Q, Yang H, Li Y, et al. Toxicological evaluation of ethanolic extract from Stevia rebaudiana Bertoni leaves: Genotoxicity and subchronic oral toxicity. *Regul Toxicol Pharmacol.* 2017;86:253-259.

49. Ramos-Tovar E, Hernández-Aquino E, Casas-Grajales S, et al. Stevia Prevents Acute and Chronic Liver Injury Induced by Carbon Tetrachloride by Blocking Oxidative Stress through Nrf2 Upregulation. *Oxid Med Cell Longev.* 2018;2018:1-12.

50. Samuel P, Ayoob KT, Magnuson BA, et al. Stevia leaf to stevia sweetener: Exploring its science, benefits, and fruture potential. *J Nutr.* 2018;148(7):1186S-1205S.

51. Chen J, Xia Y, Sui X, et al. Steviol, a natural product inhibits proliferation of the gastrointestinal cancer cells intensively. *Oncotarget.* 2018;9(41):26299-26308.

52. Sievenpiper JL, Chan CB, Dworatzek PD, et al. 2018 Clinical Practice Guidelines Nutrition Therapy Diabetes Canada Clinical Practice Guidelines Expert Committee. *Canadian Journal Diabetes.* 2018;42 Suppl 1:S64-S79.

53. Fitch C, Keim K. Position of the Academy of Nutrition and Dietetics: Use of Nutritive and Non-nutritive Sweeteners. *J Acad Nutr Diet.* 2012;112(5):739-58.

54. American Diabetes Association. Low-Calorie Sweeteners: American Diabetes Association®. http://www.diabetes.org/food-and-fitness/food/what-can-i-eat/understanding-carbohydrates/artificial-sweeteners/. 2014. Accessed January 22, 2019.

55. Sharma A, Amarnath S, Thulasimani M, Ramaswamy S. Artificial sweeteners as a sugar substitute: Are they really safe? *Indian J Pharmacol.* 2016;48(3):237-240.

56. Pearlman M, Obert J, Casey L. The association between artificial sweeteners and obesity. *Curr Gastroenterol Rep.* 2017;19(12):64.

57. Suez J, Korem T, Zilberman-Schapira G, et al. Non-caloric artificial sweeteners and the microbiome: findings and challenges. *Gut Microbes.* 2015;6(2):149-155.

58. Suez J, Korem T, Zeevi D, et al. Artificial sweeteners induce glucose intolerance by altering the gut microbiota. *Nature.* 2014;514(7521):181-186.

59. Swithers SE. Artificial sweeteners produce the counterintuitive effect of inducing metabolic derangements. *Trends Endocrinol Metab.* 2014;24(9):431-441.

60. Mattes RD, Popkin BM. Nonnutritive sweetener consumption in humans: effects on appetite and food intake and their putative mechanisms. *Am J Clin Nutr.* 2009;89(1):1-14.

61. Takata Y, Shu X-O, Gao Y-T, et al. Red meat and poultry intakes and risk of total and cause-specific mortality: Results from cohort studies of Chinese adults in Shanghai. *PLoS One.* 2013;8(2):e56963.

62. Yang Q. Gain weight by "going diet?" Artificial sweeteners and the neurobiology of sugar cravings: Neuroscience 2010. *Yale J Biol Med.* 2010;83(2):101-108.

63. Slavin J. Fiber and Prebiotics: Mechanisms and Health Benefits. *Nutrients.* 2013;5(4):1417-1435.

64. Fuller S, Beck E, Salman H, Tapsell L. New horizons for the study of dietary fiber and health: A review. *Plant Foods Hum Nutr.* 2016;71(1):1-12.

65. Anderson JW, Baird P, Davis Jr RH, et al. Health benefits of dietary fiber. *Nutr Rev.* 2009;67(4):188-205.

66. Gray J. *Dietary Fiber: Definition, Analysis, Physiology and Health.* ILSI Europ. Brussels, Belgium: ILSI Europe; 2006.

67. Cummings JH, Stephen AM. Carbohydrate terminology and classification. *Eur J Clin Nutr.* 2007; 61 Suppl 1(S1):S5-18.

68. Englyst KN, Liu S, Englyst HN. Nutritional characterization and measurement of dietary carbohydrates. *Eur J Clin Nutr*. 2007;61(S1):S19-S39.

69. Weickert MO, Pfeiffer AFH. Impact of dietary fiber consumption on insulin resistance and the prevention of type 2 diabetes. *J Nutr*. 2018;148(1):7-12.

70. Hoy K, Goldman JD. *Fiber intake of the U.S. population. What we eat in America. HANES 2009-2010. Food Surveys Research Group Dietary Data Brief No. 12. September 2014.*

71. Prebiotin/Prebiotic. Fiber Content Of Foods. https://www.prebiotin.com/prebiotin-academy/fiber-content-of-foods/. Accessed January 22, 2019.

72. The Daily Fiber Chart – Your Secret Key To Better Health. http://www.puristat.com/fiber/fiber-chart2.aspx. Accessed January 22, 2019.

73. U.S. Department of Agriculture. Agriculture Research Service. Nutrient Data Library. USDA National Nutrition Database for Standard Reference, Legacy Version Current: April 2018. https://ndb.nal.usda.gov/ndb/search/list.

74. Konner M, Eaton SB. Paleolithic Nutrition. *Nutr Clin Pract*. 2010;25(6):594-602.

75. Shah M, Chandalia M, Adams-Huet B, et al. Effect of a high-fiber diet compared with a moderate-fiber diet on calcium and other mineral balances in subjects with type 2 diabetes. *Diabetes Care*. 2009;32(6):990-995.

76. Jenkins DJ, Wolever TM, Taylor RH, et al. Glycemic index of foods: a physiological basis for carbohydrate exchange. *Am J Clin Nutr*. 1981;34(3):362-366.

77. Brand-Miller JC, Stockmann K, Atkinson F, et al. Glycemic index, postprandial glycemia, and the shape of the curve in healthy subjects: analysis of a database of more than 1000 foods. *Am J Clin Nutr*. 2009;89(1):97-105.

78. Atkinson FS, Foster-Powell K, Brand-Miller JC. International Tables of Glycemic Index and Glycemic Load Values: 2008. *Diabetes Care*. 2008;31(12):2281-2283.

79. Gell P. From jelly beans to kidney beans: what diabetes educators should know about the glycemic index. *Diabetes Educ*. 2001;27(4):505-508.

80. Livesey G, Taylor R, Livesey H, Liu S. Is there a dose-response relation of dietary glycemic load to risk of type 2 diabetes? Meta-analysis of prospective cohort studies. *Am J Clin Nutr*. 2013;97(3):584-596.

81. Foster-Powell K, Holt SH, Brand-Miller JC. International table of glycemic index and glycemic load values: 2002. *Am J Clin Nutr*. 2002;76(1):5-56.

82. Östman E, Granfeldt Y, Persson L, Björck I. Vinegar supplementation lowers glucose and insulin responses and increases satiety after a bread meal in healthy subjects. *Eur J Clin Nutr*. 2005;59(9):983-988.

83. Shishehbor F, Mansoori A, Shirani F. Vinegar consumption can attenuate postprandial glucose and insulin responses; a systematic review and meta-analysis of clinical trials. *Diabetes Res Clin Pract*. 2017;127:1-9.

84. Mitrou P, Petsiou E, Papakonstantinou E, et al. Vinegar consumption increases insulin-stimulated glucose uptake by the forearm muscle in humans with type 2 diabetes. *J Diabetes Res*. 2015;2015:175204.

85. Tremblay F, Lavigne C, Jacques H, Marette A. Role of dietary proteins and amino acids in the pathogenesis of insulin resistance. *Annu Rev Nutr*. 2007;27(1):293-310.

86. Duke University Medical Center. Too Much Protein, Eaten Along With Fat, May Lead To Insulin Resistance -- ScienceDaily. ScienceDaily, 9 April 2009. https://www.sciencedaily.com/releases/2009/04/090407130905.htm. Accessed January 22, 2019.

CHAPTER 6

1. Malik VS, Li Y, Tobias DK, et al. Dietary protein intake and risk of type 2 diabetes in us men and women. *Am J Epidemiol*. 2016;183(8):715-728.

2. Shang X, Scott D, Hodge AM, et al. Dietary protein intake and risk of type 2 diabetes: results from the Melbourne Collaborative Cohort Study and a meta-analysis of prospective studies. *Am J Clin Nutr*. 2016;104(5):1352-1365.

3. Virtanen HEK, Koskinen TT, Voutilainen S, et al. Intake of different dietary proteins and risk of type 2 diabetes in men: the Kuopio Ischaemic Heart Disease Risk Factor Study. *Br J Nutr*. 2017;117(06):882-893.

4. Levine ME, Suarez JA, Brandhorst S, et al. Low protein intake is associated with a major reduction in IGF-1, cancer, and overall mortality in the 65 and younger but not older population. *Cell Metab*. 2014;19(3):407-417.

5. Barnard ND, Cohen J, Jenkins DJA, et al. A low-fat vegan diet and a conventional diabetes diet in the treatment of type 2 diabetes: A randomized, controlled, 74-wk clinical trial. *Am J Clin Nutr*. 2009;89(5):1588-1596.

6. Kahleova H, Tura A, Hill M, Holubkov R, Barnard ND. A plant-based dietary intervention improves beta-cell function and insulin resistance in overweight adults: A 16-week randomized clinical trial. *Nutrients*. 2018;10(2).

7. Kahleova H, Matoulek M, Malinska H, et al. Vegetarian diet improves insulin resistance and oxidative stress markers more than conventional diet in subjects with Type 2 diabetes. *Diabet Med*. 2011;28(5):549-559.

8. Dunaief DM, Fuhrman J, Dunaief JL, Ying G. Glycemic and cardiovascular parameters improved in type 2 diabetes with the high nutrient density (HND) diet. *Open J Prev Med*. 2012;2(3):364-371.

9. Institute of Medicine. *Dietary Reference Intakes for Energy, Carbohydrate, Fiber, Fat, Fatty Acids, Cholesterol, Protein, and Amino Acids (Macronutrients)*. Washington, D.C.: National Academies Press; 2005.

10. WHO. *WHO | Diet, Nutrition and the Prevention of Chronic Diseases*. Vol No.916. Rome: World Health Organization; 2003. https://www.who.int/dietphysicalactivity/publications/trs916/en/. Accessed January 22, 2019.

11. Eckel RH, Jakicic JM, Miller NH, et al. 2013 AHA / ACC Guideline on Lifestyle Management to Reduce Cardiovascular Risk A Report of the American College of Cardiology / American Heart Association Task Force on Practice Guidelines. *Circulation*. 2013:1-46.

12. U.S. Deparment of Agriculture. Agriculture Research Service. Nutrient Data Library. USDA National Nutrition Database for Standard Reference, Legacy Version Current: April 2018. https://ndb.nal.usda.gov/ndb/search/list.

13. Santoro N, Caprio S, Giannini C, et al. Oxidized Fatty acids: a potential pathogenic link between Fatty liver and type 2 diabetes in obese adolescents? *Antioxid Redox Signal*. 2014;20(2):383-389.

14. Codoñer-Franch P, Navarro-Ruiz A, Fernández-Ferri M, Arilla-Codoñer Á, Ballester-Asensio E, Valls-Bellés V. A matter of fat: insulin resistance and oxidative stress. *Pediatr Diabetes*. 2012;13(5):392-399.

15. Das UN. Essential fatty acids: Biochemistry, physiology and pathology. *Biotechnol J*. 2006;1(4):420-439.

CHAPTER 7

1. World Cancer Research Fund, American Institute for Cancer Research. *Food, Nutrition, Physical Activity and the Prevention of Cancer: A Global Perspective*. Washington, D.C.; 2007.

2. Winter CK, Davis SF. Organic Foods. *J Food Sci.* 2006;71(9):R117-R124.

3. Young JE, Zhao X, Carey EE, et al. Phytochemical phenolics in organically grown vegetables. *Mol Nutr Food Res.* 2005;49(12):1136-1142.

4. Crinnion WJ. Organic foods contain higher levels of certain nutrients, lower levels of pesticides, and may provide health benefits for the consumer. *Altern Med Rev.* 2010;15(1):4-12.

5. Getahun SM, Chung FL. Conversion of glucosinolates to isothiocyanates in humans after ingestion of cooked watercress. *Cancer Epidemiol Biomarkers Prev.* 1999;8(5):447-451.

6. Conaway CC, Getahun SM, Liebes LL, et al. Disposition of glucosinolates and sulforaphane in humans after ingestion of steamed and fresh broccoli. *Nutr Cancer.* 2000;38(2):168-178.

7. Shapiro TA, Fahey JW, Wade KL, Stephenson KK, Talalay P. Chemoprotective Glucosinolates and Isothiocyanates of Broccoli Sprouts : Metabolism and Excretion in Humans. Cancer Epidemiol Biomarkers Prev. 2001;10(5):501-508.

8. Vermeulen M, van den Berg R, Freidig AP, van Bladeren PJ, Vaes WHJ. Association between consumption of cruciferous vegetables and condiments and excretion in urine of isothiocyanate mercapturic acids. *J Agric Food Chem.* 2006;54(15):5350-5358.

9. Ferracane R, Pellegrini N, Visconti A, et al. Effects of different cooking methods on antioxidant profile, antioxidant capacity, and physical characteristics of artichoke. *J Agric Food Chem.* 2008;56(18):8601-8608.

10. Miglio C, Chiavaro E, Visconti A, et al. Effects of different cooking methods on nutritional and physicochemical characteristics of selected vegetables. *J Agric Food Chem.* 2008;56(1):139-147.

11. Dewanto V, Wu X, Adom KK, Liu RH. Thermal Processing Enhances the Nutritional Value of Tomatoes by Increasing Total Antioxidant Activity. *J Agric Food Chem.* 2002;50(10):3010-3014.

12. Porrini M, Riso P, Testolin G. Absorption of lycopene from single or daily portions of raw and processed tomato. *Br J Nutr.* 1998;80(4):353-361.

13. Gärtner C, Stahl W, Sies H. Lycopene is more bioavailable from tomato paste than from fresh tomatoes. *Am J Clin Nutr.* 1997;66(1):116-122.

14. Livny O, Reifen R, Levy I, et al. Beta-carotene bioavailability from differently processed carrot meals in human ileostomy volunteers. *Eur J Nutr.* 2003;42(6):338-345.

15. Prince MR, Frisoli JK. Beta-carotene accumulation in serum and skin. *Am J Clin Nutr.* 1993; 57(2):175-181.

16. Jalal F, Nesheim MC, Agus Z, et al. Serum retinol concentrations in children are affected by food sources of beta-carotene, fat intake, and anthelmintic drug treatment. *Am J Clin Nutr.* 1998; 68(3):623-629.

17. van het Hof KH, West CE, Weststrate JA, Hautvast JGAJ. Dietary factors that affect the bioavailability of carotenoids. *J Nutr.* 2000;130(3):503-506.

18. Brown MJ, Ferruzzi MG, Nguyen ML, et al. Carotenoid bioavailability is higher from salads ingested with full-fat than with fat-reduced salad dressings as measured with electrochemical detection. *Am J Clin Nutr.* 2004;80(2):396-403.

19. Unlu NZ, Bohn T, Clinton SK, Schwartz SJ. Carotenoid absorption from salad and salsa by humans is enhanced by the addition of avocado or avocado oil. *J Nutr.* 2005;135(3):431-436.

20. Maiani G, Castón MJP, Catasta G, et al. Carotenoids: actual knowledge on food sources, intakes, stability and bioavailability and their protective role in humans. *Mol Nutr Food Res.* 2009;53 Suppl 2(S2):S194-218.

21. Rock CL, Lovalvo JL, Emenhiser C, et al. Bioavailability of beta-carotene is lower in raw than in processed carrots and spinach in women. *J Nutr.* 1998;128(5):913-916.

22. McEligot AJ, Rock CL, Shanks TG, et al. Comparison of serum carotenoid responses between women consuming vegetable juice and women consuming raw or cooked vegetables. *Cancer Epidemiol Biomarkers Prev.* 1999;8(3):227-231.

23. Reboul E, Richelle M, Perrot E, et al. Bioaccessibility of carotenoids and vitamin E from their main dietary sources. *J Agric Food Chem.* 2006;54(23):8749-8755.

24. Katina K, Liukkonen K, Kaukovirta-norja A, et al. Fermentation-induced changes in the nutritional value of native or germinated rye. *Journal of Cereal Science.* 2007;46(3):348-355.

25. Lee SU, Lee JH, Choi SH, et al. Flavonoid content in fresh, home-processed, and light-exposed onions and in dehydrated commercial onion products. *J Agric Food Chem.* 2008;56(18):8541-8548.

26. Fahey JW, Zhang Y, Talalay P. Broccoli sprouts: an exceptionally rich source of inducers of enzymes that protect against chemical carcinogens. *Proc Natl Acad Sci USA.* 1997;94(19): 10367-10372.

27. Yang F, Basu TK, Ooraikul B. Studies on germination conditions and antioxidant contents of wheat grain. *Int J Food Sci Nutr.* 2001:52(4);319-330.

28. Calzuola I, Marsili V, Gianfranceschi GL. Synthesis of Antioxidants in Wheat Sprouts. *J Agric Food Chem.* 2004;52(16):5201-5206.

29. Marsili V, Calzuola I, Gianfranceschi GL. Nutritional relevance of wheat sprouts containing high levels of organic phosphates and antioxidant compounds. *J Clin Gastroenterol.* 2004;38(6 Suppl):S123-6.

30. Liukkonen K-H, Katina K, Wilhelmsson A, et al. Process-induced changes on bioactive compounds in whole grain rye. *Proc Nutr Soc.* 2003;62(1):117-122.

31. Randhir R, Ms YL, Shetty K. Phenolics , their antioxidant and antimicrobial activity in dark germinated fenugreek sprouts in response to peptide and phytochemical elicitors. 2004;13(April):295-307.

32. Fahey JW, Haristoy X, Dolan PM, et al. Sulforaphane inhibits extracellular, intracellular, and antibiotic-resistant strains of Helicobacter pylori and prevents benzo[a]pyrene-induced stomach tumors. *Proc Natl Acad Sci USA.* 2002;99(11):7610-7615.

33. Galan M V, Kishan AA, Silverman ANNL. Oral broccoli sprouts for the treatment of helicobacter pylori infection : A preliminary report. 2004;49:1088-1090.

34. Bahadoran Z, Tohidi M, Nazeri P, et al. Effect of broccoli sprouts on insulin resistance in type 2 diabetic patients: a randomized double-blind clinical trial. *Int J Food Sci Nutr.* 2012;63(7): 767-771.

35. Boddupalli S, Mein JR, Lakkanna S, James DR. Induction of phase 2 antioxidant enzymes by broccoli sulforaphane: perspectives in maintaining the antioxidant activity of vitamins a, C, and e. *Front Genet.* 2012;3:7.

36. Mishra C, Singh B, Singh S, et al. Role of phytochemicals in diabetes lipotoxicity: an overview. 4(4):1604-1610.

37. Firdous SM. Guest Editorial: phytochemicals for treatment of diabetes. *EXCLI Journal.* 2014;13: 451-453.

38. Heather Hausenblas. Resveratrol in Diabetes Care. *Natural Medicine Journal.* 2014;6(2).

39. Axelsson AS, Tubbs E, Mecham B, et al. Sulforaphane reduces hepatic glucose production and improves glucose control in patients with type 2 diabetes. *Sci Transl Med.* 2017;9(394):eaah4477.

40. Son MJ, Miura Y, Yagasaki K. Mechanisms for antidiabetic effect of gingerol in cultured cells and obese diabetic model mice. *Cytotechnology.* 2015;67(4):641-652.

41. Bansode T, Salalkar B, Dighe P, et al. Comparative evaluation of antidiabetic potential of partially purified bioactive fractions from four medicinal plants in alloxan-induced diabetic rats. *AYU (An Int Q J Res Ayurveda)*. 2017;38(2):165.

42. Gebel E. Resveratrol: A Miracle Molecule? *Diabetes Forecast*. 2009;62(5):50-1.

43. Gonzalez-Abuin N, Pinent M, Casanova-Marti A, et al. Procyanidins and their healthy protective effects against type 2 diabetes. *Curr Med Chem*. 2015;22(1):39-50.

44. Turrini E, Ferruzzi L, Fimognari C. Possible effects of dietary anthocyanins on diabetes and insulin resistance. *Curr Drug Targets*. 2017;18(6):629-640.

45. Khan N, Mukhtar H. Tea polyphenols in promotion of human health. *Nutrients*. 2018;11(1).

46. Sluijs I, Cadier E, Beulens JWJ, et al. Dietary intake of carotenoids and risk of type 2 diabetes. *Nutr Metab Cardiovasc Dis*. 2015;25(4):376-381.

47. Roohbakhsh A, Karimi G, Iranshahi M. Carotenoids in the treatment of diabetes mellitus and its complications: A mechanistic review. *Biomed Pharmacother*. 2017;91:31-42.

48. Guo H, Ling W. The update of anthocyanins on obesity and type 2 diabetes: Experimental evidence and clinical perspectives. *Rev Endocr Metab Disord*. 2015;16(1):1-13.

49. Fabricio G, Malta A, Chango A, De Freitas Mathias PC. Environmental Contaminants and Pancreatic Beta-Cells. *J Clin Res Pediatr Endocrinol*. 2016;8(3):257-263.

50. Yokoi K, Konomi A. Toxicity of so-called edible hijiki seaweed (Sargassum fusiforme) containing inorganic arsenic. *Regul Toxicol Pharmacol*. 2012;63(2):291-297.

51. Mania M, Rebeniak M, Szynal T, et al. Total and inorganic arsenic in fish, seafood and seaweeds--exposure assessment. *Rocz Panstw Zakl Hig*. 2015;66(3):203-210.

52. Nachman KE, Ginsberg GL, Miller MD, Murray CJ, Nigra AE, Pendergrast CB. Mitigating dietary arsenic exposure: Current status in the United States and recommendations for an improved path forward. *Sci Total Environ*. 2017;581-582:221-236.

53. Cubadda F, Jackson BP, Cottingham KL, et al. Human exposure to dietary inorganic arsenic and other arsenic species: State of knowledge, gaps and uncertainties. *Sci Total Environ*. 2017;579:1228-1239.

54. Smith-Spangler C, Brandeau ML, Hunter GE, et al. Are Organic Foods Safer or Healthier Than Conventional Alternatives? *Ann Intern Med*. 2012;157(5):348.

55. Mie A, Andersen HR, Gunnarsson S, et al. Human health implications of organic food and organic agriculture: a comprehensive review. *Environ Heal*. 2017;16(1):111.

56. Hurtado-Barroso S, Tresserra-Rimbau A, Vallverdú-Queralt A, Lamuela-Raventós RM. Organic food and the impact on human health. *Crit Rev Food Sci Nutr*. 2019:59(4):704-714.

57. Yang T, Doherty J, Zhao B, et al. Effectiveness of Commercial and Homemade Washing Agents in Removing Pesticide Residues on and in Apples. *J Agric Food Chem*. 2017;65(44):9744-9752.

58. Birlouez-Aragon I, Saavedra G, Tessier FJ, et al. A diet based on high-heat-treated foods promotes risk factors for diabetes mellitus and cardiovascular diseases. *Am J Clin Nutr*. 2010;91(5):1220-1226.

59. Liu G, Zong G, Wu K, et al. Meat cooking methods and risk of type 2 diabetes: Results from three prospective cohort studies. *Diabetes Care*. 2018;41(5):1049-1060.

60. Sugimura T, Wakabayashi K, Nakagama H, Nagao M. Heterocyclic amines: Mutagens/carcinogens produced during cooking of meat and fish. *Cancer Sci*. 2004;95(4):290-299.

61. Khan MR, Busquets R, Saurina J, et al. Identification of Seafood as an Important Dietary Source of Heterocyclic Amines by Chemometry and Chromatography–Mass Spectrometry. *Chem Res Toxicol*. 2013;26(6):1014-1022.

62. Lee Y-N, Lee S, Kim J-S, et al. Chemical analysis techniques and investigation of polycyclic aromatic hydrocarbons in fruit, vegetables and meats and their products. *Food Chem*. 2019;277:156-161.

63. Zhang Q, Qin W, Lin D, et al. The changes in the volatile aldehydes formed during the deep-fat frying process. *J Food Sci Technol*. 2015;52(12):7683-7696.

64. Goldberg T, Cai W, Peppa M, et al. Advanced glycoxidation end products in commonly consumed foods. *J Am Diet Assoc*. 2004;104(8):1287-1291.

65. Chen G, Scott Smith J. Determination of advanced glycation endproducts in cooked meat products. *Food Chem*. 2015;168:190-195.

66. Semla M, Goc Z, Martiniaková M, et al. Acrylamide: a common food toxin related to physiological functions and health. *Physiol Res*. 2017;66(2):205-217.

67. Hamidi EN, Hajeb P, Selamat J, Abdull Razis AF. Polycyclic Aromatic Hydrocarbons (PAHs) and their Bioaccessibility in Meat: a Tool for Assessing Human Cancer Risk. *Asian Pac J Cancer Prev*. 2016;17(1):15-23.

68. Dobarganes C, Márquez-Ruiz G. Possible adverse effects of frying with vegetable oils. *Br J Nutr*. 2015;113(S2):S49-S57.

69. Sansano M, Juan-Borrás M, Escriche I, et al. Effect of pretreatments and air-frying, a novel technology, on acrylamide generation in fried potatoes. *J Food Sci*. 2015;80(5):T1120-T1128.

70. Yaacoub R, Saliba R, Nsouli B, Khalaf G, Birlouez-Aragon I. Formation of lipid oxidation and isomerization products during processing of nuts and sesame seeds. *J Agric Food Chem*. 2008; 56(16):7082-7090.

71. Provenzano LF, Stark S, Steenkiste A, Piraino B, Sevick MA. Dietary sodium intake in type 2 diabetes. *Clin Diabetes*. 2014;32(3):106-112.

72. Harnack LJ, Cogswell ME, Shikany JM, et al. Sources of sodium in us adults from 3 geographic regions. *Circulation*. 2017;135(19):1775-1783.

73. U.S. Department of Agriculture. Agriculture Research Service. Nutrient Data Library. USDA National Nutrition Database for Standard Reference, Legacy Version Current: April 2018. https://ndb.nal.usda.gov/ndb/search/list.

74. Lee Y-J, Wang M-Y, Lin M-C, Lin P-T. Associations between vitamin B-12 status and oxidative stress and inflammation in diabetic vegetarians and omnivores. *Nutrients*. 2016;8(3):118.

75. Bell DSH. Metformin-induced vitamin B12 deficiency presenting as a peripheral neuropathy. *South Med J*. 2010;103(3):265-267.

76. Liu Q, Li S, Quan H, Li J. Vitamin B12 status in metformin treated patients: systematic review. Pietropaolo M, ed. *PLoS One*. 2014;9(6):e100379.

77. Institute of Medicine (US) Standing Committee on the Scientific Evaluation of Dietary Reference Intakes and its Panel on Folate OBV and C. *Dietary Reference Intakes for Thiamin, Riboflavin, Niacin, Vitamin B6, Folate, Vitamin B12, Pantothenic Acid, Biotin, and Choline*. National Academies Press (US); 1998.

78. Forrest KYZ, Stuhldreher WL. Prevalence and correlates of vitamin D deficiency in US adults. *Nutr Res*. 2011;31(1):48-54.

79. Nakashima A, Yokoyama K, Yokoo T, Urashima M. Role of vitamin D in diabetes mellitus and chronic kidney disease. *World J Diabetes*. 2016;7(5):89.

80. Wei Z, Yoshihara E, He N, et al. Vitamin D Switches BAF Complexes to Protect b Cells. *Cell*. 2018;173(5):1135-1149.e15.

81. Kalaany NY, Sabatini DM. Tumours with PI3K activation are resistant to dietary restriction. *Nature*. 2009;458(7239):725-731.

82. Wacker M, Holick MF. Sunlight and Vitamin D: A global perspective for health. *Derm Endocrinol.* 2013;5(1):51-108.

83. National Institutes of Health Office of Dietary Supplements. *Vitamin D - Health Professional Fact Sheet.*; 2018. https://ods.od.nih.gov/factsheets/VitaminD-HealthProfessional/.

84. Odegaard AO, Jacobs DR, Sanchez OA, et al. Oxidative stress, inflammation, endothelial dysfunction and incidence of type 2 diabetes. *Cardiovasc Diabetol.* 2016;15(1):1-12.

85. Rains JL, Jain SK. Oxidative stress, insulin signaling, and diabetes. *Free Radic Biol Med.* 2011; 50(5):567-575.

86. Wilson R, Willis J, Gearry R, et al. Inadequate vitamin C status in prediabetes and type 2 diabetes mellitus: associations with glycaemic control, obesity, and smoking. *Nutrients.* 2017;9(9):997.

87. Jaffe R. Phytonutrients in Diabetes Management. In *Bioactive Food as Dietary Interventions for Diabetes.* Watson, RR and Preddy VR. Elsevier Inc. 2013:339-353.

88. Cefalu WT, Hu FB. Role of chromium in human health and in diabetes. *Diabetes Care.* 2004;27(11): 2741-2751.

89. Roussel AM, Andriollo-Sanchez M, Ferry M, et al. Food chromium content, dietary chromium intake and related biological variables in French free-living elderly. *Br J Nutr.* 2007;98(2):326-331.

90. National Institutes of Health Office of Dietary Supplements. Dietary Supplement Fact Sheet: Chromium — Health Professional Fact Sheet. 2018. https://ods.od.nih.gov/factsheets/Chromium-HealthProfessional/. Accessed January 23, 2019.

91. Mooren FC. Magnesium and disturbances in carbohydrate metabolism. *Diabetes, Obes Metab.* 2015;17(9):813-823.

92. Barbagallo M, Dominguez LJ. Magnesium and type 2 diabetes. *World J Diabetes.* 2015;6(10): 1152-1157.

93. Institute of Medicine. *Dietary Reference Intakes for Calcium, Phosphorus, Magnesium, Vitamin D, and Fluoride.* Washington, D.C.: National Academies Press; 1997.

94. National Academy of Sciences, Engineering, and Medicine. *Dietary Reference Intakes for Sodium and Potassium.* Washington, D.C.: National Academies Press; 2019.

95. Rizzo NS, Jaceldo-Siegl K, Sabate J, Fraser GE. Nutrient profiles of vegetarian and nonvegetarian dietary patterns. *J Acad Nutr Diet.* 2013;113(12):1610-1619.

96. Weaver CM. Potassium and health. *Adv Nutr.* 2013;4(3):368S-77S.

97. Polsky S, Akturk HK. Alcohol consumption, diabetes risk, and cardiovascular disease within diabetes. *Curr Diab Rep.* 2017;17(12):136.

98. Joosten MM, Chiuve SE, Mukamal KJ, Hu FB, Hendriks HFJ, Rimm EB. Changes in alcohol consumption and subsequent risk of type 2 diabetes in men. *Diabetes.* 2011;60(1):74-79.

99. Heianza Y, Arase Y, Saito K, et al. Role of alcohol drinking pattern in type 2 diabetes in Japanese men: the Toranomon Hospital Health Management Center Study 11 (TOPICS 11). *Am J Clin Nutr.* 2013;97(3):561-568.

100. Seike N, Noda M, Kadowaki T. Alcohol consumption and risk of type 2 diabetes mellitus in Japanese: a systematic review. *Asia Pac J Clin Nutr.* 2008;17(4):545-551.

101. American Addiction Centers. Alcoholism and Health Issues: Cholesterol, Triglycerides, the Liver, and More. https://americanaddictioncenters.org/alcoholism-treatment/health-issues. Published 2018. Accessed January 23, 2019.

102. Varela-Rey M, Woodhoo A, Martinez-Chantar M-L, et al. Alcohol, DNA methylation, and cancer. *Alcohol Res.* 2013;35(1):25-35.

CHAPTER 9

1. Christakis NA, Fowler JH. The spread of obesity in a large social network over 32 years. *N Engl J Med.* 2007;357(4):370-379.

2. Colberg SR, Sigal RJ, Yardley JE, et al. Physical activity/exercise and diabetes: A position statement of the American Diabetes Association. *Diabetes Care.* 2016;39(11):2065-2079.

3. Johannsen DL, Welk GJ, Sharp RL, Flakoll PJ. Differences in Daily Energy Expenditure in Lean and Obese Women: The Role of Posture Allocation. *Obesity.* 2008;16(1):34-39.

4. National Institutes of Health. How is the body affected by sleep deprivation? | NICHD - Eunice Kennedy Shriver National Institute of Child Health and Human Development. https://www.nichd.nih.gov/health/topics/sleep/conditioninfo/sleep-deprivation. Published 2016. Accessed September 2, 2018.

5. Khandelwal D, Dutta D, Chittawar S, Kalra S. Sleep Disorders in Type 2 Diabetes. *Indian J Endocrinol Metab.* 2017;21(5):758-761.

6. Anothaisintawee T, Reutrakul S, Van Cauter E, Thakkinstian A. Sleep disturbances compared to traditional risk factors for diabetes development: Systematic review and meta-analysis. *Sleep Med Rev.* 2016;30:11-24.

7. Gerdts J, Brace EJ, Sasaki Y, et al. SARM1 activation triggers axon degeneration locally via NAD destruction. *Science.* 2015;348(6233):453-457.

8. Reutrakul S, Van Cauter E. Interactions between sleep, circadian function, and glucose metabolism: implications for risk and severity of diabetes. *Ann N Y Acad Sci.* 2014;1311(1):151-173.

9. Hirshkowitz M, Whiton K, Albert SM, et al. National Sleep Foundation's sleep time duration recommendations: methodology and results summary. *Sleep Heal.* 2015;1(1):40-43.

10. Hackett RA, Kivimäki M, Kumari M, Steptoe A. Diurnal Cortisol Patterns, Future Diabetes, and Impaired Glucose Metabolism in the Whitehall II Cohort Study. *J Clin Endocrinol Metab.* 2016;101(2):619-625.

11. Misra M, Bredella MA, Tsai P, Mendes N, Miller KK, Klibanski A. Lower growth hormone and higher cortisol are associated with greater visceral adiposity, intramyocellular lipids, and insulin resistance in overweight girls. *Am J Physiol Endocrinol Metab.* 2008;295(2):E385-92.

12. Joseph JJ, Golden SH. Cortisol dysregulation: the bidirectional link between stress, depression, and type 2 diabetes mellitus. *Ann NY Acad Sci.* 2017;1391(1):20-34.

13. Mayo Clinic. Need stress relief? Try the 4 A's - Mayo Clinic. https://www.mayoclinic.org/healthy-lifestyle/stress-management/in-depth/stress-relief/art-20044476. Published 2016. Accessed September 3, 2018.

14. Holt-Lunstad J, Smith TB, Layton JB. Social relationships and mortality risk: A meta-analytic review. *PLoS Med.* 2010;7(7):e1000316.

15. Laugesen K, Baggesen LM, Schmidt SAJ, et al. Social isolation and all-cause mortality: A population-based cohort study in Denmark. *Sci Rep.* 2018;8(1):4-11.

Index

inflammation and, 102
ketosis and, 27
macronutrients and, *34*
Marshallese people and, 24
micronutrients in, lack of, *35*
Neu5Gc and, *37*, 51, 102, *103*
oxidative stress and, 102
PAHs and, 117
pathogenic effects and, *36*, 53
phytochemicals and, lack of, *103*
plant sterols in, lack of, *103*
POPs and, *37*, 50, 116
pre- or probiotics in, lack of, *103*
protein and, 101–102
purines in, 138
replacements for, 102–103, 125
risk of diabetes and, 35, 39
saturated fat and, 49, 102, *103, 109*
TMAO and, *37*, 102
trans-fatty acids in, *36*, 107
as unhealthful, 126
vitamin B$_{12}$ and, 121
anthocyanins, as protective, *114*
antibodies, LADA and, 3
antifungal, allicin as, 44
antimicrobial, sulforaphane as, 113
antioxidants/antioxidant effect. *See also*
    specific types of
animal protein and, *103*
colorful plant foods and, 113
detoxification and, 65
fat (dietary) and, 105, 114
in fruits, 82, 134
GI/GL and, 98
grains and, 141
green vegetable juice and, 68
herbs and/or spices and, 83, 145
as important, 121–122
in legumes, 47
low-carb diets and, 33, *34*
maximizing, 113–114
nuts and/or seeds and, 143, 144
oils (dietary) and, *107*
oxidative stress and, 9, *10*
phytochemicals and, 112
plant-based diet and, *34*, 71, 102, *103*,
    105, 111
as protective, 44–45, 112–113
in sample menu, 169
in starchy vegetables, 139
study and, 24

superstar foods for, 114, *114–115*
tea and, 44, 165
vegetable juices and, 114, 131
in whole grains, 141
antiviral, allicin as, 44
appetite
calorie-free beverages and, 68
cortisol and, 65
meal timing & frequency and, 176
medications and, 16, 58
processed foods and, 13, 60
sugar/sweeteners and, 67, 74, 80, 87
apple(s), 35, 44, *89, 115*
    Pie Oats, 200
arsenic, in foods, *37, 50*, 116, 139
artery disease/problems
antioxidants and, *34*
arteriosclerosis, 8, 11
atherosclerosis, 6, 11, 52
Carlos (patient) and, *25*
low-carb diet and, 31
peripheral artery disease (PAD), 6,
    11, *25*, 121, 156
phytochemicals and, *34*
arthritis, antioxidants and, *34*
artificial sweeteners
bacteria and, 88
in beverages, 68
calories and, 67
FDA and, 86
pathogenic effects and, 53, 67
weight loss and, 64
Asia/Asians
alcohol consumption study and, 124
BMI and, 58
dairy products' study and, 55
fish study and, 54
insulin resistance/weight and, 8
legumes and, 136
refined grains' study and, 55
aspartame, 86
atherosclerosis, 6, 11, 52
Atkins diet, 27
Australian studies, 30, 55, 102
author's father, health and, 147–148
avocado(s)
avocado oil, carotenoid absorption
    and, 113
as calorically dense healthy whole
    food, 66
fat (dietary) and, 28, 105

GI/GL and, 104
as high-fat food, 104
in low-carb diets, 27
plant sterols/stanols in, *34, 45*

B

bacon, 35, 98, 102
bacteria
dysbiosis and, 12
endotoxins and, *37, 52*
fiber and, 88
fructose and, 77
inflammation and, 9
phytochemicals and, *34*, 112
polyphenols and, 45
pre- and probiotics and, 45, 88
sugar alcohols and, 85
bad breath, very low-carb diet and, 31
baked beans, 137
baked potatoes, 98, 140
baking foods, vitamins and, 132
banana(s)
calories and, 133
carbohydrates and, 28, 133
GI and, 97
in Marshallese diet, 23
and Nut Butter Wrap, Ezekiel, 202
pesticides and, 116
potassium and, 82, 123
prebiotics and, 45
bariatric surgery, reversal of diabetes
    and, 17
barley
Bowl, Spiced Creamy, 199
brown rice vs., 140
cooking, *187*
fiber and, 97
as food friend, *146*
in soup recipe, as variation, *206*
Barnard, Neal, 20–21
batch cooking, *181*
bean(s)
age of, 137
baked potatoes and, 140
batch cooking and, 137, *181*
bean pasta, 135
carbohydrates and, 74
cleaning, 182
cooking, 137, 182–185, *186*
dips/dressings/spreads and, 136

TMA and, 51

H

hamburger, endotoxins and, 52
Harvard School of Public Health studies, 35, 38
HbA1C (or A1C)
    CVD and, 52
    diet and, 18, 20, 21, 22, 23, 30, 31
    Marshallese study and, 24
    reversal of diabetes and, 16
    sleep and, lack of, 156
    test, 5
HCAs (heterocyclic amines), 37, 50, 117
HCF (high-carbohydrate, high-fiber) diet, 19
HDL cholesterol
    diet and, 18, 30, 31
    fructose and, 75
    GI and, 94
    sugar (dietary) and, 75
    trans-fatty acids and, 49
headaches, 31, 123
Health Professionals Follow-Up Study, 38
healthful plant-based diet index (hPDI), 38
healthy foods, sources of, 178, 182
heart disease. See cardiovascular (heart) disease
heavy metals, 37, 49, 50, 65, 116
Helicobacter pylori (*H. pylori*), sulforaphane and, 113
hemagglutinin, in kidney beans, 182
heme iron, 23, 37, 52, *103*
hemicelluloses, *89*
hemp seeds
    in breakfast recipe, *197*
    in dressing recipe, *221*
    as food friend, *146*
    omega-3 and/or omega-6 and, 45, 110, *110*, 128
    salad dressing and, *107*
herbs and/or spices
    antioxidants in, *34*, 44, 83, 114, 145
    beans and, 185
    benefits of, 68
    blood glucose (blood sugar) and, 144
    breakfast and, 145, *201*
    in broth base recipe, *203*

choosing, 144–145
cooking, 145
dehydrating, 68
dried vs. fresh, 145
as food friend, *146*
freezing, 68
glucose and, 68
growing your own, 68
herbal tea, 68, 145
inflammation and, 64, 68, 144
intestinal gas and, 137
metabolism and, 68
as pantry staples, *184*
phytochemicals in, 83, 114
in protocol for kicking diabetes, *127*
salad dressings and, 145
in sautéing liquid, *181*
servings and, 144
sodium (salt) and, 120, 180
soups and, 145, *205*
storing, 145
as sugar (dietary) alternative, 83
hesperidin, antioxidants/phytochemicals and, *115*
heterocyclic amines (HCAs), *37, 50,* 117
hexane, 138
HFCS-42/55/90, *79*
hierarchy of grains, *140*
high blood pressure, Carlos (patient) and, *25*
high blood sugar. See hyperglycemia (high blood sugar)
high energy density, 65
high nutrient density (HND) diet/foods, 18, *18,* 66
high-carbohydrate, high-fiber (HCF) diet, 19
high-carbohydrate foods, GI and, 99
high-fat diet/foods, 51, 64, 104
high-fructose corn syrup/sweeteners, 77, 78, 79, *79,* 82
high-intensity sweeteners, 85–86
high-protein diet, TMAO and, 51
high-temperature cooking
    leaky gut and, 64–65
    pathogenic effects and, *37,* 50–51, 117–118
    plant-based diet and, 111
    poultry and, 54
    vitamin/mineral loss and, 132
hijiki seaweed, arsenic in, 116

Hispanic Americans, 2, 121
HND (high nutrient density) diet/foods, 18, *18,* 66
HOMA-IR test, 24, 47
home-prepared foods, 70, 118, 120, 135, 137
honey, 77, 79, 82, *83, 100*
hormones
    adrenaline (fight-or-flight hormone), 158
    animal products and, 53
    contaminants and, *37, 49, 60,* 116
    cortisol, 65, 158
    exercise (physical activity) and, 65
    food allergies and, 65
    inflammation and, 64
    phytochemicals and, 112
    plant-based diet and, 46, 65
    processed foods and, 53
    sex hormones, 65
    stress hormones, 65
    supplements and, 65
    thyroid hormones, 65
    weight loss and, 65
hot dogs, risk of diabetes and, 35
hPDI (healthful plant-based diet index), 38
hsCRP test, 24, 94
hummus, 135, 176
hunger
    alternative sweeteners and, 87
    diet and, 163, 176
    drinking water and, 69, 176
    emotions and, 60, 176
    environmental chemicals and, 60
    fiber and, 42
    food/environmental components and, 60
    fruit as snack to alleviate, 134
    fullness and, 69
    high-intensity sweeteners and, 87
    increased, as symptom, 1, 4, *4*
    listening to signals about, 69
    meal timing & frequency and, 176
    overeating and, 69
    polyphagia, 4, *4*
    satiety, 22, 68, 69, 74, 139
    as signal, 69
    skipping meals and, 69
    snacks and, 176
    stimulants to, 176

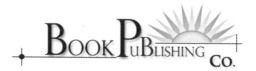

BookPublishing Co.

books that educate, inspire, and empower

To find your favorite books on plant-based cooking and nutrition,
raw-foods cuisine, and healthy living, visit:

BookPubCo.com

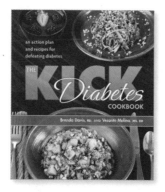

The Kick Diabetes Cookbook

Brenda Davis, RD
Vesanto Melina, MS, RD

978-1-57067-359-7 • $24.95

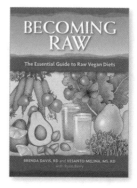

Becoming Raw

Brenda Davis, RD
Vesanto Melina, MS, RD

978-1-57067-238-5 • $24.95

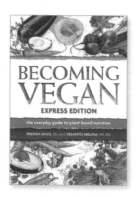

**Becoming Vegan
Express Edition**

Brenda Davis, RD
Vesanto Melina, MS, RD

978-1-57067-295-8 • $19.95

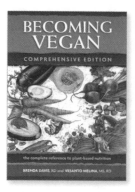

**Becoming Vegan
Comprehensive Edition**

Brenda Davis, RD
Vesanto Melina, MS, RD

978-1-57067-297-2 • $29.95

Purchase these titles from your favorite book source or buy them directly from:

Book Publishing Company • PO Box 99 • Summertown, TN 38483 • 1-888-260-8458

Free shipping and handling on all orders